Manual of Adolescent Substance Abuse Treatment

Manual of Adolescent Substance Abuse Treatment

Edited by

Todd Wilk Estroff, M.D.

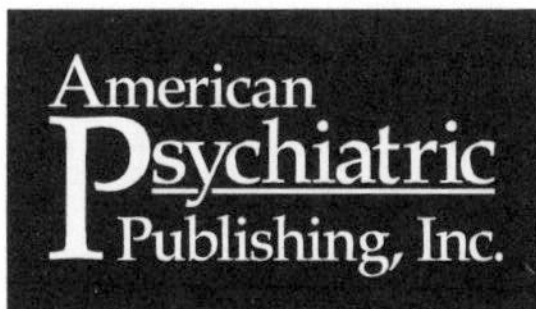

Washington, DC
London, England

Manufactured in the United States of America on acid-free paper

04 03 02 01 4 3 2 1
First Edition

American Psychiatric Publishing, Inc.
1400 K Street, N.W.
Washington, DC 20005
www.appi.org

Library of Congress Cataloging-in-Publication Data

Manual of adolescent substance abuse treatment / edited by Todd Wilk Estroff.-- 1st ed.

p. cm.
Includes bibliographical references and index.
ISBN 0-88048-712-7
1. Substance abuse--Treatment. 2. Teenagers--Substance use. 3. Teenagers--Drug use. 4. Drug abuse--Treatment. I. Estroff, Todd Wilk.
RJ506.D78 M36 2001
616.86'06'0835--dc21

2001022179

British Library Cataloguing in Publication Data
A CIP record is available from the British Library.

Contents

Contributors ix

Acknowledgements xi

1 Epidemiology 1

Patricia A. Harrison, Ph.D.

2 Predisposing Factors 13

Patricia A. Harrison, Ph.D.

3 Routes of Abuse and Specific Drugs 35

Todd Wilk Estroff, M.D.

4 Diagnosis of Adolescent Substance Abuse Disorders. 51

Peter R. Cohen, M.D.

Todd Wilk Estroff, M.D.

5 Comorbidity and Adolescent Substance Abuse 69

Oscar G. Bukstein, M.D., M.P.H.

6 Medical Evaluation of Substance-Abusing Adolescents 91

Anthony H. Dekker, D.O.

Todd Wilk Estroff, M.D.

Norman G. Hoffmann, Ph.D.

7 **Psychiatric and Substance Abuse Evaluation of Adolescents** .99

R. Jeremy A. Stowell, M.D.

Todd Wilk Estroff, M.D.

8 **Treatment Planning and Case Management** 129

Linda Semlitz, M.D.

9 **Outpatient Treatment** 155

Todd Wilk Estroff, M.D.

10 **Inpatient Programs** 165

R. Jeremy A. Stowell, M.D.

Todd Wilk Estroff, M.D.

11 **Use of Medications With Substance-Abusing Adolescents** 187

Steven L. Jaffe, M.D.

Todd Wilk Estroff, M.D.

12 **Adolescent Psychiatry and 12-Step Treatment** . . .205

J. Calvin Chatlos, M.D.

Todd Wilk Estroff, M.D.

13 **Spirituality** 229

Martha A. Morrison, M.D.

Norman G. Hoffmann, Ph.D.

Sara S. DeHart, Ph.D.

Todd Wilk Estroff, M.D.

Paul King, M.D.

14 **Family Treatment** 235

Susan D. Wallace

Todd Wilk Estroff, M.D.

15 **Relapse** 253

Steven L. Jaffe, M.D.

Todd Wilk Estroff, M.D.

16 **Adolescent Development and Substance Abuse** . . 265

Stuart A. Copans, M.D.

Jean Kinney, M.S.W.

Todd Wilk Estroff, M.D.

17 **Untreatable Substance-Abusing Adolescents** 273

Todd Wilk Estroff, M.D.

Index 285

Contributors

Oscar G. Bukstein, M.D., M.P.H.
Associate Professor of Psychiatry, Department of Psychiatry, Western Psychiatric Institute and Clinic, University of Pittsburgh School of Medicine, Pittsburgh, Pennsylvania

J. Calvin Chatlos, M.D.
Director, Substance Abuse Services, Carrier Clinic, Belle Meade, New Jersey

Peter R. Cohen, M.D.
Medical Director, Behavioral Health Services, Washington County Hospital System, Hagerstown, Maryland

Stuart A. Copans, M.D.
Adjunct Associate Professsor, Department of Psychiatry, Dartmouth Medical School, Brattleboro, Vermont

Sara S. DeHart, Ph.D.
Affiliate Associate Professor, School of Nursing, University of Washington, Seattle, Washington

Anthony H. Dekker, D.O.
Associate Director, Phoenix Indian Medical Center; Director, Ambulatory Care and Community Health, Phoenix, Arizona

Todd Wilk Estroff, M.D.
Private practice, Atlanta Georgia

Patricia A. Harrison, Ph.D.
Co-Director, Health Care Research Division, Minnesota Department of Human Services, St. Paul, Minnesota

Norman G. Hoffmann, Ph.D.
Clinical Associate Professor, Department of Community Health, Brown University, Providence, Rhode Island; President, Evince Clinical Assessments, Smithfield, Rhode Island

Steven L. Jaffe, M.D.
Professor of Child and Adolescent Psychiatry, Emory School Of Medicine; Clinical Professor Of Psychiatry, Morehouse School of Medicine, Atlanta, Georgia

Paul King, M.D.
Clinical Assistant Professor of Psychiatry, University Of Tennessee, Memphis, Tennessee; Medical Director, Parkwood Hospital, Olive Branch, Mississippi

Jean Kinney, M.S.W.
Lecturer in Community and Family Medicine, Dartmouth Medical School, Hanover, Vermont

Martha A. Morrison, M.D.
Atlanta, Georgia

Linda Semlitz, M.D.
Senior Consultant, Child and Adolescent Psychiatry, Adam Road Hospital, Singapore

R. Jeremy A. Stowell, M.D.
Medical Director, Substance Abuse Division, Norfolk Community Services Board, Norfolk, Virginia; Private Practice, Virginia Beach, Virginia

Susan D. Wallace
Executive Director, Caritas Inc., Pawtucket, Rhode Island

Acknowledgements

The editor wishes to thank Norman and Linda Hoffmann, for their constant advice and encouragement to complete the book, and his family—Maria, Emmanuelle, and Esther—for putting up with the enormous amount of time the book took away from family activities.

1 Epidemiology

Patricia A. Harrison, Ph.D.

Substance use among adolescents is particularly dangerous because adolescence is a period of critical physical, mental, emotional, and social development. Substance use is associated with the three highest causes of mortality among young people: injury, suicide, and homicide. It is also associated with sexually transmitted diseases (including HIV infection and hepatitis), teenage pregnancy, and mental health problems (Sells and Blum 1996). In addition, substance abuse at an early age is more likely to lead to substance dependence and its associated problems than when substance abuse begins at a later age (Anthony and Petronis 1995; Grant and Dawson 1997; Kandel et al. 1992).

Sources of Data

Epidemiological data on substance use behaviors are typically collected through household or school surveys. Researchers using such data must rely on self-reported information. Two major federally funded population-based surveys are the source of most of the information on adolescent substance use in the United States. The National Household Survey on Drug Abuse was instituted in 1971 and has been administered periodically since then; it has been conducted annually since 1991. The 1999 administration included interviews with 25,357 adolescents between the ages of 12 and 17 (Office of Applied Studies 2000a).

School surveys have the advantage of easy and inexpensive administration to large samples of students. The best long-term source of annual data on adolescent substance use in the United States is the Monitoring the Future study. This school-based survey has been administered since 1975 to a nationally representative sample of high school seniors in both public and private schools (Johnston et al. 1999). Because of concerns about increasing substance use among younger students, eighth- and tenth-grade students were included beginning in 1991. The annual sample size includes 14,000–18,000 students at each grade level.

One advantage of the household survey over the school survey is that the household sample may include school dropouts or chronic truants missed by the school surveys. However, an advantage of the school survey over the household survey is the apparently higher degree of perceived privacy associated with the former (Weinberg et al. 1998). Analyses of age-matched samples from the National Household Survey on Drug Abuse and Monitoring the Future have found higher reports of substance use in the school setting (Gfroerer et al. 1997). It is likely that both household and school surveys produce conservative estimates of adolescent substance abuse. This is because youth with higher rates of substance use, especially problem use, are more likely to be missed in one or both settings. Substance use has been found to be higher among school dropouts, chronic truants and absentees, homeless youth, delinquent youth, and youth in juvenile correctional or clinical settings (Bates et al. 1997; Beauvais 1996; Dembo et al. 1994; Forst 1994; Harrison 1997).

Because annual information is available from Monitoring the Future for a 26-year period, these data are used in this chapter to compare trends over time (Johnston et al. 2001). This survey collects substance information in three time frames. *Lifetime prevalence* of use measures the number of use occasions at any point in the past. *Annual prevalence* of use measures the number of use occasions in the past 12 months. *Current prevalence* of use measures the number of use occasions in the past 30 days. Twenty or more use occasions during the past 30 days is used as an indicator of daily use.

General Trends of Substance Abuse Over Time

Lifetime Use

Lifetime use is a commonly reported measure of trends over time, because any lifetime use is an indicator of changes in use initiation. That is, the lifetime prevalence measures whether adolescents have *ever* tried a particular substance. Figure 1–1 illustrates the trends in lifetime prevalence rates for high school seniors for alcohol, cigarettes, marijuana, amphetamines, inhalants, hallucinogens, and cocaine. Because patterns of use vary somewhat for different substances, a brief summary is provided for each substance or class of substances. Because long-term data are available only for high school seniors (twelfth graders), the long-term trend summary focuses only on this age group.

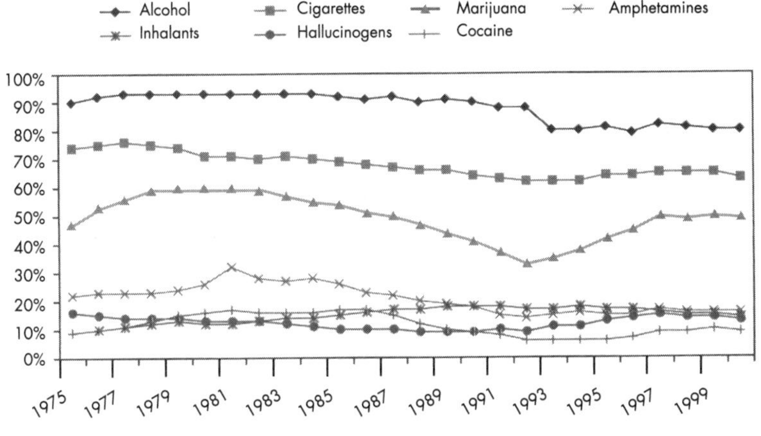

Figure 1–1. Lifetime use prevalence of various substances for twelfth graders. Decrease in alcohol use beginning in 1993 resulted from a change in the question that defined a drink as "more than a few sips" at that point.

Alcohol

Of all substances, the lifetime use rates for high school seniors are consistently the highest for alcohol. Alcohol lifetime prevalence rates ranged from about 90% to 93% between 1975 and 1989. A small decline in 1990 led to the first lifetime alcohol use prevalence rate below 90%. The rate continued to drop, reaching 87% in 1993. At that point, the alcohol question in the survey was reworded to specify "more than a few sips." A subsample of survey respondents who answered the newly phrased question in 1993 reported a lower lifetime prevalence rate (80%) than those answering the question about any alcohol. The rates for responses to this revised question remained between 80% and 82% through 2000.

Tobacco

Cigarettes are the next most commonly used substance after alcohol. In the late 1970s, 74%–76% of high school seniors reported having smoked cigarettes. This rate slowly but steadily dropped over the next decade, from 71% in 1980 to 66% in 1989. In the 1990s and in the year 2000, the rate remained relatively low, ranging from 62% to 65%. The low point occurred in 1992, and the highest recent rates were seen between 1997 and 1999. In 2000, the rate decreased to 63% from 65% in 1999.

Data on the use of smokeless tobacco by adolescents have been available only since 1986. The lifetime use rate of smokeless tobacco for high school seniors ranged from 29% to 32% between 1986 and 1996 and then gradually declined to 23% in 2000.

Any Illicit Drug

The lifetime use of any illicit drug (a substance other than alcohol or tobacco) increased from 55% in 1975 to a peak of 66% in 1981. This rapid increase was followed by a steady decline over the next decade, with lifetime use reaching a low of 41% in 1992. The first increase after this long decline was seen in 1993, and the rate continued to rise to 55% in 1999. In 2000, a small decline was seen, with a prevalence rate of 54%.

Marijuana

Most of the change in the illicit drug use prevalence rate over time can be attributed to change in marijuana use prevalence. Lifetime use of marijuana rose from 47% in 1975 to a high of 60% in 1979. A decline began in 1980 that continued until the mid-1980s. The low was reached in 1992, with 33% of high school seniors reporting that they had tried marijuana. Since that time, lifetime marijuana use has increased fairly rapidly, resulting in lifetime use prevalence rates of 50% in 1999 and 49% in 2000.

Amphetamines

Among illicit drugs, amphetamines historically have been the next most prevalently used among high school seniors after marijuana. The survey question about amphetamines in Monitoring the Future excludes prescription use. In 1975, 22% of seniors reported amphetamine use. This rate increased to a high of 32% in 1981. Amphetamine use rates then declined by more than half, to a low of 14% in 1992. A small increase in amphetamine use to 16% was evident between 1997 and 2000.

Methamphetamine use has been tracked separately only since 1990. The lifetime use prevalence rate for methamphetamine has risen from about 3% between 1990 and 1994 to 8% by 2000.

Inhalants

Inhalant use has not followed the same pattern over time as have marijuana and stimulant use. The 10% rate first recorded in 1976 increased to a high of 18% between 1989 and 1991. Since then, lifetime inhalant use has dropped very slowly, decreasing to 14% in 2000. It is interesting to note that between 1990 and 1996 the lifetime prevalence use rate for inhalants was higher than that for amphetamines.

Hallucinogens

Hallucinogens include drugs such as lysergic acid diethylamide (LSD) and phencyclidine hydrochloride (PCP). Lifetime prevalence of hallucinogen use dropped from a high of 16% in 1975 to a low of 9% from 1988 to 1990. In the 1990s, hallucinogen use increased again to 15% in 1997 then dropped to 13% by 2000.

Cocaine

The lifetime prevalence rate for cocaine (including crack cocaine) use increased from 9% in 1975 to its peak of 17% in 1985 and 1986. Beginning in the mid-1980s, lifetime cocaine use declined among high school seniors to about 6% from 1992 to 1995. However, a slight increase in the lifetime use prevalence rate has been apparent in recent years, with the cocaine use rate reaching 10% in 1999 and 9% in 2000.

Heroin and Other Opiates

Heroin use is relatively rare among adolescents. The lifetime use prevalence rate for heroin among high school seniors was over 2% in 1975 but declined to less than 1% in 1991. However, heroin use rose again to 2% in 1997 and remained there through 2000. The use of other opiates generally remained between 9% and 10% from 1975 through 1988. Then the rate began to decline, reaching a low of 6% in 1992. The use of other opiates began to rise again, reaching 11% in 2000.

Annual Use

The percentage of high school seniors reporting use of any illicit drug in the previous 12 months ranges from about 10% to 15% lower in any given year than the percentage who report lifetime use. Annual use as a proportion of lifetime use differs considerably for different substances and can be used as a rough measure of the likelihood that the youth will maintain rather than discontinue use.

An example of a class of substances for which discontinuance rates are relatively high is the inhalants. The prevalence of use in the past 12 months is less than half the lifetime use prevalence reported by students in 2000. In contrast, alcohol is associated with a much higher likelihood of use maintenance. In Monitoring the Future, a very high proportion of students (over 90%) who reported lifetime alcohol use also reported use in the past 12 months.

Current Use/Daily Use

Current use, or use within the past 30 days, is most useful as a measure of use frequency. The shorter time interval compared with the measures of lifetime and annual use allows for a more precise measure of how frequently students use a particular substance. So-called daily use measures are based on this recent 30-day interval.

Although alcohol is the most prevalent substance used on a lifetime or annual basis, it is not the substance high school students are most likely to use on a daily basis. At its peak, daily alcohol use was reported by 7% of high school seniors. Since 1988, daily alcohol use has remained at or below 4%. The substance most often used daily is cigarettes. Daily cigarette use peaked for high school seniors at about 29% in 1976 and 1977 and then began to decline, reaching a low of 17% in 1992. However, daily cigarette use increased to 25% in 1997 before dropping off to 21% in 2000.

After cigarettes, marijuana is the next substance most commonly used on a daily basis. Daily marijuana use peaked among high school seniors in 1978 at 11% and declined steadily to just under 2% in 1992. However, daily use increased to 6% in 1999 and 2000.

Daily use of other substances is quite low (typically about 0.1%–0.3%). However, daily use of alcohol or illicit drugs is indicative of a serious problem and is likely to lead to school difficulties such as absenteeism, truancy, and dropping out. Daily users are therefore underrepresented in a school survey when compared with substance users in general.

Quantity of Use

Quantity of use is difficult to measure in surveys of illegal drugs because packaging and dosages of the psychoactive ingredients are not standardized.

However, measures do exist for alcohol and tobacco.

In Monitoring the Future (and in most national surveys), *binge drinking* is defined as five or more drinks in a row in the previous 2 weeks. The prevalence of binge drinking among high school seniors peaked at about 41% between 1978 and 1983 and then slowly began to decline. At its low, binge drinking was reported by 28% of seniors from 1992 to 1994. Since then, binge drinking has increased, with 30% of seniors in 2000 reporting binge drinking.

Smoking a half a pack of cigarettes or more daily is clearly associated with health risks. For high school seniors, this level of heavy smoking peaked at 19% between 1976 and 1978 and then declined to a low of 10% in 1992. Heavy smoking subsequently increased to 14% in 1997 and then decreased to 11% in 2000.

Substance Use Among Younger Students

Monitoring the Future data are available for eighth and tenth graders from 1991 through 2000. As with twelfth graders, survey responses showed an increase in use in recent years with peaks in use generally seen during 1996 or 1997. These were followed by slight decreases through 2000. In 2000, lifetime prevalence of alcohol use was reported by over half (52%) of eighth graders and 71% of tenth graders (compared with 80% of twelfth graders). Lifetime prevalence of cigarette smoking was reported by 41% of eighth graders, 55% of tenth graders, and 63% of twelfth graders. Lifetime prevalence of any illicit drug use was reported by 27% of eighth graders, 46% of tenth graders, and 54% of twelfth graders.

The substances reported used most often by eighth graders in 2000 were, in order, alcohol (52%), cigarettes (41%), marijuana (20%), inhalants (18%), smokeless tobacco (13%), amphetamines (10%), hallucinogens (5%), cocaine (5%), tranquilizers (5%), methamphetamines (4%), steroids (3%), and heroin (2%). For tenth graders, the corresponding lifetime prevalence rates were alcohol (71%), cigarettes (55%), marijuana (40%), smokeless tobacco (19%), inhalants (17%), amphetamines (16%), hallucinogens (9%), tranquilizers (8%), cocaine (7%), methamphetamines (7%), steroids (4%), and heroin (2%).

In 2000, one-fourth (25%) of eighth graders and almost one-half (49%) of tenth graders said that they had been drunk at some point in their lives (compared with 62% of twelfth graders). Seven percent of eighth graders and

14% of tenth graders reported daily smoking (compared with 21% of twelfth graders).

Perceived Availability of Substances

Long-term trends in the perceived availability of various substances are available for high school seniors. Perceived availability of barbiturates and tranquilizers peaked in the first year of the Monitoring the Future survey (1975), and the perceived availability of amphetamines peaked in 1982. The proportion who believed that obtaining amphetamines would be fairly easy or very easy decreased from 71% in 1982 to 57% by 2000. The perceived ease of obtaining barbiturates and tranquilizers has declined even more over time. This corresponds to the profound decrease in the number of legal prescriptions for barbiturates and more highly addicting sedative hypnotics. Perceived availability of barbiturates decreased from 60% in 1975 to 37% in 2000, and perceived availability of tranquilizers decreased by more than half, from 72% in 1975 to 34% in 2000.

The perceived availability of cocaine peaked in 1989 at 59% and was reported at 48% in 2000. Perceived availability of LSD peaked at 54% in 1995, the same year that use levels rose above the high recorded in 1975, and was at 47% in 2000. Perceived availability of marijuana peaked in 1998 at 90% and remained at 89% in 1999 and 2000. Perceived availability of heroin also reached a peak in 1998 at 36%, rising much faster than the reported increase in use. Perceived availability of other opiates peaked at 44% in 2000, which far outstripped use rate increases.

Perceived Harmfulness and Disapproval of Substances

Among twelfth-grade students, the perceived harmfulness of alcohol and most drugs peaked in 1990 and 1991. Two notable exceptions are cigarettes and smokeless tobacco, for which perceived harmfulness peaked in 2000, perhaps as a result of the increased media attention to this issue following the settlement of the states' lawsuit against the tobacco companies. Decreases in perceived harmfulness generally precede declines in use. Perceived disapproval of substance use (a measure of social norms) varied more by individual substances but generally peaked between 1987 and 1993. Increases in perceived disapproval also precede declines in use.

Gender, Race/Ethnicity, and Regional Comparisons

The National Household Survey on Drug Abuse provides data on adolescents ages 12–17. Annual prevalence of use data are available for 1999 and can be used to examine differences between males and females, adolescents in different racial/ethnic groups, and adolescents in different parts of the United States (Office of Applied Studies 2000). In 1999, any alcohol use in the past month, binge drinking, and heavy drinking were all more common among males than females. Past-month alcohol use was higher among American Indians or Alaska Natives (21%), whites (20%), and Hispanics (20%) than among blacks and Asians (13% each). Past-month alcohol use was most prevalent in the Northeast (20%), followed by the Midwest and West (19% each) and the South (18%).

Past-year illicit drug use was similar for males (21%) and females (20%) in 1999. The highest rates were reported for American Indians or Alaska Natives (31%). The rates for whites and Hispanics (21% each) and blacks (19%) were higher than the rate for Asians (14%). Annual illicit drug use was highest in the West (22%), followed by the Northeast and Midwest (20% each) and the South (19%).

Past-month cigarette smoking in 1999 was similar for females and males. American Indians or Alaska Natives had the highest rate of current smoking (27%). Whites (17%) and Hispanics (12%) had substantially higher rates than blacks (9%) and Asians (8%). The Midwest had the highest rate (18%), followed by the Northeast and South (15% each) and the West (12%).

According to data from the National Household Survey on Drug Abuse for the years 1994–1996, adolescents with serious emotional problems (as measured by self-report) were nearly four times more likely to be dependent on alcohol or illicit drugs than adolescents with low levels of emotional problems. The association with serious behavioral problems was even stronger; adolescents who reported serious behavioral problems were more than seven times more likely to report alcohol or illicit drug dependence than those with low levels of behavioral problems (Office of Applied Studies 1999).

Substance Abuse Treatment Admissions

A standardized national reporting system on substance abuse treatment admissions was developed only within the past decade. According to these data, adolescent (under age 18) treatment admissions rose by almost 50%

between 1993 and 1998. In 1998, approximately 148,000 adolescents were admitted to treatment compared with 99,000 admitted in 1993 (Office of Applied Studies 2000b). In 1993, treatment admissions for individuals under age 18 made up 6.3% of total admissions. This proportion increased to 9.5% in 1998. Marijuana was the primary substance of abuse, accounting for most adolescent admissions into treatment (57%). This was followed by alcohol (25%), amphetamines (3%) and cocaine (3%) (Office of Applied Studies 2000b).

An International Perspective

The increases in substance use seen among adolescents in the 1990s in the United States were consistent with those seen in most developed countries, including Canada, Western Europe, and Australia (Bauman and Phongsavan 1999). Changes in adolescent substance use prevalence must be considered within the context of the home, school, and broader social environments to which young people are exposed. The regulations and legislation enacted in an attempt to control use and the prevention efforts under way in different areas and at different points in time are other factors that should also be considered when comparing different populations of adolescent substance abusers (Bauman and Phongsavan 1999).

Understanding Changes in Prevalence of Adolescent Substance Use

No single explanation can account for the increases and decreases seen in substance use among adolescents. Changes in attitudes and social norms clearly account for some increases and decreases in use prevalence. Drug use among young people increases when fewer believe that it is dangerous and fewer peers disapprove of use. The Monitoring the Future study showed that changes in perceived harmfulness of drug use and social disapproval of substance use precede changes in the prevalence of use, suggesting that these factors may be causally related to use (Bachman et al. 1998).

Experts also believe that, in periods of declining substance use, attention to the problem wanes, and resources devoted to prevention efforts diminish. This may be what occurred when drug use among adolescents steadily and dramatically declined through the 1980s and into the early 1990s. Complacency may have set in so that the youngest segment of the population was not exposed to sufficient drug prevention messages and strategies. There is evidence that news coverage related to drug abuse and antidrug advertisements decreased as substance abuse decreased (Bachman et al. 1998).

Another possibility that might explain reversals in substance use declines is that as drug use becomes less prevalent, fewer young people directly observe the adverse consequences of use, especially among their peers. This may contribute to their minimization of the hazards of use and lead to a greater willingness to experiment with drugs (Bachman et al. 1998). Some experts also speculate that because the current generation of parents of adolescents is the first among whom drug use was widespread, the parents may feel some ambivalence or sense of hypocrisy when they attempt to warn their children about drugs. They may not be as comfortable or effective in communicating antidrug messages as older generations of parents before them. Complicating the antidrug message further may be the public acknowledgment that illicit drugs were used by many of today's successful public figures. Whatever the explanation, it is clear that in recent years, many of the earlier gains in reducing adolescent substance use have been reversed, and as we approach the start of a new decade, this is an issue that demands more creative responses.

References

Anthony JC, Petronis KR: Early-onset drug use and risk of later drug problems. Drug Alcohol Depend 40:9–15, 1995

Bachman JG, Johnston LD, O'Malley PM: Explaining recent increases in students' marijuana use: impacts of perceived risks and disapproval, 1976 through 1996. Am J Public Health 88:887–892, 1998

Bates SC, Plemons BW, Jumper-Thurman P, et al: Volatile solvent use: patterns by gender and ethnicity among school attenders and dropouts. Drugs and Society 10:61–78, 1997

Bauman A, Phongsavan P: Epidemiology of substance use in adolescence: prevalence, trends and policy implications. Drug Alcohol Depend 55:187–207, 1999

Beauvais F: Trends in drug use among American Indian students and dropouts, 1975 to 1994. Am J Public Health 86:1594–1598, 1996

Dembo R, Williams L, Wothke W, et al: The relationships among family problems, friends' troubled behavior, and high risk youths' alcohol/other drug use and delinquent behavior: a longitudinal study. International Journal of the Addictions 29:1419–1442, 1994

Forst ML: A substance use profile of delinquent and homeless youths. J Drug Educ 24:219–231, 1994

Gfroerer J, Wright D, Kopstein A: Prevalence of youth substance use: the impact of methodological differences between two national surveys. Drug Alcohol Depend 47:19–30, 1997

Grant BF, Dawson DA: Age at onset of alcohol use and its association with DSM-IV alcohol abuse and dependence: results from the National Longitudinal Alcohol Epidemiologic Survey. J Subst Abuse 9:100–103, 1997

Harrison PA: Substance Use in Adolescence: Patterns and Profiles. St. Paul, Minnesota Department of Human Services, 1997

Johnston LD, O'Malley PM, Bachman JG: National Survey Results on Drug Use From the Monitoring the Future Study, 1975–2000, Vol 1: Secondary School Students (NIH Publ No 01-4924). Rockville, MD, National Institute on Drug Abuse, 2001

Kandel DB, Yamaguchi K, Chen K: Stages of progression in drug involvement from adolescence to adulthood: further evidence for the gateway theory. J Stud Alcohol 53:447–457, 1992

Office of Applied Studies: The Relationship Between Mental Health and Substance Abuse Among Adolescents (DHHS Publ No [SMA] 99–3286). Rockville, MD, Substance Abuse and Mental Health Services Administration, 1999

Office of Applied Studies: Summary of Findings from the 1999 National Household Survey on Drug Abuse (DHHS Publ No [SMA] 00-3466). Rockville, MD, Substance Abuse and Mental Health Services Administration, 2000a

Office of Applied Studies: Treatment Episode Data Set (TEDS): 1992–1997 (DHHS Publ No [SMA] 00-3465). Rockville, MD, Substance Abuse and Mental Health Services Administration, 2000b

Sells CW, Blum R: Current trends in adolescent health, in Handbook of Adolescent Risk Behavior. Edited by DiClemente RJ, Hansen WB, Ponton WB. New York, Plenum, 1996, pp 5–29

Weinberg NZ, Rahdert E, Colliver JD, et al: Adolescent substance abuse: a review of the past 10 years. J Am Acad Child Adolesc Psychiatry 37:252–61, 1998

2 Predisposing Factors

Patricia A. Harrison, Ph.D.

Identifying risk factors for alcohol and drug abuse among adolescents is essential to successful prevention and early intervention efforts. Although alcohol and other drugs pose dangers for users of all ages, the potential for physical and psychosocial harm to adolescents is heightened because of the magnified effects of these substances on developing minds and bodies (Czechowicz 1988; Stowell and Estroff 1992). Alcohol and other drugs are readily available to most young people, either in their own homes or through friends (Harrison et al. 2000). In addition, the price of many illicit drugs, such as marijuana or lysergic acid diethylamide (LSD), is within the reach of adolescent budgets. The popular media frequently associate alcohol and other drug use with fun, sex, and success. In American society, experimentation with alcohol and other drugs is viewed as a rite of passage into adulthood (Baumrind 1985; Kandel 1982). For these reasons all young people in American society are at risk for problems with alcohol and other drugs. It is important to remember that the degree of risk varies as a result of factors intrinsic and extrinsic to the individual (Hawkins et al. 1992).

Various rationalizations may lead a young person to experiment with alcohol and other drugs, and once initiated into substance use, he or she continues to use because of the pleasurable feelings associated with it (Marlatt et al. 1988). Alcohol and other drugs are also appealing because they can alleviate painful states (Crowley 1988), an effect that may be especially attractive during adolescence when some young people experience a turbulent transition into adulthood. Although adolescents may intellectually know the risks associated with alcohol and other drugs, they tend to distort the acts by believing they are personally invulnerable to such harm (Botvin and Wills 1985). When this illusion is combined with the inexperience, poor judgment, and recklessness of youth, tragic consequences frequently result. Alcohol and other drug use, particularly among young people, is associated with delinquency, violence, victimization, and the early onset of sexual behavior (Cherpitel 1992; Durant et al. 1997; Kandel 1990; Kingery et al. 1992; Martin 1992; Pihl and Peterson 1993; Stinson et al. 1993; Swanson 1993). Substance abuse has also been found to be associated with suicide attempts (Martin et al. 1997) and completed suicides (Brent et al. 1993) among adolescents.

Assessing risk factors for alcohol and drug abuse among young people can be problematic because any amount of use can legitimately be defined as abuse. In fact, federal policymakers recommend using the term *abuse* for any illicit drug and alcohol use among people under the legal drinking age. Although this makes sense in terms of a clear and consistent message of "zero tolerance" for substance use among adolescents, it often blurs the distinction between patterns of use involving varying amounts and frequencies of use. In diagnostic classifications, abuse is typically distinguished by the occurrence of harmful consequences that typically result from excessive use, such as an arrest for driving under the influence. Because most social, medical, and economic costs are associated with abuse rather than use, it is useful to carefully note such distinctions (Kumpfer 1989). Generally, risk factors are most evident among users whose use patterns deviate most widely from those of their peers—this includes the youngest users and older adolescents who use much more frequently or in greater amounts than others their age (Harrison and Luxenberg 1995).

Early age of onset of substance use is a predictor of progression to more serious drugs and adverse use consequences (Bailey et al. 1992; Kandel and Yamaguchi 1993; Kumpfer 1989). It is frequently indicative of concomitant problems (Harrison and Luxenberg 1995). Early onset of alcohol use is strongly associated with a diagnosis of alcohol dependence among adults (Grant and Dawson 1997). In contrast, initiation of drug and alcohol use in late adolescence does not necessarily lead to abuse nor is it causally associated with other problems or risk factors. Not all adolescents who initiate drug use continue to use. Not all adolescents who continue use escalate to more frequent use, use larger amounts of drugs, or experience apparent adverse consequences (Bailey et al. 1992). In fact, most adolescents who drink heavily moderate their use later in life (Donovan et al. 1983; Fillmore and Midanik 1984; Kandel and Logan 1984). Similarly, most young people who try marijuana do not progress to regular use (Kandel et al. 1992). Etiological factors implicated in the initiation of drug and alcohol use differ from those that explain continuance, escalation, or addiction (Baumrind 1985; Hawkins et al. 1985; Robins and Przybeck 1985; Scheier and Newcomb 1991; Scheier et al. 1997; Simcha-Fagan et al. 1986; Weber et al. 1989).

As use escalates toward abuse, warning signs appear in many areas of the adolescent's life. As young people get into trouble with alcohol or other drugs they give more rationalizations for their use and thus justify their increase in the quantity and frequency of use and the frequency of intoxication. They also tend to try a greater number of different kinds of drugs and experience more adverse consequences (Harrison et al. 1998; Kandel et al. 1992).

General school surveys and studies of special populations of adolescents all support the contention that substance abuse is not a random phenomenon. High rates of coexisting problems are seen among adolescents referred to or admitted for treatment of alcohol and drug problems. These include psychological distress, learning difficulties, poor self-image, social alienation, antisocial behavior, and histories of sexual and physical abuse (Grilo et al. 1996; Harrison et al. 1989a, 1989b; Mezzich et al. 1997; Whitmore et al. 1997; Young et al. 1995). Elevated rates of these same problems are also seen among alcohol- and drug-abusing adolescents in alternative schools, correctional settings, and residential programs for adolescents with emotional and behavioral problems (Dembo et al. 1990; Fulkerson et al. 1999a, 1999b; Hedger et al. 1999) and among runaways and homeless youth (Fors and Rojek 1991; Smart and Adlaf 1991).

Behavioral Correlates

Conduct Disorders

One of the most consistently identified risk factors for alcohol and other drug abuse among adolescents is antisocial behavior (Clayton 1981; Donovan and Jessor 1985; Jessor and Jessor 1975; Kingery et al. 1992; Robins 1978). Some specific factors predictive of later drug use have been identified in childhood, including impulsiveness, aggressiveness, and rebelliousness (Brook et al. 1992). A longitudinal study of children through early adulthood found that childhood aggression is a precursor of adolescent drug use

(Brook et al. 1992) and that drug use during early adolescence predisposes children to delinquency throughout adolescence and into young adulthood (Brook et al. 1996).

The association of substance abuse with antisocial behaviors and conduct disorders begs the question of etiology, however. In fact, it is now generally agreed that substance abuse is merely one of a variety of behaviors that make up a problem behavior syndrome (Jessor and Jessor 1975). The predictors of alcohol and other drug abuse are similar to the predictors of other maladaptive behaviors including delinquency and academic failure (Newcomb and Bentler 1989). Genetic or family factors have been strongly implicated in the development of antisocial behavior and delinquency among children and adolescents. Absence of or inconsistency in parental discipline, parental substance abuse, parental antisocial behavior, disparaging and blaming parental communication patterns, and family disruption have all been found to be associated specifically with adolescent substance abuse (Baumrind 1985; Kandel 1982; Loeber and Dishion 1983; Robins 1978). Childhood physical abuse has been implicated more generally in conduct disorders and adolescent delinquency (Cavaiola and Schiff 1988; Livingston 1987; McCord 1983). Overall, alienation from important adults has been found to be a key contributor to the development of alcohol and drug problems among young people (Hawkins et al. 1986).

Novelty seeking, doing dangerous things "just for kicks," and other physically risky behavior such as hitchhiking or carrying a weapon are significantly associated with substance use among adolescents (Fe Caces et al. 1991; Kandel and Davies 1996; Kingery et al. 1992; Wills et al. 1994); greater frequency of drinking and drug use is accompanied by an increased tendency to engage in risky behavior. Early initiation into sexual activity is also strongly correlated with alcohol and other drug use (Kandel 1990).

Attention-Deficit/Hyperactivity Disorder

Childhood attention-deficit/hyperactivity disorder (ADHD) has been associated with alcohol, opiate, and cocaine abuse in adulthood as well as adolescent substance abuse (Carroll and Rounsaville 1993; DeMilio 1989; Eyre et al. 1982; Whitmore et al. 1997; Windle 1993). Childhood ADHD has been found to be associated with the early onset of substance abuse in a clinical sample (Wilens et al. 1997) and a nonclinical sample (Windle 1993). The risk for early onset of substance abuse appears higher when ADHD is comorbid with conduct disorder (Milberger et al. 1997). In one longitudinal study, children with concurrent diagnoses of ADHD and conduct disorder were more likely than those with ADHD alone to abuse alcohol and other drugs 8 years later (Barkley et al. 1990). Because of the considerable overlap between diagnostic criteria for conduct disorder and ADHD, many children meet diagnostic criteria for both (Bukstein et al. 1989). It has been speculated that it is conduct disorder or specific behaviors, such as aggression, that predict substance abuse rather than ADHD (Pihl and Peterson 1991); one study reported that ADHD did not predict substance abuse in the absence of aggression (Halikas et al. 1990).

School Performance

Like antisocial behavior, poor school performance has been found in longitudinal studies to be an antecedent to drug use (Jessor and Jessor 1977; Kandel 1981). Student surveys have also found that absenteeism, truancy, and poor academic performance are significantly related to substance abuse (Harrison and Luxenberg 1995; Kandel and Davies 1996). Poor school performance may not lead to substance use, but the same factors that lead to school difficulties may also lead to drug use. The relationship between alcohol and drug use and poor school performance is frequently a downward spiral leading to a cycle of failure (Brook et al. 1977; Jessor and Jessor 1977; Kandel 1982). Substance use is also a predictor of school dropout (Annis and Watson 1975; Johnson and Solis 1983). Adolescents who drop out have a higher rate of substance abuse than those still enrolled in school (Guagliardo et al. 1998). School failure may involve more than academic performance, however. Adolescents who do not believe teachers and friends care very much about them are also at elevated risk to develop substance abuse (Harrison and Luxenberg 1995).

Peer Influences

Association with alcohol- or drug-using peers is consistently found to be among the strongest correlates of adolescent substance use and abuse (Dinges and Oetting 1993; Dishion et al. 1995; Jessor et al. 1980; Kandel and Davies 1996; Loveland-Cherry et al. 1996; Rachal et al. 1982; Smart et al. 1978). The influence of peers greatly increases during adolescence (Glynn 1987), and the use of alcohol and other drugs is frequently encouraged by peers (Botvin and Wills 1985).

Children and adolescents do not always freely choose their peer groups. Some young persons are rejected by non-drug-using social groups and turn away from them and associate with other individuals on the "outside." These youth may engage in deviant behavior in their search for social acceptance.

Gravitation toward deviant peers may be a consequence of family conflict, school failure, or isolation. Young people who come from families characterized by hostility, discord, violence, or sexual abuse are likely to withdraw from the family (Barnes and Farrell 1992). They may have a particularly hard time establishing healthy friendships. Association with delinquent and drug-using peers is more likely in the absence of strong bonds to family, religion, and school and with noninvolvement in school, family, and work activities (Buckhalt et al. 1992; Elliott et al. 1982). Peer influences clearly interact with family influences (Barnes and Farrell 1992; Farrell and White 1998) and in some cases can even counteract the best family influences.

Expectations

Whether the effects of alcohol or drugs are experienced as positive or negative is highly influenced by the abuser's beliefs and expectations (Rohsenow 1983; Sher 1985; Zinberg 1984). Drug and alcohol abusers are more likely than other users to expect positive consequences of use and to minimize negative consequences. Positive expectations include increased social and physical pleasure, improved sexual performance or responsiveness, reduction of tension or stress, and improved ability to deal with negative feelings (Brown et al. 1985; Christiansen and Goldman 1983; Christiansen et al. 1982, 1985; Mann et al. 1987; Oei and Jones 1986). These expectations may antedate drinking or drug use and predict later use (Christiansen et al. 1989). Expectations of alcohol and drug abuse can be heavily influenced by the adolescent's drinking history and level of intoxication (Southwick et al. 1981). Adolescents whose parents abuse alcohol are more likely to believe that alcohol has positive effects (Brown et al. 1987).

Self-Esteem

Many young people experience a heightened and even painful sense of self-consciousness during adolescence. This is particularly true with respect to personal appearance and doubts about personal qualities and abilities (Elkind 1978). However, findings have been contradictory with respect to the relationship of self-esteem to the increased likelihood of substance use (e.g., Barnes 1984; Emery et al. 1993; Labouvie and McGee 1986; Newcomb and Bentler 1986). A review of prospective studies concluded that low self-esteem is not more common among adolescent illicit drug users (Petraitis et al. 1998). The failure to find consistent relationships may result from differences in defining self-esteem and differences in the level of substance use examined (e.g., any use versus regular use). When substance abuse was defined as three or more adverse consequences of use, a student survey found strong associations between substance abuse and low self-esteem, but the relationship was stronger for younger adolescents than for older adolescents (Harrison and Luxenberg 1995).

Psychiatric Disturbances

Epidemiological and clinical studies of adults have found a very high rate of comorbidity of mental disorders with substance abuse (Regier et al. 1990); the same has held true for adolescents (Stowell and Estroff 1992; Substance Abuse and Mental Health Services Administration 1999). Adolescents in treatment for substance abuse exhibit elevated rates of depression and anxiety (Stowell and Estroff 1992) as well as posttraumatic stress disorder, especially females (Deykin and Buka 1997). The severity of major depressive disorder has also been found to be associated with the severity of substance abuse (Whitmore et al. 1997). Elevated rates of substance abuse have been reported among patients with eating disorders, particularly bulimia (Newman and Gold 1992). Psychopathology among young people has been found to be both an antecedent to and a consequence of substance abuse (Friedman et al. 1987). Epidemiological studies also find a strong correlation between affective disturbances and substance abuse (Harrison and Luxenberg 1995; Kandel and Davies 1986; Substance Abuse and Mental Health Services Administration 1999). Specifically, depressive mood is associated with both the onset of marijuana use and the progression from marijuana to other illicit drugs (Paton et al. 1977). Crack cocaine abuse is associated with the lowest levels of psychosocial functioning among adolescents (Kandel and Davies 1996).

Suicidal Behavior

Suicides among adolescents have increased greatly over recent decades and the increase may be attributable in part to the increase in substance abuse among this age group (McKenry et al. 1983; Shaffer 1988; Shafii et al. 1985). Substance abuse can lead directly to feelings of depression and hopelessness and can impair judgment and lessen inhibitions against suicidal behavior. Substance abuse can also exacerbate preexisting psychiatric conditions that pose an increased risk for suicide. A student survey found that adolescents who reported three or more negative consequences of substance use were much more likely to have attempted suicide than substance users with fewer consequences or nonusers, with the risk greatest among younger students (Harrison and Luxenberg 1995). A study of adolescent suicide completers found an association with substance abuse, especially when comorbid with depression (Brent et al. 1993).

Individual Risk Factors

Genetics/Family History

Research to date has not discovered an "addiction gene," although there is little argument that alcoholism and drug abuse run in families—that is, the prevalence of substance abuse is higher among family members of an identified substance abuser than among the general population (Clark et al. 1998). Research has also shown that there may be risk factors present that predict a specific class of drug abuse as well as general risk factors that predispose the adolescent to substance use disorders in general (Merikangas et al. 1998). The magnitude of the genetic contribution to alcoholism has not been established, and it is highly likely that both genetic and environmental factors influence the development of alcohol dependence (Schuckit 1994, 1998). Although the mechanism for genetic influence has not yet been identified, there may be a gene (or combination of genes) that contributes to an unusually strong positive response to alcohol or other drugs, thus increasing the desire for consumption. On the other hand, a gene or group of genes may reduce the adverse effects associated with alcohol or other drugs, such as a hangover, which would minimize the deterrents to excessive use (Pickens and Svikis 1988). Other possibilities include more indirect heritability. Genes may determine personality characteristics, which might increase the probability of exposure to drugs or to excessive use patterns (Pickens and Svikis 1988), or familial clustering of substance use disorders could result from a genetic transmission of psychopathology that may underlie the development of substance abuse (Rounsaville 1988).

Research into genetic vulnerability has included animal studies, family incidence studies, twin studies, adoption studies, and high-risk population studies, and all support the heritability of alcoholism. Most research with human subjects has examined alcoholism rather than drug addiction. However, animal studies support heritability of both alcohol and drug addiction (Meisch and George 1988).

Most twin studies have found a higher concordance rate for alcoholism in identical twins (approximately 60%) than in fraternal twins (approximately 30%), providing evidence that genes are more important than environment in determining alcoholism (Schuckit 1985a, 1985b). Adoption studies reach similar conclusions. Adopted-away children of alcoholic biological parents have rates of alcoholism three to four times higher than adoptees raised in alcoholic households. Being raised by an alcoholic adoptive parent does not increase the risk of alcoholism for an adopted child (Cloninger 1988; Cloninger et al. 1981; Gabrielli and Plomin 1985; Goodwin 1984; Schuckit 1985a, 1985b).

In the search for genetic markers, children of alcoholic parents have been compared with children of nonalcoholic parents to look for differences that cannot be attributed to their own use of alcohol (Begleiter et al. 1984; Moss et al. 1989; Propping et al. 1981; Schaeffer et al. 1984; Schuckit 1984; Schuckit et al. 1987). Some studies have found a decreased intensity of reaction to modest doses of alcohol in children of alcoholics. Such a characteristic could be related to a greater likelihood of alcoholism because the lessened response makes it more difficult to know when to stop drinking (Schuckit 1985a). Such a lowered response measured at around age 20 has been found to be predictive of subsequent alcoholism among sons of alcoholics studied over 10–15 years (Schuckit 1998). In other lines of investigation, electroencephalographic and other brain wave studies have found differences between children of alcoholics and children of nonalcoholics that may be related to a difficulty in focusing attention associated with learning deficits (Begleiter and Porjesz 1988; Pollock et al. 1983; Schuckit 1985a, 1987). Differences have also been found in muscle-tension response to alcohol in young men with family histories of alcoholism (Schuckit et al. 1981).

Parent–Child Relationships

Poor parent–child relationships, turbulent marital relationships, and general family disharmony have been consistently associated with delinquent behavior among young people. This includes substance abuse (Gove and Crutchfield 1982; Simcha-Fagan et al. 1986; Webb and Baer 1995). Other forms of child maltreatment by parents, such as psychological unavailability and neglect, lack of warmth and affection, and rejection, predict problems such as substance abuse among offspring (Egeland et al. 1983; Parker 1979). Unfair, inconsistent, and harsh discipline has been found to influence the development of both alcoholism and depression (Holmes and Robins 1987, 1988). Parental permissiveness is also positively correlated with alcohol use among young adolescents (Loveland-Cherry et al. 1996). Parents of adolescent drug users use drugs themselves more extensively than do the parents of nonusers (Kandel and Davies 1996). In a panel study involving parents and children in a clinical and community sample, the presence of parental substance use disorders and parental affective disorders were both found to increase adolescent substance use disorders (Su et al. 1997).

Sexual and Physical Abuse

Rates of sexual and physical abuse among adolescents in treatment for substance abuse are much higher than rates reported in epidemiological studies (Cavaiola and Schiff 1988, 1989; Harrison et al. 1989a, 1989b; Rohsenow et al. 1988). In student surveys, adolescents who report a history of sexual or physical abuse have higher rates of alcohol and other drug use, are much more likely to use a variety of drugs, and more often report using substances to escape from personal problems or cope with negative affect (Harrison et al. 1997; Watts and Ellis 1993). These findings are consistent with clinical reports of abuse victims in treatment for chemical dependency (Harrison et al. 1989a, 1989b) and the elevated rates of posttraumatic stress disorders reported by adolescents in substance abuse treatment (Deykin and Buka 1997). Because trauma victims often experience both heightened feeling states (such as anxiety and aggression) and constriction of emotions, they may be at particularly high risk for experimenting with drugs and continuing use in an attempt to distance themselves from their experiences (Hussey and Singer 1993; van der Kolk 1987).

Gender Differences in Substance Use Disorders

Epidemiological studies of adult populations consistently find higher rates of alcohol and drug abuse and dependence among men than women. In the most methodologically rigorous and extensive lifetime prevalence study conducted to date, adult male–female ratios approximate 5:1 for alcohol use disorders and 2:1 for drug use disorders (Regier et al. 1988; Robins et al. 1984). Although little difference is seen in rates of problem use among young adolescents, by age 18 substance-abusing males outnumber substance-abusing females. Male adolescents are more likely than female adolescents to use illicit drugs, and the differences increase at higher use frequency levels. Males also predominate among heavy drinkers at this age (O'Malley et al. 1993). According to one definition of substance dependence used in a household survey of adolescents, male and female rates were similar (Substance Abuse and Mental Health Services Administration 1999). However, in a clinical population in which the diagnostic criteria were presumably more stringent, males who met diagnostic threshold outnumbered females by a ratio of 2:1 (Stowell and Estroff 1992).

None of the genetic research to date can explain the male predominance of alcohol use disorders (Helzer 1987); psychosocial factors probably account for the higher rate seen in males. Social constraints against heavy drinking remain stronger for females (Cloninger et al. 1978), and young women more readily accept parental drinking norms than do young men (Wilks and Callan 1988). Young males frequently drink in the company of other young males and often derive their concept of "normal" drinking from these limited and biased comparisons. The social network perspective has also been found to explain gender differences in marijuana use (Wister and Avison 1982).

Another important factor in understanding gender prevalence rates for substance use disorders is the limitations of diagnosis. Alcohol and drug abuse and dependence are diagnosed not by laboratory tests but by behavior patterns. Males have generally higher rates of the socially irresponsible behaviors and legal complications that support a substance use disorder diagnosis. Young males typically report higher-volume and higher-frequency drinking than females, and more males disregard the risks of drinking and driving. More males also report destructive and assaultive behaviors regardless of whether or not they have been drinking or using drugs. Because social and vocational consequences of drinking and drug use are integral to the diagnostic determination of substance use disorders, abuse and dependence diagnoses based on associated behaviors may be more sensitive to male manifestations of alcohol and drug problems.

Summary

Alcohol and other drug use initiation, continuance, and abuse are typically the result of a complex interaction of parental and peer influences, life events, other sociocultural and environmental factors, outcome expectancies, psychological vulnerability to the effects or perceived effects of use, and genetic or biological vulnerabilities including psychiatric disorders and different pharmacological responses. Young people at higher than average risk for substance abuse problems are not as likely as their peers to be deterred by broad-based prevention efforts. Interventions targeted to their special needs may be essential to reducing their high rates of alcohol and drug problems.

References

Annis HM, Watson C: Drug use and school dropouts: a longitudinal study. Canadian Counselor 6:155–162, 1975

Bailey SL, Flewelling RL, Rachal JV: Predicting continued use of marijuana among adolescents: the relative influence of drug-specific and social context factors. Journal of Health and Social Behavior 33:51–66, 1992

Barkley RA, Fischer M, Edelbrock C, et al: The adolescent outcome of hyperactive children diagnosed by research criteria, I: an 8-year prospective follow-up study. J Am Acad Child Adolesc Psychiatry 29:546–557, 1990

Barnes GM: Adolescent alcohol abuse and other problem behaviors: their relationship and common parental influences. Journal of Youth and Adolescence 13:329–348, 1984

Barnes GM, Farrell MP: Parental support and control as predictors of adolescent drinking, delinquency, and related problem behaviors. Journal of Marriage and the Family 54:763–776, 1992

Baumrind D: Familial antecedents of adolescent drug use: a developmental perspective, in Etiology of Drug Abuse: Implications for Prevention (NIDA Res Monogr 56; DHHS Publ No [ADM]-85-1335). Washington, DC, U.S. Government Printing Office, 1985, pp 13–44

Begleiter H, Porjesz B: Potential biological markers in individuals at high risk for developing alcoholism. Alcohol Clin Exp Res 12:488–493, 1988

Begleiter H, Porjesz B, Bihari B, et al: Event-related brain potentials in boys at risk for alcoholism. Science 225:1493–1495, 1984

Botvin GJ, Wills TA: Personal and social skills training: cognitive-behavioral approaches to substance abuse prevention, in Prevention Research: Deterring Drug Abuse Among Children and Adolescents (NIDA Res Monogr 63; DHHS Publ No [ADM]-85-1334). Washington, DC, U.S. Government Printing Office, 1985, pp 8–49

Brent DA, Perper JA, Moritz G, et al: Psychiatric risk factors for adolescent suicide: a case-control study. J Acad Child Adolesc Psychiatry 32:521–529, 1993

Brook JS, Lukoff IF, Whiteman M: Peer, family, and personality domains as related to adolescents' drug behavior. Psychol Rep 41:1095–1102, 1977

Brook JS, Whiteman MM, Finch S: Childhood aggression, adolescent delinquency, and drug use: a longitudinal study. J Genet Psychol 153:369–383, 1992

Brook JS, Whiteman M, Finch SJ, et al: Young adult drug use and delinquency: childhood antecedents and adolescent mediators. J Acad Child Adolesc Psychiatry 35:1584–1592, 1996

Brown SA, Goldman MS, Christiansen BA: Do alcohol expectancies mediate drinking patterns of adults? J Consult Clin Psychol 53:512–519, 1985

Brown SA, Creamer VA, Stetson BA: Adolescent alcohol expectancies in relation to personal and parental drinking patterns. J Abnorm Psychol 96:117–121, 1987

Buckhalt JA, Halpin G, Noel R, et al: Relationship of drug use to involvement in school, home, and community activities: results of a large survey of adolescents. Psychol Rep 70:139–146, 1992

Bukstein OG, Brent DA, Kamminer Y: Comorbidity of substance abuse and other psychiatric disorders in adolescents. Am J Psychiatry 146:1131–1141, 1989

Carroll KM, Rounsaville BJ: History and significance of childhood attention deficit disorder in treatment-seeking cocaine abusers. Compr Psychiatry 34:75–82, 1993

Cavaiola AA, Schiff M: Behavioral sequelae of physical and/or sexual abuse in adolescents. Child Abuse Negl 12:181–188, 1988

Cavaiola AA, Schiff M: Self-esteem in abused chemically dependent adolescents. Child Abuse Negl 13:327–334, 1989

Cherpitel CJ: The epidemiology of alcohol-related trauma. Alcohol Health Res World 16:191–196, 1992

Christiansen BA, Goldman MS: Alcohol-related expectancies vs demographic/background variables in the prediction of adolescent drinking. J Consult Clin Psychol 51:249–257, 1983

Christiansen BA, Goldman MS, Inn A: The development of alcohol-related expectancies in adolescents: separating pharmacological from social learning influences. J Consult Clin Psychol 50:336–344, 1982

Christiansen BA, Goldman MS, Brown SA: The differential development of adolescent alcohol expectancies may predict adult alcoholism. Addict Behav 10:299–306, 1985

Christiansen BA, Roehling PV, Smith GT, et al: Using alcohol expectancies to predict adolescent drinking behavior after one year. J Consult Clin Psychol 57:93–99, 1989

Clark DB, Kirisci L, Moss HB: Early adolescent gateway drug use in sons of fathers with substance use disorders. Addict Behav 23:561–566, 1998

Clayton RR: The delinquency and drug use relationship among adolescents: a critical review, in Drug Abuse and the American Adolescent (NIDA Res Monogr 38; DHHS Publ No [ADM] 81-1166). Washington, DC, U.S. Government Printing Office, 1981, pp 82–103

Cloninger CR: Etiological factors in substance abuse: an adoption study perspective, in Biological Vulnerability to Drug Abuse (NIDA Res Monogr 89; DHHS Publ No [ADM] 88-1590). Washington, DC, U.S. Government Printing Office, 1988, pp 52–72

Cloninger CR, Christiansen KO, Reich T, et al: Implications of sex differences in the prevalence of antisocial personality, alcoholism, and criminality for familial transmission. Arch Gen Psychiatry 35:941–951, 1978

Cloninger CR, Bohman M, Sigvardsson S: Inheritance of alcohol abuse: cross-fostering analysis of adopted men. Arch Gen Psychiatry 38:861–868, 1981

Crowley TJ: Learning and unlearning drug abuse in the real world: clinical treatment and public policy, in Learning Factors in Substance Abuse (NIDA Res Monogr 84; DHHS Publ No [ADM] 88-1576). Washington, DC, U.S. Government Printing Office, 1988, pp 100–121

Czechowicz D: Adolescent alcohol and drug abuse and its consequences—an overview. Am J Drug Alcohol Abuse 14:189–197, 1988

Dembo R, Williams L, La Voie L, et al: A longitudinal study of the relationships among alcohol use, marijuana/hashish use, cocaine use, and emotional/psychological functioning problems in a cohort of high-risk youths. International Journal of the Addictions 25:1341–1382, 1990

DeMilio L: Psychiatric syndromes in adolescent substance abusers. Am J Psychiatry 146:1212–1214, 1989

Deykin EY, Buka SL: Prevalence and risk factors for posttraumatic stress disorder among chemically dependent adolescents. Am J Psychiatry 154:752–757, 1997

Dinges MM, Oetting ER: Similarity in drug use patterns between adolescents and their friends. Adolescence 28:253–266, 1993

Dishion TJ, Capaldi D, Spracklen KM, et al: Peer ecology of male adolescent drug use. Dev Psychopathol 7:803–824, 1995

Donovan JE, Jessor R: Structure of problem behavior in adolescence and young adulthood. J Consult Clin Psychol 53:890–904, 1985

Donovan JE, Jessor R, Jessor L: Problem drinking in adolescence and young adulthood: a follow-up study. J Stud Alcohol 44:109–136, 1983

Durant RH, Knight J, Goodman E: Factors associated with aggressive and delinquent behaviors among patients attending an adolescent medicine clinic. J Adolesc Health 21:303–308, 1997

Egeland B, Sroufe LF, Erickson M: The developmental consequences of different patterns of maltreatment. Child Abuse Neglect 7:459–469, 1983

Elkind D: Understanding the young adolescent. Adolescence 8:127–134, 1978

Elliott DS, Huizinga D, Ageton SS: Explaining Delinquency and Drug Use (BRI Report No 21). Boulder, CO, Behavioral Research Institute, 1982

Emery EM, McDermott RJ, Holcomb DR, et al: The relationship between youth substance use and area-specific self-esteem. Journal of School Health 63:224–228, 1993

Eyre SL, Rounsaville BJ, Kleber HD: History of childhood hyperactivity in a clinic population of opiate addicts. J Nerv Ment Dis 170:522–529, 1982

Farrell AD, White KS: Peer influences on drug use among urban adolescents: family structure and parent-adolescent relationship as protective factors. J Consult Clin Psychol 66:248–258, 1998

Fe Caces M, Stinson FS, Harford TC: Alcohol use and physically risky behavior among adolescents. Alcohol Health Res World 15:228–233, 1991

Fillmore KM, Midanik L: Chronicity of drinking problems among men: a longitudinal study. J Stud Alcohol 45:228–236, 1984

Fors SW, Rojek DG: A comparison of drug involvement between runaways and school youths. J Drug Educ 21:13–25, 1991

Friedman AS, Utada AT, Glickman NW: Psychopathology as an antecedent to and as a "consequence" of substance use in adolescence. J Drug Educ 17:233–244, 1987

Fulkerson JA, Harrison PA, Hedger SA: 1998 Minnesota Student Survey Alternative Schools and Area Learning Centers. St Paul, Minnesota Department of Human Services, 1999a

Fulkerson JA, Harrison PA, Hedger SA: 1998 Minnesota Student Survey Juvenile Correctional Facilities. St Paul, Minnesota Department of Human Services, 1999b

Gabrielli WF, Plomin R: Drinking behavior in the Colorado adoptee and twin sample. J Stud Alcohol 46:24–31, 1985

Glynn TJ: From family to peer: transitions of influence among drug-using youth, in Drug Abuse and the American Adolescent (NIDA Res Monogr 38; DHHS Publ No [ADM]-81-1166). Washington, DC, U.S. Government Printing Office, 1987, pp 57–81

Goodwin DW: Studies of familial alcoholism: a review. J Clin Psychiatry 45 (No 12, Sec 2):14–17, 1984

Gove WR, Crutchfield RD: The family and juvenile delinquency. Sociological Quarterly 23:301–319, 1982

Grant BF, Dawson DA: Age at onset of alcohol use and its association with DSM-IV alcohol abuse and dependence: results from the National Longitudinal Alcohol Epidemiologic Survey. J Subst Abuse 9:103–110, 1997

Grilo CM, Becker DF, Fehon DC, et al: Conduct disorder, substance use disorders, and co-existing conduct and substance use disorders in adolescent inpatients. Am J Psychiatry 153:914–920, 1996

Guagliardo MF, Huang Z, Hicks J, et al: Increased drug use among old-for-grade and dropout urban adolescents. Am J Prev Med 15:42–48, 1998

Halikas J, Melles J, Morse C, et al: Predicting substance abuse in juvenile offenders: attention deficit disorder versus aggressivity. Child Psychiatry Hum Dev 21:49–55, 1990

Harrison PA, Luxenberg MG: Comparisons of alcohol and other drug problems among Minnesota adolescents in 1989 and 1992. Arch Pediatr Adolesc Med 149:137–144, 1995

Harrison PA, Hoffmann NG, Edwall GE: Differential drug use patterns among sexually abused adolescent girls in treatment for chemical dependency. International Journal of the Addictions 24:499–514, 1989a

Harrison PA, Hoffmann NG, Edwall GE: Sexual abuse correlates: similarities between male and female adolescents in chemical dependency treatment. Journal of Adolescent Research 4:385–399, 1989b

Harrison PA, Fulkerson JA, Beebe TJ: Multiple substance use among adolescent physical and sexual abuse victims. Child Abuse Negl 21:529–539, 1997

Harrison PA, Fulkerson JA, Beebe TJ: DSM-IV substance use disorder criteria for adolescents: a critical examination based on a statewide school survey. Am J Psychiatry 155:486–492, 1998

Harrison PA, Fulkerson JA, Park E: The relative importance of social versus commercial sources in youth access to tobacco, alcohol, and other drugs. Preventive Medicine 31:39–48, 2000

Hawkins JD, Lishner DM, Catalano RF: Childhood predictors and the prevention of adolescent substance abuse, in Etiology of Drug Abuse: Implications for Prevention (NIDA Res Monogr 56; DHHS Publ No [ADM]-85–1335). Washington, DC, U.S. Government Printing Office, 1985, pp 75–126

Hawkins JD, Lishner DM, Catalano RF, et al: Childhood predictors of adolescent substance abuse: towards an empirically grounded theory. Journal of Children in Contemporary Society 18:1–65, 1986

Hawkins JD, Catalano RF, Miller JY: Risk and protective factors for alcohol and other drug problems in adolescence and early adulthood: implications for substance abuse prevention. Psychol Bull 112:64–105, 1992

Hedger SA, Harrison PA, Fulkerson JA: 1998 Minnesota Student Survey: Residential Behavioral Treatment Facilities. St Paul, Minnesota Department of Human Services, 1999

Helzer JE: Epidemiology of alcoholism. J Consult Clin Psychol 55:284–292, 1987

Holmes SJ, Robins LN: The influence of childhood disciplinary experience on the development of alcoholism and depression. J Child Psychol Psychiatry 28:399–415, 1987

Holmes SJ, Robins LN: The role of parental disciplinary practices in the development of depression and alcoholism. Psychiatry 51:24–36, 1988

Hussey DL, Singer M: Psychological distress, problem behaviors, and family functioning of sexually abused adolescent inpatients. J Acad Child Adolesc Psychiatry 32:954–961, 1993

Jessor R, Jessor SL: Adolescent development and the onset of drinking: a longitudinal study. J Stud Alcohol 36:27–51, 1975

Jessor R, Jessor SL: Problem Behavior and Psychosocial Development: A Longitudinal Study of Youth. New York, Academic Press, 1977

Jessor R, Chase JA, Donovan JE: Psychosocial correlates of marijuana use and problem drinking in a national sample of adolescents. Am J Public Health 70:604–613, 1980

Johnson CA, Solis J: Comprehensive Community Programs for Drug Abuse Prevention (NIDA Res Monogr 47; DHHS Publ No [ADM]-83–1280). Washington, DC, U.S. Government Printing Office, 1983, pp 76–114

Kandel DB: Drug use by youth: an overview, in Drug Abuse and the American Adolescent (NIDA Res Monogr 38; DHHS Publ No (ADM) 81-1166). Washington, DC, U.S. Government Printing Office, 1981, pp 1–24

Kandel DB: Epidemiological and psychosocial perspectives on adolescent drug use. Journal of the American Academy of Child Psychiatry 21:328–347, 1982

Kandel DB: Early onset of adolescent sexual behavior and drug involvement. Journal of Marriage and the Family 52:783–798, 1990

Kandel DB, Davies M: Adult sequelae of adolescent depressive symptoms. Arch Gen Psychiatry 43:255–262, 1986

Kandel DB, Davies M: High school students who use crack and other drugs. Arch Gen Psychiatry 53:71–80, 1996

Kandel DB, Logan JA: Patterns of drug use from adolescence to young adulthood: periods of risk for initiation, continued use, and discontinuation. Am J Public Health 74:660–666, 1984

Kandel D, Yamaguchi K: From beer to crack: developmental patterns of drug involvement. Am J Public Health 83:851–855, 1993

Kandel DB, Yamaguchi K, Chen K: Stages of progression in drug involvement from adolescence to adulthood: further evidence for the gateway theory. J Stud Alcohol 53:447–457, 1992

Kingery PM, Pruitt BE, Hurley RS: Violence and illegal drug use among adolescents: evidence from the US National Adolescent Student Health Survey. International Journal of the Addictions 27:1445–1464, 1992

Kumpfer KL: Prevention of alcohol and drug abuse: a critical review of risk factors and prevention strategies, in Prevention of Mental Disorders, Alcohol and Other Drug Use in Children and Adolescents (Office for Substance Abuse Prevention Monogr 2; DHHS Publ No [ADM]-89-1646). Washington, DC, U.S. Government Printing Office, 1989, pp 309–371

Labouvie EW, McGee CR: Relationship of personality to alcohol and drug use in adolescents. J Consult Clin Psychol 54:289–293, 1986

Livingston R: Sexually and physically abused children. J Am Acad Child Adolesc Psychiatry 26:413–415, 1987

Loeber R, Dishion T: Early predictors of male delinquency: a review. Psychol Bull 93:68–99, 1983

Loveland-Cherry CJ, Leech S, Laetz VB, et al: Correlates of alcohol use and misuse in fourth-grade children: psychosocial, peer, parental, and family factors. Health Education Quarterly 23:497–511, 1996

Mann LM, Chassin L, Sher KJ: Alcohol expectancies and the risk for alcoholism. J Consult Clin Psychol 55:411–417, 1987

Marlatt GA, Baer JS, Donovan DM, et al: Addictive behaviors: etiology and treatment. Annual Reviews in Psychology 39:223–252, 1988

Martin CA, Milich R, Martin WR, et al: Gender differences in adolescent psychiatric outpatient substance use: associated behaviors and feelings. J Am Acad Child Adolesc Psychiatry 36:486–494, 1997

Martin SE: The epidemiology of alcohol-related interpersonal violence. Alcohol Health Res World 16:230–237, 1992

McCord J: A forty-year perspective on effects of chlid abuse and neglect. Child Abuse and Neglect 7:265–270, 1983

McKenry PC, Tishler CL, Kelley C: The role of drugs in adolescent suicide attempts. Suicide Life Threat Behav 13:166–175, 1983

Meisch RA, George FR: Influence of genetic factors on drug-reinforced behavior in animals, in Biological Vulnerability to Drug Abuse (NIDA Res Monogr 89; DHHS Publ No [ADM] 88-1590). Washington, DC, U.S. Government Printing Office, 1988, pp 9–24

Merikangas KR, Stolar M, Stevens DE, et al: Familial transmission of substance use disorders. Arch Gen Psychiatry 55:973–979, 1998

Mezzich AC, Giancola PR, Tarter RE, et al: Violence, suicidality, and alcohol/drug use involvement in adolescent females with a psychoactive substance use disorder and controls. Alcohol Clin Exp Res 21:1300–1307, 1997

Milberger S, Biederman J, Faraone SV, et al: Associations between ADHD and psychoactive substance use disorders. Am J Addict 6:318–329, 1997

Moss HB, Yao JK, Maddock JM: Responses by sons of alcoholic fathers to alcoholic and placebo drinks: perceived mood, intoxication, and plasma prolactin. Alcoholism (NY) 13:252–257, 1989

Newcomb MD, Bentler PM: Frequency and sequence of drug use: a longitudinal study from adolescence to young adulthood. J Drug Educ 16:101–120, 1986

Newcomb MD, Bentler PM: Substance use and abuse among children and teenagers. Am Psychol 44:242–248, 1989

Newman MM, Gold MS: Preliminary findings of patterns of substance abuse in eating disorder patients. Am J Drug Alcohol Abuse 18:207–211, 1992

Oei TPS, Jones R: Alcohol-related expectancies: have they a role in the understanding and treatment of problem drinking? Advances in Alcoholism and Substance Abuse 6:89–105, 1986

O'Malley PM, Johnston LD, Bachman JG: Adolescent substance use and addictions: epidemiology, current trends, and public policy. Adolesc Med 4:227–248, 1993

Parker G: Parental characteristics in relation to depressive disorders. Br J Psychiatry 134:138–147, 1979

Paton S, Kessler R, Kandel D: Depressive mood and adolescent illicit drug use: a longitudinal analysis. J Genet Psychol 131:267–289, 1977

Petraitis J, Flay BR, Miller TQ, et al: Illicit substance use among adolescents: a matrix of prospective predictors. Subst Use Misuse 33:2561–2604, 1998

Pickens RW, Svikis DS: Genetic vulnerability to drug abuse, in Biological Vulnerability to Drug Abuse (NIDA Res Monogr 89; DHHS Publ No [ADM] 88-1590). Washington, DC, U.S. Government Printing Office, 1988, pp 1–8

Pihl RO, Peterson JB: Attention-deficit hyperactivity disorder, childhood conduct disorder, and alcoholism: is there an association? Alcohol Health Res World 15:25–30, 1991

Pihl RO, Peterson JB: Alcohol/drug use and aggressive behavior, in Mental Disorder and Crime. Edited by Hodgins S. London, Sage, 1993, pp 263–283

Pollock VE, Volavka J, Goodwin DW, et al: The EEG after alcohol administration in men at risk for alcoholism. Arch Gen Psychiatry 40:857–861, 1983

Propping P, Krueger J, Mark N: Genetic predisposition to alcoholism: an EEG study in alcoholics and relatives. Hum Genet 59:51–59, 1981

Rachal JV, Maisto SA, Guess LL, et al: Alcohol use among youth, in Alcohol Consumption and Related Problems (Alcohol and Health Monogr 1). Rockville, MD, National Institute on Alcohol Abuse and Alcoholism, 1982, pp 55–95

Regier DA, Boyd JH, Burke JD, et al: One-month prevalence of mental disorders in the United States. Arch Gen Psychiatry 45:977–986, 1988

Regier DA, Farmer ME, Rae DS, et al: Comorbidity of mental disorders with alcohol and other drug abuse. JAMA 264:2511–2518, 1990

Robins LN: Sturdy childhood predictors of adult antisocial behavior: replications from longitudinal studies. Psychol Med 8:611–622, 1978

Robins LN, Przybeck TR: Age of onset of drug use as a factor in drug and other disorders, in Etiology of Drug Abuse: Implications for Prevention (NIDA Res Monogr 56; DHHS Publ No [ADM]-85–1335). Washington, DC, U.S. Government Printing Office, 1985, pp 178–192

Robins LN, Helzer JE, Weissman MM, et al: Lifetime prevalence of specific psychiatric disorders in three sites. Arch Gen Psychiatry 41:949–958, 1984

Rohsenow DJ: Drinking habits and expectancies about alcohol's effects for self versus others. J Consult Clin Psychol 51:752–756, 1983

Rohsenow DJ, Corbett R, Devine D: Molested as children: a hidden contribution to substance abuse? J Subst Abuse Treat 5:13–18, 1988

Rounsaville BJ: The role of psychopathology in the familial transmission of drug abuse, in Biological Vulnerability to Drug Abuse (NIDA Res Monogr 89; DHHS Publ No [ADM] 88-1590). Washington, DC, U.S. Government Printing Office, 1988, pp 108–119

Schaeffer KW, Parsons OQ, Yohman JR: Neuropsychological differences between male familial and nonfamilial alcoholics and nonalcoholics. Alcoholism Clin Exp Res 8:347–358, 1984

Scheier LM, Newcomb MD: Differentiation of early adolescent predictors of drug use versus abuse: a developmental risk-factor model. J Subst Abuse 3:277–299, 1991

Scheier LM, Botvin GJ, Baker E: Risk and protective factors as predictors of adolescent alcohol involvement and transitions in alcohol use: a prospective analysis. J Stud Alcohol 58:652–667, 1997

Schuckit MA: Subjective response to alcohol in sons of alcoholics and controls. Arch Gen Psychiatry 41:879–884, 1984

Schuckit MA: Genetics and the risk for alcoholism. JAMA 254:2614–2617, 1985a

Schuckit MA: Studies of populations at high risk for alcoholism. Psychiatric Developments 3:31–63, 1985b

Schuckit MA: Biological vulnerability to alcoholism. J Consult Clin Psychol 55:301–309, 1987

Schuckit MA: A clinical model of genetic influences in alcohol dependence. J Stud Alcohol 55:5–17, 1994

Schuckit MA: Biological, psychological and environmental predictors of the alcoholism risk: a longitudinal study. J Stud Alcohol 59:485–494, 1998

Schuckit MA, Engstrom D, Alpert R, et al: Differences in muscle-tension response to ethanol in young men with and without family histories of alcoholism. J Stud Alcohol 42:918–924, 1981

Schuckit MA, Gold E, Risch SC: Changes in blood prolactin levels in sons of alcoholics and controls. Am J Psychiatry 144:854–859, 1987

Shaffer D: The epidemiology of teen suicide: an examination of risk factors. J Clin Psychiatry 49 (No 9, Suppl):36–41, 1988

Shafii M, Carrigan S, Whittinghill JR, et al: Psychological autopsy of completed suicide in children and adolescents. Am J Psychiatry 142:1061–1064, 1985

Sher KJ: Subjective effects of alcohol: the influence of setting and individual differences in alcohol expectancies. J Stud Alcohol 46:137–146, 1985

Simcha-Fagan O, Gersten JC, Langner TS: Early precursors and concurrent correlates of patterns of illicit drug use in adolescence. Journal of Drug Issues 16:7–28, 1986

Smart RG, Adlaf EM: Substance use and problems among Toronto street youth. British Journal of Addiction 86:999–1010, 1991

Smart RG, Gray G, Bennett C: Predictors of drinking and signs of heavy drinking among high school students. International Journal of the Addictions 13:1079–1094, 1978

Southwick LL, Steele CM, Marlatt GA, et al: Alcohol-related expectancies: defined by phase of intoxication and drinking experience. J Consult Clin Psychol 49:713–721, 1981

Stinson FS, Dufour MC, Steffens RA, et al: Alcohol-related mortality in the United States, 1979–1989. Alcohol Health Res World 17:251–260, 1993

Stowell RJA, Estroff TW: Psychiatric disorders in substance-abusing adolescent inpatients: a pilot study. J Am Acad Child Adolesc Psychiatry 31:1036–1040, 1992

Su SS, Hoffmann JP, Gerstein DR, et al: The effect of home environment on adolescent substance use and depressive symptoms. Journal of Drug Issues 4:851–878, 1997

Substance Abuse and Mental Health Services Administration: The Relationship Between Mental Health and Substance Abuse Among Adolescents (DHHS Publ No [SMA]-99–3286). Rockville, MD, Substance Abuse and Mental Health Services Administration, 1999

Swanson JW: Alcohol abuse, mental disorder, and violent behavior. Alcohol Health Res World 17:123–132, 1993

van der Kolk BA: The psychological consequences of overwhelming life experiences, in Psychological Trauma. Edited by van der Kolk BA. Washington, DC, American Psychiatric Press, 1987, pp 1–30

Watts WD, Ellis AM: Sexual abuse and drinking and drug use: implications for prevention. Journal of Drug Education 23:183–200, 1993

Webb JA, Baer PE: Influence of family disharmony and parental alcohol use on adolescent social skills, self-efficacy, and alcohol use. Addict Behav 20:127–135, 1995

Weber MD, Graham JW, Hansen WB, et al: Evidence for two paths of alcohol use onset in adolescents. Addict Behav 14:399–408, 1989

Whitmore EA, Mikulich SK, Thompson LL, et al: Influences on adolescent substance dependence: conduct disorder, depression, attention deficit hyperactivity disorder, and gender. Drug Alcohol Depend 47:87–97, 1997

Wilens TE, Biederman J, Mick E, et al: Attention deficit hyperactivity disorder (ADHD) is associated with early onset substance use disorders. J Nerv Ment Dis 185:475–482, 1997

Wilks J, Callan VJ: Expectations about appropriate drinking contexts: comparisons of parents, adolescents and best friends. British Journal of Addiction 83:1055–1062, 1988

Wills TA, Vaccaro D, McNamara G: Novelty-seeking, risk taking, and related constructs as predictors of adolescent substance use: an application of Cloninger's theory. J Subst Abuse 6:1–20, 1994

Windle M: A retrospective measure of childhood behavior problems and its use in predicting adolescent problem behaviors. J Stud Alcohol 54:422–431, 1993

Wister AV, Avison WR: "Friendly persuasion": a social network analysis of sex differences in marijuana use. International Journal of the Addictions 17:523–541, 1982

Young SE, Mikulich SK, Goodwin MB, et al: Treated delinquent boys' substance use: onset, pattern, relationship to conduct and mood disorders. Drug Alcohol Depend 37:149–162, 1995

Zinberg NE: Drugs, Set, Setting: The Basis for Controlled Intoxicant Use. New Haven, CT, Yale University Press, 1984

3 Routes of Abuse and Specific Drugs

Todd Wilk Estroff, M.D.

Adolescents are usually not as sophisticated or knowledgeable about drug abuse as adults. They are not as discriminating when choosing their drug. Many are so inexperienced that they do not even have a drug of choice. This lack of experience leads to a great deal of experimentation with a wide variety of different substances (Millman et al. 1978). Inexperienced multiple-drug-abusing adolescents will therefore ingest almost any substance available that may induce euphoria (DeMilio et al. 1986). Simultaneous abuse of more than one substance is also common. The most typical combination is alcohol with some other drug, usually marijuana, cocaine, inhalants, or hallucinogens (Martin et al. 1995). The specific patterns and combinations of adolescent drug abuse vary with price and availability and also vary over time (Brasseux et al. 1998).

Routes of Abuse

The route of abuse can make a tremendous difference in the abuse potential and the intensity of the high produced. The different routes of abuse can be viewed as brain delivery systems. Some routes deliver the drugs very slowly, producing low but steadily rising blood levels over a period of several minutes to hours, whereas other routes deliver the drug to the brain within 8 seconds. Individual drugs can produce vastly different effects depending on their chemical form and how they are ingested.

Oral

Most drugs of abuse can be abused orally as tablets, powder, or liquid. Sedative hypnotics and barbiturates are usually taken in tablet form. Cocaine and heroin can be used orally as either a powder or a liquid. Lysergic acid diethylamide (LSD) is usually taken orally by licking dried blotter paper soaked with the drug. Even marijuana and hashish can be eaten alone or mixed with food. Absorption tends to be smooth and without a dramatic rise in blood levels. This produces a less intense euphoria. Cocaine in the form of coca leaves can also be chewed or made into an herbal tea known as *mate*. This tea is used throughout South America as a remedy for altitude sickness. Freud's own papers on cocaine describe the effects on himself of oral cocaine use.

Intranasal

Many drugs can be ingested intranasally. To be absorbed by the body, the drugs must be water soluble; such drugs include amphetamines, cocaine, and heroin. When any of these drugs are deposited on mucous membranes they dissolve rapidly and are slowly absorbed into the bloodstream. The result is a relatively smooth onset of euphoria that peaks slowly and then gradually diminishes back to the baseline state.

Intranasal use of cocaine, heroin, and amphetamines is less dangerous and addicting than intravenous use. In addition, the slower absorption rates mean that much less total drug can be absorbed by the limited intranasal mucous membrane surface.

The use of heroin among adolescents is rising. Unfortunately, at the same time, the purity of the heroin has increased from 5% 25 years ago to 80%–90% today (Bruner and Fishman 1998). This heroin is more easily absorbed and thus makes needle injection unnecessary. As a result, many individuals, especially adolescents, are using heroin intranasally to avoid needle-transmitted exposure to AIDS. Today's heroin is so pure that it is possible to produce respiratory arrest, shock, and seizures as well as subsequent central nervous system infarction in opiate-naïve adolescents (Zuckerman et al. 1996).

Other Mucous Membranes

Other mucous membranes can be used for drug abuse. Drugs can be ingested anywhere mucous membranes exist in the body. This includes the rectum and the vagina. In all cases the absorption of cocaine is limited because of the intense vasoconstriction it produces. Drug abuse through alternative mucous membranes is more easily concealed than when it is abused intranasally. Adolescent drug abusers will not talk about these unusual routes of abuse unless they are asked specific questions.

Smoking

Heroin, opium, marijuana, and hashish have been ingested by smoking for many centuries and have caused addiction via this route. Smoking remains the fastest way to deliver drugs to the substance abuser's brain, even faster than intravenous injection, because the drug is directly absorbed into the bloodstream from the lungs and is pumped to the brain 8 seconds later. Intravenous injections require 14 seconds to arrive at the brain. Thus, smoking a shorter-acting drug produces the same pattern of euphoria and dysphoria as injecting it intravenously. Cocaine in particular produces rapid, very intense onset of euphoria followed by an equally rapid onset of dysphoria when it is smoked as crack.

The entire cycle from euphoria to dysphoria is usually over within 15–20 minutes. The more rapid the onset of the euphoria, the more intense it is, and the subsequent dysphoria is equally intense. As a general rule, as the euphoria and dysphoria become more intense and the drug's duration of action lessens, the drug's addictiveness increases. It is disconcerting to realize that smokable crack cocaine and pure heroin are available to wide segments of the adolescent population in the United States. Worse, these drugs are available in small quantities and at low prices.

Inhalation

Some individuals abuse volatile hydrocarbons (e.g., glue, paint, Freon, toluene, correction fluid, carburetor cleaner) by inhaling them. Adolescent substance abusers call this "huffing." These compounds do not need to be heated in order to be inhaled. Delivery of these substances to the brain is similar to what occurs after smoking, and the duration of the high depends on the solubility and duration of action of the particular inhalant being used. There was a trend between 1991 and 1995 toward increased use among adolescents ages 12–17 years (Neumark et al. 1998), but use has since decreased slightly.

Subcutaneous/Intramuscular

Some individuals turn to subcutaneous or intramuscular injection as a means of avoiding intravenous abuse. This is sometimes known as "skin popping." It is most frequently used by opiate abusers who wish to avoid the risks of intravenous abuse. Cocaine can also be abused in this fashion but almost never is because it causes uncomfortable local anesthesia and the vasoconstriction limits its own absorption. Anabolic steroids are often abused by intramuscular injection. This problem is likely to occur among athletes from around the world (Franchini et al. 1998).

Adults can become addicted to intramuscular opiates by their own physicians. They are especially prone to abuse Talwin (pentazocine) and Demerol (meperidine). In many cases, these individuals will inject so much medication with such frequency that severe fibrosis occurs around the injection sites. I have never encountered this kind of addiction in an adolescent.

Intravenous

An intense high is usually produced whenever a drug of abuse is injected intravenously. The onset of euphoria occurs in approximately 14 seconds. The intense high peaks about 15 minutes after injection and can last up to several hours with opiates and amphetamines because of their long duration of action. On the other hand, intravenous cocaine is potentially more addicting because it has an extremely short duration of action; the short, intense high rapidly changes to dysphoria and intense cocaine cravings within 15–30 minutes after injection.

Progression to intravenous drug use is one of the most ominous developments in adolescent substance abuse. In my opinion, this form of abuse signifies a condition that is virtually untreatable on an outpatient basis. One of the most frightening aspects of intravenous drug use is the greater risk of developing AIDS from shared needles.

Specific Drugs of Abuse

This section is not meant to be a comprehensive review of all the substances that can be abused, their mechanisms of action, or their medical complications. Numerous reviews of this material already exist and need not be repeated (Ciraulo and Shader 1991). Instead, the focus here is on the usual ways adolescents use individual drugs and on the unusual and dangerous ways these drugs can affect the adolescent drug abuser.

Inhalants

Volatile Hydrocarbons

Volatile hydrocarbons are most likely to be abused by children and younger adolescents because they are cheap and easily available (Bowers and Sage 1983; Neumark et al. 1998; Watson 1984; Westermeyer 1987). They can be purchased in a wide variety of products, including paints, glues, gasoline, correction fluid, and carburetor cleaners. Purchases of these items by youngsters are rarely questioned. Adolescents often have legitimate reasons for using these items. When the product is poured or sprayed into a plastic or paper bag, the hydrocarbon can be inhaled directly from the bag. Alternatively, a rag soaked in hydrocarbons is placed in the bag and the vapors are inhaled. As mentioned earlier, adolescents refer to this practice as "huffing" or "sniffing" (Prockop et al. 1974). Ether is also a volatile hydrocarbon; since it became available in 1848 for use as the first anesthetic, it has also been a drug of abuse.

Volatile hydrocarbons can cause medical complications such as encephalopathy, peripheral neuropathy, glomerulonephritis, distal renal acidosis, and sudden death (Capurro and Capurro 1979; Lindstrom and Wickstrom 1983; Struwe and Wennberg 1983; Struwe et al. 1983; Westermeyer 1987; Wyse 1973). Lead poisoning has occurred when children or adolescents have huffed leaded gasoline. This problem has been declining in the United States since the introduction of unleaded gasoline, but it may persist in countries where leaded gasoline is still widely available. Psychiatric symptoms of huffing can include severe depression, neurologic damage, and hallucinations, particularly visual hallucinations.

Amyl Nitrate (Poppers)

Amyl nitrate, or "poppers," has been popular as a sexual stimulant in male homosexual communities. It is reported to give a pleasurable "rush" and to increase the intensity of orgasm. Many adolescents may use or abuse amyl nitrate to obtain a rush from it, but they use it less frequently for sexual stimulation unless they are homosexual males (Israelstram et al. 1978; Westermeyer 1987). Amyl nitrate is not an illegal drug and it is sold commercially across the country in many "head shops." Many adolescents looking for an inexpensive way to achieve a high will buy and experiment with it. The chief danger with amyl nitrate use is that it may lead to use of more potent and addicting substances. There are no reported cases of addiction to amyl nitrate, which is probably why it is not regulated at present.

Nitrous Oxide

Nitrous oxide (laughing gas) is also a volatile hydrocarbon but it must be considered separately because it is available only in a gaseous form packaged in a pressurized cylinder. It is a favorite drug of abuse because of its low price, but it is also less available because a commercial dealer must be located in order to make a purchase (Schwartz and Calihan 1984).

Cannabis Products

Marijuana

Self-reported lifetime marijuana use by adolescents and young adults increased dramatically among high school seniors from 5% in 1967 to between 64% and 68% in 1980–1982. These numbers have declined to 49% in the year 2000. However marijuana use has increased so much that it is now regarded as a normal part of adolescent behavior (Johnston et al. 1997; Kandel 1984). Over the same period, great strides have been made in the selection, breeding, and genetic manipulation of the cannabis plant. This has led to tremendous increases in the concentration of delta-9-tetrahydrocannabinol (THC), the active component in marijuana. The concentration of THC has increased from 1%–3% to 10%–13% since the 1960s (MacDonald and Newton 1981). Marijuana is available everywhere today. Its use is accepted and it is available inexpensively to any adolescent willing to make a few inquiries. Adolescents often obtain marijuana from their own parents.

Hashish

Hashish is the resin of the marijuana plant. It is collected as a sticky substance secreted by the leaves of the marijuana plant. It is then solidified into lumps of brownish resin known as hashish. It can be smoked directly by heating the resin in a pipe and inhaling it directly into the lungs. Hashish is a more concentrated form of cannabis and contains more of the active component THC. It has fallen into relative disuse over recent years because of the improved THC concentration in marijuana.

Alcohol

Alcohol has always been abused by adolescents. It is available from various sources, including parents' liquor cabinets, older friends who buy and share it, and unscrupulous liquor dealers. Stealing alcohol is another popular practice. Beer or other alcoholic beverages stored in a neighbor's garage can easily be removed with little chance of detection. Alcohol is a particular favorite of adolescents because it is cheap and widely available and its abuse is more acceptable to their parents, who are more likely to abuse it themselves.

Adolescents who develop an alcohol abuse problem are more likely to have a severe course. This is especially true if they have significant genetic loading. They are also more likely to develop psychiatric symptoms with aggressive tendencies and criminal behavior (Buydens-Branchey et al. 1989). This behavior, if it begins before age 20, is referred to as type 2 alcoholism. These early alcoholics are "twice as likely to have been incarcerated for crimes involving physical violence, three times as likely to be depressed and four times as likely to have attempted suicide as patients with a later onset of alcohol abuse" (Buydens-Branchey et al. 1989, p. 225). Type 2 alcoholism may be related to a genetically inherited biochemical deficit (Buydens-Branchey et al. 1989). Buydens-Branchey et al. (1989) argued that adolescent substance abuse disorders may be different from substance abuse disorders of later life and that adolescent substance abuse treatment is likely to be a cost-effective intervention providing lifelong health care savings with regard to medical, psychiatric, and drug abuse treatment coverage. Early detection and treatment of adolescent alcoholism and drug abuse may prevent later addiction, criminal behavior, depression, and suicide attempts.

Phencyclidine Hydrochloride (PCP)

PCP was developed as a general anesthetic and is still used extensively in veterinary medicine. It is no longer used in humans because of extreme reactions that occurred when patients woke up from the anesthetic. It is now manufactured for veterinary use only. It is easily synthesized from simple chemicals in clandestine home laboratories. Because it is so inexpensive to manufacture, it is often used as an adulterant for other more expensive drugs, especially cannabis products. Undetected PCP abuse has been responsible for many otherwise unexplained psychoses among adolescents. PCP is sold on the street as "angel dust."

Sedative Hypnotics, Benzodiazepines, Barbiturates, Methaqualone

Abusable oral medications are more expensive and less available to adolescents and adults because they must be obtained by prescription or stolen from a legitimate patient or a pharmacy. These medications include sedative hypnotics such as Doriden (glutethimide) and Placidyl (ethchlorvynol); Quaalude (methaqualone); benzodiazopines such as Valium (diazepam), Librium (chlordiazepoxide), Xanax (alprazolam), and Ativan (lorazepam); and less commonly used barbiturates (DeBard 1979; Dysken and Chan 1977; Flemenbaum and Gunby 1971; Heston and Hastings 1980; Preskorn and Denner 1977). These pharmacuticals are most commonly obtained through theft; adolescents often steal them from family members' medicine cabinets. These drugs can also be purchased on the street. Less frequently, an adolescent may devise an elaborate scheme to persuade a sympathetic pediatrician, family doctor, or emergency department doctor to prescribe them. Prescription of these medications is almost never indicated for adolescents.

These medications include several drugs that can produce medically dangerous withdrawal reactions. Barbiturate, Doriden, or Placidyl abusers must be watched. Failure to detect and treat a sedative hypnotic withdrawal can be life threatening.

"Look-Alike Drugs"

Several so-called "look-alike drugs" came on the market in the 1980s. They were designed to resemble illegal drugs as closely as possible by using compounds approved for over-the-counter sale. Most contained phenylpropanolamine, ephedrine, and/or caffeine. None of the compounds is addicting, but some cases of disturbing medical side effects have been noted. Phenylpropanolamine is structurally very similar to amphetamine, and its abuse has rarely been associated with psychosis.

Amphetamines and Other Stimulants

Amphetamine and Methamphetamine

Amphetamines such as dextroamphetamine have legitimate medical uses, such as in the treatment of attention-deficit/hyperactivity disorder (ADHD), narcolepsy, and refractory depression. A questionable but still acceptable use of dextroamphetame is as a diet pill prescribed by weight control physicians. The prescription of methamphetamine is rare, but it is abused more than amphetamine or dextroamphetamine. It is sold on the street as "speed" or "crank" and is inexpensive. Its low price and easy availability favor its use by adolescents.

Amphetamines are usually ingested orally as a capsule or through smoking or snorting. Methamphetamine experienced a renewed popularity starting in the late 1980s. It is a less expensive alternative to cocaine and is increasingly more available. When released from prison, former manufacturers of illegal methamphetamine often begin manufacturing the drug again in new clandestine laboratories.

As an adolescent uses more amphetamine, there is a great danger that the abuse will progress to intravenous injection. Intravenous methamphetamine is not quite as addicting as intravenous or crack cocaine, but it is nevertheless very addicting. Use of intravenous methamphetamine ("crystal meth") has the potential to progress to as much as several grams a day. It is also medically and psychiatrically dangerous. It is so powerful that psychosis may result when large doses are ingested by a normal individual (Griffith et al. 1970). The decline in its use is directly associated with the recognition in the 1960s that "Speed Kills."

During the late 1980s, a "new" drug, ice, was promoted on the street. In fact, ice is nothing more than methamphetamine in smokable form. Its abuse is similar to intravenous methamphetamine abuse and cocaine freebasing. It produces a longer high than cocaine and is, for that reason, slightly less addicting. Adolescents are particularly vulnerable to amphetamine addiction because of the drug's low cost, ease of manufacture, and ready availability.

Ecstasy

Methylenedioxymethamphetamine (MDMA), also known as ecstasy, was a widely available drug that was easily manufactured and enjoyed widespread popularity. This activity was sharply curtailed on July 1, 1985, when the Drug Enforcement Administration reclassified it as a schedule one controlled substance. MDMA is very similar to methylenedioxyamphetamine (MDA); it differs only by one methyl group (Climko et al. 1986). Both of these drugs have a chemical resemblance to mescaline. MDA is noted to be hallucinogenic and also has stimulant properties. Because the availability of MDMA has been limited, it is likely that other hallucinogenic amphetamines will be synthesized to overcome the Drug Enforcement Administration's prohibition on MDMA (Climko et al. 1986). Research on nonhuman primates indicates that MDMA can damage the fine serotonergic neurons of the dorsal raphe (Ricaurte et al. 1988). These neurons may play a major role in the control of the affective state.

Cocaine

Cocaine still represents a significant risk to adolescents. Cocaine abuse can rapidly lead to severe addiction. It is available in four forms and is abusable by five different routes. The Indians of Peru chew coca plant leaves and often add a little alkaline ash to increase its absorption through the mucous membranes. The Spanish noted that chewing coca leaves helped the Indians work longer and harder at high altitudes and decreased their hunger. The cocaine concentration of coca leaves is very low, and its absorption is slow and produces a slight effect. As mentioned previously, oral cocaine has a gradual onset with a gradual decrease in its stimulatory effects, and the coca leaves can brewed into a tea called *mate* or *mate de cocoa* that is often used to treat altitude sickness. This form of cocaine ingestion is the least likely to cause addiction.

More concentrated forms of cocaine may be prepared by harvesting the leaves of the coca plant and mixing them with an organic solvent such as kerosene and sulfuric acid. This process extracts the cocaine from leaves; the cocaine sinks to the bottom of the solution in the form of a paste called *basa* or *pasta* in South America. This mixture is approximately one-third cocaine sulfate, one-third cocaine hydrochloride, and one-third cocaine freebase. It can be smoked in the form of a cigarette, a form that is widely and inexpensively available in South America. There are many cocaine addicts who abuse this form of cocaine in Peru, Bolivia, and Colombia.

Cocaine Hydrochloride

Further processing of the cocaine paste turns it into cocaine hydrochloride, which is prepared by dissolving the paste in a water solution and adding acid. It is extremely soluble. One gram of cocaine hydrochloride powder will dissolve in 0.4 mL of water. It is also easily dissolved in water for intravenous use. This is the form of cocaine most frequently abused intranasally or by injection. It is unstable at high temperatures and cannot be smoked because of its relatively high melting point of 190°C. If it is smoked, it simply burns up without producing any effect.

Cocaine hydrochloride is rapidly dissolved and is absorbed upon contact with any mucous membrane. It can be ingested through the mucous membranes of the nose, mouth, rectum, or vagina. Most commonly it is inhaled, lands on the mucous membranes of the nasal pharynx, dissolves immediately, and is absorbed.

Crack Cocaine

Crack cocaine is the freebase form of cocaine. It can be prepared directly from cocaine paste or cocaine hydrochloride by dissolving either form in a water base or by using an organic solvent and adding a base such as sodium hydroxide or sodium bicarbonate. Crack cocaine is very different in its chemical properties than cocaine hydrochloride. It is not soluble in water. In addition, it will vaporize at 90°C (less than the boiling point of water) and thus can be smoked. It takes only 8 seconds to reach the brain after ingestion. It is widely and cheaply available in "rock" form. It is sold inexpensively on the street in small preprocessed quantities. It is the most addicting form of cocaine and one of the most addicting forms of any drug.

Heroin and Other Opiates

It is rare to find adolescents who are addicted to heroin (Millman et al. 1978). Their opiate use and abuse is usually limited to oral medications such as codeine and oxycodone. Heroin is sometimes used intranasally, but adolescents who have tried intravenous heroin are rare. This has been especially true since the AIDS epidemic began. Most adolescent drug abusers have enough judgment to realize that intravenous heroin is a step toward severe addiction, and thus they avoid it even when they are addicted to other substances.

Hallucinogens

Hallucinogens include LSD, mescaline, peyote, psilocybin-containing mushrooms, and the amphetamines STP and DOM. These drugs are enjoying a resurgence of popularity among adolescents. However, many products are labeled and sold as acid or LSD when they are, in fact, something else.

LSD can be manufactured by anyone with a basic knowledge of organic chemistry. It is active in very small quantities. It can be placed onto a piece of paper as a "microdot," making it easily transportable and concealable. LSD is often popular among young adolescent males because they view taking acid as a particularly brave and sophisticated action.

The venom of the Colorado River toad (*Bufo alvarius*) contains bufotenine, a hallucinogenic chemical and a schedule one drug. This venom can be milked from the toad, dried, and smoked. Its effects are reported to be more powerful than LSD ("Missionary for Toad Venom Facing Charges" 1994).

Questionable Addictions

There are several disorders that are labeled as addictions largely because they are severe, repetitive, and compulsive, and many of the individuals afflicted with them respond well to 12-step self-help programs. The repetitive compulsive behaviors are harmful to these individuals and their behavior closely resembles that of an addict. The major difference is that there is usually no euphorogenic substance involved. It is important when confronted with these individuals to perform the same thorough and complete diagnostic evaluation that is outlined in this book for clear-cut addictions.

Anabolic Steroids

The estimated prevalence of anabolic steroid use among male high school seniors is high. Among athletes and nonathletes surveyed, 6.6% had used anabolic steroids at some time in their lives. (Buckley et al. 1988). This abuse started before age 16 in two-thirds of the subjects. The steroids were supplied by a health care professional in 21% of the subjects, and 38% had injected the steroids intramuscularly. Improvement of athletic performance was the most common reason for abuse (47.1%), followed by appearance in 26.7%.

A study of 41 anabolic steroid–abusing adult males revealed that 12.2% met DSM-III-R (American Psychiatric Association 1987) criteria for psychotic symptoms while abusing the steroids (Pope and Katz 1988). An additional 12.2% met criteria for a manic episode, and 19.5% fell just short of that diagnosis; 12.5% developed major depression. Reports have been made of unexpected steroid-induced violence (Pope and Katz 1990), and there is speculation that anabolic steroid abuse may be a previously unrecognized drug dependency disorder (Kashkin and Kleber 1989). Significantly more depression, anger, vigor, and total disturbance was found among adolescent male athletes using steroids than among those not using steroids (Burnett and Kleiman 1994).

Gamma-Hydroxybutyrate (GHB, Georgia Home Boy)

Another drug associated with body building is gamma-hydroxybutyrate (GHB). It was once sold openly in health food stores as a nonsteroidal way of building muscles. Its sale is now banned by the U.S. Food and Drug Administration, although taking GHB is not illegal (Centers for Disease Control 1990, 1997; Mamelak 1989; Vayer et al. 1987). It is most often used by males ages 16–24. It can produce a high but has a small margin of safety. Overdose occurs swiftly, producing life-threatening coma and respiratory depression usually resulting in admission to hospital emergency departments and intensive care units. The effects wear off abruptly, and the patient and his or her family usually leave the hospital setting as quickly as possible. Because GHB is not commonly recognized as a drug of abuse, appropriate psychiatric and substance abuse referrals are usually not made (Smolowe 1993).

Gambling

Gambling is a compulsive disorder that resembles drug addiction in many ways. The major difference is no substances are involved. Despite this, one of the best methods for treating pathological gambling is through Gamblers Anonymous, a 12-step self-help group similar to Alcoholics Anonymous. Hospitalization and medication are rarely, if ever, indicated to treat a gambling disorder. Psychiatric evaluation is indicated to rule out a psychiatric illness that can resemble pathological gambling, such as bipolar disorder in its manic phase. Little is known about adolescent gambling disorders because they are rarely seen or diagnosed. Whether this is because adolescent gambling disorders do not occur or because they are not recognized or diagnosed when they do occur is unknown.

Sexual

Compulsive sexual activity and behavior has also been labeled as an addictive illness. It has been treated using 12-step programs, which has helped a number of individuals. However, many psychiatrists believe that if the behavior is examined more closely, several causative psychiatric illnesses will be found. The most common are posttraumatic stress disorder (due to past sexual or physical abuse), manic-phase bipolar disorder, drug abuse disorders, and severe personality disorders, especially borderline personality disorder. In any case, if a given treatment works and helps control the abnormal behavior it is hard to argue against it, especially if the argument is based solely on theoretical grounds. Adolescent compulsive sexual disorders are rarely diagnosed and little is known about them.

Food/Eating Disorders

Severe exogenous obesity can be viewed as an addiction to food. It most resembles an addiction when an individual weighs 200%–300% of his or her ideal body weight and has unsuccessfully tried tens or even hundreds of diet and exercise programs. These individuals may have had intestinal bypass surgery or gastric stapling procedures. They may have life-threatening illnesses yet still cannot lose weight. Sometimes these individuals respond well and lose weight when their obesity is treated as an addictive illness using 12-step techniques. However, the biggest problem with labeling eating disorders as an addiction is that food, the abused substance, does not induce euphoria and is necessary to sustain life. When treating drug and alcohol abuse, the offending agent can be eliminated entirely. Food, even if addicting, must be consumed; abstinence is not an option. Limited use and moderation are the only choices.

It is an even larger leap to include anorexia nervosa and bulimia as addictive disorders. Many medical disorders can mimic eating disorders, particularly obesity and anorexia nervosa. It is especially important to perform complete evaluations on adolescents with eating disorders before deciding that their disorder should be treated as an addiction.

Summary

In conclusion, the route of abuse and the properties of the substance used can powerfully influence the seriousness of an adolescent's substance abuse and how it should be treated. Knowledge of these individual differences adds diagnostic precision to their evaluation.

References

American Psychiatric Association: Diagnostic and Statistical Manual of Mental Disorder, 3rd Edition Revised. Washington, DC, American Psychiatric Association, 1987

Bowers AJ, Sage LR: Solvent abuse in adolescents: the who? what? and why? Child Care Health Dev 9:169–178, 1983

Brasseux C, D'Angelo L, Guadgliardo M, et al: The changing pattern of substance abuse in urban adolescents. Arch Pediatr Adolesc Med 153:234–237, 1998

Bruner AE, Fishman M: Adolescents and illicit drug use. JAMA 280:597–598, 1998

Buckley WE, Yesalis CE, Fried L, et al: Estimated prevalence of anabolic steroid use among male high school seniors. JAMA 260:3441–3445, 1988

Burnett KF, Kleiman ME: Psychological characteristics of adolescent steroid users. Adolescence 29:81–89, 1994

Buydens-Branchey L, Branchey MH, Noumair D: Age of alcoholism onset, I: relationship to psychopathology. Arch Gen Psychiatry 46:225–230, 1989

Capurro PU, Capurro C: Solvent exposure and mental depression. Clin Toxicol 15:193–195, 1979

Centers for Disease Control and Prevention: Multistate outbreak of poisonings associated with illicit use of gamma hydroxy butyrate. MMWR Morb Mortal Wkly Rep 39:861–863, 1990

Centers for Disease Control and Prevention: Gamma hydroxy butyrate use—New York and Texas 1995–1996. MMWR Morb Mortal Wkly Rep 46:861–863, 1997

Ciraulo DA, Shader RI (eds): Clinical Manual of Chemical Dependence. Washington, DC, American Psychiatric Press, 1991

Climko R, Roehrich H, Sweeney DR, et al: Ecstasy: a review of MDMA and MDA. Int J Psychiatry Med 16:359–372, 1986

DeBard ML: Diazepam withdrawal syndrome: a case with psychosis, seizure, and coma. Am J Psychiatry 136:104–105, 1979

DeMilio L, Gold MS, Martin D: Evaluation of the substance abuser, in Diagnostic and Laboratory Testing in Psychiatry. Edited by Gold MS, Pottash ALC. New York, Plenum, 1986, pp 235–247

Dysken MW, Chan CH: Diazepam withdrawal psychosis: a case report. Am J Psychiatry 134:573, 1977

Flemenbaum A, Gunby B: Ethchlorvynol (Placidyl) abuse and withdrawal: review of clinical picture and report of 2 cases. Diseases of the Nervous System 32:188–192, 1971

Franchini F, Calabri GB, Casini T, et al: L'abuso di sostanze anabolizzanti nell'adolescente che fa sport. Pediatr Med Chir 20:219–221, 1998

Griffith JD, Cavanaugh JH, Held J, et al: Experimental psychosis induced by the administration of a d-amphetamine, in Amphetamines and Related Compounds. Edited by Costa E, Garattini S. New York, Raven, 1970, pp 897–904

Heston LL, Hastings D: Psychosis with withdrawal from ethchlorvynol. Am J Psychiatry 137:249–250, 1980

Israelstram S, Lambert S, Oki G, et al: A new recreational drug craze. Canadian Psychiatric Association Journal 23:493–495, 1978

Johnston LD, Bachman JG, O'Malley PM: Monitoring the Future: Questionnaire Responses from the Nation's High School Seniors 1995. Ann Arbor, MI, Institute for Social Research, 1997

Kandel DB: Marijuana users in young adulthood. Arch Gen Psychiatry 41:200–209, 1984

Kashkin KB, Kleber HD: Hooked on hormones? An anabolic steroid addiction hypothesis. JAMA 262:3166–3170, 1989

Lindstrom K, Wickstrom G: Psychological function changes among maintenance house painters exposed to low levels of organic solvent mixtures. Acta Psychiatr Scand 67:81–91, 1983

MacDonald DI, Newton M: The clinical syndrome of adolescent drug abuse. Adv Pediatr 28:1–25, 1981

Mamelak M: Gamma hydroxy butyrate: an endogenous regulator of energy metabolism. Neurosci Biobehav Rev 13:187–198, 1989

Martin CS, Kaczynski NA, Maisto SA, et al: Patterns of DSM-IV alcohol abuse and dependence symptoms in adolescent drinkers. J Stud Alcohol 56:672–680, 1995

Millman RB, Kuhri ET, Nyswander ME: Therapeutic detoxification of adolescent heroin addicts. Ann N Y Acad Sci 311:153–164, 1978

Missionary for toad venom facing charges. New York Times 19 Feb 1994

Neumark YD, Delva J, Anthony JC: The epidemiology of adolescent inhalant drug involvement. Arch Pediatr Adolesc Med 152:781–786, 1998

Pope HG Jr, Katz DL: Affective and psychotic symptoms associated with anabolic steroid abuse. Am J Psychiatry 145:487–490, 1988

Pope HG Jr, Katz DL: Homicide and near-homicide by anabolic steroid users. J Clin Psychiatry 51:28–31, 1990

Preskorn SH, Denner LJ: Benzodiazepines and withdrawal psychosis. JAMA 237:36–38, 1977

Prockop LD, Alt M, Tison J: Huffer's neuropathy. JAMA 229:1083–1084, 1974

Ricaurte GA, Forno LS, Wilson MA, et al: 3,4-Methylenedioxy methamphetamine selectively damages central serotonergic neurons in central serotonergic neurons in non human primates. JAMA 260:51–55, 1988

Schwartz RH, Calihan M: Nitrous oxide: a potentially lethal euphoriant inhalant. Am Fam Physician 30:171–172, 1984

Smolowe J: Choose your own poison. Time July 26, 1993, pp 56–57

Struwe G, Wennberg A: Psychiatric and neurological symptoms in workers occupationally exposed to organic solvents: results of a differential epidemiological study. Acta Psychiatr Scand 67:68–80, 1983

Struwe G, Knave B, Mindus P: Neuropsychiatric symptoms in workers exposed to jet fuel: a combined epidemiological and causative study. Acta Psychiatr Scand 67:55–67, 1983

Vayer P, Mandel P, Maitre M: Gamma hydroxy butyrate, a possible neurotransmtter. Life Sci 41:1547–1557, 1987

Watson JM: Solvent abuse and adolescents. Practitioner 228:487–490, 1984

Westermeyer J: The psychiatrist and solvent-inhalant abuse: recognition, assessment, and treatment. Am J Psychiatry 144:903–907, 1987

Wyse DG: Deliberate inhalation of volatile hydrocarbons: a review. Can Med Assoc J 108:71–74, 1973

Zuckerman GB, Ruiz DC, Keller IA, et al: Neurologic complications following intranasal administration of heroin in an adolescent. Ann Pharmacother 30:778–781, 1996

4 Diagnosis of Adolescent Substance Abuse Disorders

Peter R. Cohen, M.D.
Todd Wilk Estroff, M.D.

Establishing the diagnosis of substance abuse or dependence in an adolescent is perplexing and challenging. Definitions and diagnostic criteria have changed a great deal since the 1970s. Enormous resources, effort, and money have been spent in both the private and public sectors in multiple attempts to identify, diagnose, and treat teenage substance abusers. These endeavors are infrequently based on research or scientific data (Geller et al. 1998). As a result, the validity and reliability of diagnostic criteria for substance abuse disorders are not as clearly established for adolescents as they are for adults. Nevertheless, we believe that there is ample clinical evidence for the existence of adolescent substance abuse disorders criteria, and physicians have a medical duty to identify and treat them. DSM-IV (American Psychiatric Association 1994) makes no age distinction when defining the difference between dependence and abuse.

Assumptions

This chapter focuses on what is known about adolescent substance abuse disorders and how they are diagnosed despite the diagnostic problems described above. Several assumptions must first be stated: 1) These disorders represent primary disease processes. This proposition is based on clinical experience and consensus. 2) The onset of each adolescent substance abuse disorder can precede, coincide with, or follow the development of other physical and psychiatric disorders. Moreover, "alcohol and drug abuse can mimic and interact with all mental illnesses" (Stowell and Estroff 1992, p. 1036). 3) The psychiatric and the chemical dependence communities often use very different diagnostic criteria and approaches when identifying and treating adolescent substance abusers. 4) These substance abuse disorders disrupt normal adolescent development.

What a Diagnosis Should Mean

Ideally, a diagnosis should not only identify a specific set of behavioral patterns but should also predict the prognosis and indicate appropriate treatments for the patient. As Bailey (1989) pointed out, "DSM-III-R [American Psychatric Association 1987] does not distinguish between childhood, adolescent and adult substance abuse and is of limited value for making the diagnosis in children and adolescents" (p. 154). Substance-abusing teenagers can display a clinical presentation different from that of adults. Valid research data about these disorders are rare (Geller et al. 1998). One consequence of this is that the DSM-IV criteria for substance use disorders do not differentiate between adults and adolescents with respect to clinical presentation (Bukstein et al. 1989).

Limitations

Diagnostic certainty is compromised by a lack of general agreement as to the definitions of *use*, *abuse*, and *dependence* for adolescents. The nature of adolescence itself makes it difficult to determine if substance use is a symptom of a primary illness, an adjustment disorder, a psychiatric disorder, or a passing behavioral phase. Adolescents in our culture tend to experiment with drugs and alcohol. They can either minimize or exaggerate their substance use and the emotional distress it causes them. Both abstinent and abusing adolescents view substance use as a private matter.

Adolescents often lie about, deny, or minimize their substance use to adults. These untruths further compromise the ability to diagnose adolescent substance abuse. Thus, it is naïve to rely too heavily on diagnostic instruments such as a checklist or a structured or semistructured diagnostic interview (see Chapter 6). Diagnosis of these disorders is best done carefully, patiently, and over time.

There are other limitations as well. Insurance and budgetary cutbacks have stifled the diagnostic process. Inpatient treatment has been shortened, allowing only a few days to a week to evaluate a troubled adolescent in a drug-free setting. Managed care companies insist that patients be discharged rapidly to a less intensive outpatient psychiatric and/or chemical dependency treatment program. The current lengths of stay are inadequate for gathering data, determining a diagnosis, confronting the patient's denial, and creating a realistic discharge plan. A provisional diagnosis of substance abuse or dependence is often insufficient to encourage a family to keep their child in treatment or to continue with an outpatient evaluation. As a result, the adolescent with poor internal controls will have great difficulty remaining abstinent and is at great risk for relapse as an outpatient.

Further compounding the problem, outpatient programs have either shrunk or disappeared altogether because they cannot be financially justified. In contrast to hospital and residential programs, it is often impossible to adequately diagnose and treat teenagers in outpatient programs because they are not under 24-hour observation and supervision. The adolescents are in treatment for only a portion of the day, so they have easy access to drugs and alcohol.

The remainder of this chapter discusses diagnostic techniques for the clinician, identifying and evaluating the potential adolescent substance abuse patient, the confused history of adolescent substance abuse diagnosis, and recommendations on how to diagnose chemical abuse and dependence based on practical realities and the present state of the art.

Clinician Techniques and Skills

Gathering of Data

Bailey (1989) emphasized that implicit in making a diagnosis of substance abuse is the "realization that all children and adolescents are at risk but some considerably more than others" (p. 154). The clinician needs to take a comprehensive diagnostic approach to determine the level of risk and commensurate interventions. Because there is no one "drug and alcohol test" for confirming a diagnosis, the clinician must rely on a careful history and qualitative and quantitative data collection. This data should be gathered from various individuals, in addition to the teenager, and from tests. Thus a full work up should include the following:

- history and mental status examination
- physical examination
- self-report
- reports of the family, peers, school, etc.
- structured interviews and standardized tests
- laboratory test results
- drug screening

Clinician Qualities

Effective diagnosis of substance abuse disorders in young people depends as much on the clinician as on the criteria. The mental health professional needs an intuitive understanding of substance abuse disorders and a flexible interviewing style that out-thinks the denying patient. Patience and tolerance for diagnostic uncertainty are essential in assessment and treatment. For the clinician in training, supervision is critical. For the trained clinician, skepticism is essential. This therapeutic distrust can take many forms.

Dedicated mental health professionals want to believe that an adolescent's emotional pleas for help are heartfelt rather than an attempt to divert the clinician's attention from the patient's substance abuse. Because adolescent substance abusers are usually not truthful, mental health professionals must not trust what the adolescent tells them. They must be able to suspect the worst and to consider what is actually taking place if the adolescent is lying. The cognitive ability to alternatively believe and disbelieve an adolescent's words and thoughts is called *double thinking*.

This process allows the diagnostician to consider and ask direct questions about worse-case scenarios before they become manifestly evident. Double thinking helps cut through the veil of lies spread by the drug abuser and is essential in the early diagnosis and later treatment of these disorders. Double thinking is a clinical skill that is not easily learned; it requires watching what adolescents do and not what they say, no matter how sincere they may appear. It requires mistrusting what teenagers and their families say and thinking the worst of them. This is particularly true when an action or statement does not make sense. In other words, the therapist must be willing to consider the question "Are these behavioral disturbances explainable by substance abuse or dependence?" This type of thinking can present a very difficult cognitive shift for mental health professionals who do not specialize in substance abuse treatment.

Adolescent Privacy Versus the Parents' Right to Know

Mistrust of what the adolescent says can take a different form when substance abuse is suspected. There is often a basic conflict between the adolescent patients' right to privacy and confidentiality and their parents' right to know. Often the evaluating physician or mental health professional is placed squarely in the middle of this dilemma. When and under what circumstances should parents demand urine or blood testing? When should parents initiate a search of their child's room, open mail, or read diaries? When should the mental health professional or physician suggest these seemingly extreme and invasive measures? How often should it be done and by whom? Should it be done secretly or with the child present?

The fundamental questions are how vigorously should one pursue the diagnosis, and when does parental concern and need to know outweigh the child's right to privacy? Denial, minimization, and lying are typical in substance abuse disorders. Therefore, to correctly diagnose these disorders, parents and treating clinicians may need to be much more intrusive in their inquiries than would ordinarily be required for other disorders.

These very difficult questions do not have easy or simple answers. Their solutions often depend on individual levels of comfort with the degree of intrusiveness and the balance of trust between parents, child, and evaluator. Nevertheless, more intrusive measures may be needed to make an objective diagnosis and to prevent a teenager from further self-harm. No diagnosis should be made until all data have been collected from all sources, carefully analyzed, and integrated.

Identifying the Potential Patient

Often the initial presentation of adolescent substance abuse disorders occurs in ways that may not at all seem to be related to drug abuse. Many parents and physicians are left puzzled and wondering if there really is a problem. Even if they decide there is one, they are often confused as to what is actually causing the symptomatic behavior. They often do not realize that the chronic telling of lies is a significant characteristic of drug abuse. Some sort of extraordinary event must occur, such as their child presenting to a local emergency department intoxicated or stuporous (Stephenson et al. 1984), after a suicide attempt, or after development of a substance abuse–related illness, or their child being arrested. These events are so unusual that even the most callous parents are alerted to the problem and must examine symptoms they may have once overlooked (Williams et al. 1989).

A growing number of mental health professionals have become aware of these disorders and have a very high index of suspicion. They recognize the necessity for rapid evaluation and referral of these disorders. Many times they are skilled at outpatient and residential treatment. Detection of substance abuse disorders in the early stages of the illness, accompanied by rapid involvement in treatment, can prevent further deterioration.

It is extremely rare for substance-abusing adolescents to request treatment on their own. They are usually responding to outside pressures from parents, school, or the legal system and believe that their autonomy is threatened. Because of their lack of motivation to tell the truth about their substance abuse, these teenagers present a significant challenge to the skills of an evaluator.

Parents

Parents can be instrumental in helping make the diagnosis if their index of suspicion is high enough and they are active and concerned enough to search for evidence of drug abuse in their children. They usually bring their children in for evaluation only after they notice extreme or outrageous acts, including coming home intoxicated, changes in friends, mood, self-care, and cooperation. Explosive outbursts, declining school performance, sexual acting out, the appearance of tattoos and unusual haircuts, or finding drugs or drug paraphernalia in their child's possession are other clues that their adolescent is abusing drugs.

School System

The school system can also be a useful source of information. Early and rapid reporting of truancy, declining grades, and disciplinary problems, which are potential signs of drug abuse, can raise the index of suspicion. If this level of suspicion that an adolescent is using or abusing drugs rises to that of double thinking, the school can provide important information that leads to early intervention.

Legal System

The legal system can help identify potential patients as well as provide the leverage to make a child and family cooperate with both evaluation and treatment. Any time a child is taken into custody or arrested for any offense, no matter how insignificant, law enforcement officials and parents should be suspicious that this is a sign of a more severe and extensive problem that the teenager is covering up with lies and half-truths. The greatest danger is that the substance-abusing adolescent is dismissed as bad, delinquent, or a young criminal; such dismissal often results in extensive involvement between the youth and the criminal justice system, in which little to no treatment is provided.

Primary Physicians

Pediatricians and family physicians treat the general population of adolescents and are, therefore, frequently asked by parents to explain their teenager's troubled and troubling behavior. Despite the limitations of time and schedule, primary physicians play a prominent role in evaluating and detecting substance abuse disorders. The symptoms of substance abuse can perplex even the most astute clinician, making diagnosis a challenge. Substance abuse disorders will eventually declare themselves over time. It is unrealistic to expect a definitive answer based on a first examination. In general, if the clinician suspects adolescent substance abuse, a referral is indicated. Drug urine screening can be easily ordered but it should be used only to confirm use. A single negative screen does not rule out drug abuse. Similarly, a positive screen does not diagnose the severity of the drug use. This is especially true when attempting to diagnose dependence. A series of tests is more useful for this purpose. Urine screens are also limited because they only measure substances used shortly before the sample was collected. It does not identify some of them consistently, such as lysergic acid diethylamide (LSD) or phencyclidine hydrochloride (PCP). Many teenagers attempt to create a false-negative test. A referral is crucial under the following circumstances: 1) continued uncertainty over the diagnosis, 2) poor compliance by the patient and/or family when recommendations are made, and 3) an amount of time spent with the patient and family that is out of proportion to the presenting medical presentation.

Psychiatrists, Psychologists, Social Workers, Psychiatric Nurses, and Counselors

Adolescent substance abusers commonly present with behavioral symptoms to a mental health professional. Substance abuse must always be ruled out first. Even when an adolescent's symptoms are classic signs of a psychotic, affective, conduct, attention-deficit, or anxiety disorder, illicit substances can cause or aggravate all of these behavioral disturbances (Estroff et al. 1985). Atypical, unusual, or bizarre symptoms such as visual hallucinations are a bold clue to an organic etiology, particularly a drug-induced one.

Peer Groups and Siblings

One valuable assessment strategy is observing how substance-abusing peers react to an adolescent substance abuser in group therapy. If the patient denies drug abuse yet is actually heavily involved in drug abuse, the other adolescents will quickly pick up on the inconsistencies and confront them about their denial and minimization. In similar fashion, the patient who pretends to be a heavy substance abuser is quickly exposed. The optimal format is to invite the adolescents being evaluated to visit group therapy for a week-long trial. A teenager who is heavily abusing drugs may be well known to the other members of the group. They may have even abused drugs together, sold drugs to each other, known the same acquaintances, or at least seen each other while intoxicated. Under these circumstances, the teenager's involvement is hard to deny and harder to avoid discussing.

Rarely will brothers, sisters, and friends show sufficient concern to coerce a teenager into an evaluation. When this does occur, these peers will become so alarmed or fearful that they will alert a parent, therapist, guidance counselor, or other school official. The information that they can provide may also be instrumental when evaluating the adolescent substance abuser or during a therapeutic intervention.

Historical Problems with Diagnosis and Terminology

Confusion of Definitions: Abuse, Dependence, Use, and Experimentation

A significant dilemma arises when attempting to define the differences between substance use, experimentation, abuse, and dependence (Winters and

Henly 1988). This confusion has been generated by the variety of diagnostic criteria proposed by organizations such as the American Psychiatric Association, the American Medical Association, the World Health Organization, and the chemical dependence treatment community. There have also been significant changes in diagnostic categories and criteria between each successive version of the DSM.

The historical confusion regarding the terminology of substance abuse disorders exists because most definitions are not standardized. Many diagnostic systems are more qualitative than quantitative. They do not clearly differentiate between more and less severe forms of substance use disorders, and they do not easily translate into treatment recommendations (Bailey 1989; Rinaldi et al. 1988). *Dependence* has many different definitions. For example, an adolescent smoking marijuana 3–4 days per week for 6 months, showing no tolerance, withdrawal, or loss of control, fits all four DSM-IV criteria for abuse but not for dependence. This is true even though he or she has drug-related school failure, arrests for reckless driving and breaking and entering, and physical fights with his or her parents. On the other hand, in a 12-step program, he or she would surely be diagnosed as chemically dependent. Is this behavior an early phase in the natural history of a substance abuse disorder? With treatment, will he or she outgrow these problems or relapse? These questions put the diagnosis of dependence in question. Finally, what difference does the diagnosis of abuse versus dependence make in determining his or her level of care and treatment modalities?

Abuse is a similarly slippery word to define. Halikas (1990) stated that "for purposes of characterizing the behavior as harmful, inappropriate, and not socially sanctioned, it is acceptable to define any use of tobacco, alcohol, or any of the psychoactive substances as abuse in [an adolescent] population" (p. 216). However, he warns that "this characterization is very different from a diagnosis for that same youngster. Diagnosis carries with it information about etiology, natural history, and clinical course" (p. 216).

Questions frequently asked by parents and clinicians include: "Do abusers automatically turn into addicts?" and "Do abusers of any substance become dependent on other drugs?" Although it is clear that those individuals who are regular users of drugs are at much higher risk of progressing to physical dependence, it is not an automatic occurrence. Most adolescents are either experimenting with or abusing drugs. They rarely become so physically dependent on drugs to the point of developing tolerance or withdrawal symptoms. However, their drug abuse can be so severe as to cause significant disturbances of social, school, and family functioning, which often result in the adolescent coming to medical attention.

Adolescent Criteria: Traditional Stages-of-Use Definitions Used by the Substance Abuse Treatment Community

When dealing with adolescents, the substance abuse treatment community has used adult definitions for substance abuse and then attempted to apply these terms to teenagers. They define levels of use along a spectrum from experimentation to dependence (Macdonald 1984; Nowinski 1990). Macdonald (1984) warned that the diagnosis of drug abuse was missed by physicians who only recognized the latter stages of this disease. In an attempt to increase the clinician's sensitivity to identifying adolescent substance abuse, he modified for adolescents an adult qualitative staging system of drug use originally proposed by Johnson (1980). Stage 1, called "learning the mood swing," is characterized by experimentation and recreational use. Stage 2 is described as "seeking the mood swing," highlighted by weekend or occasional midweek use associated with social events, and sometimes use for stress reduction. Stage 3, or "preoccupation with the mood swing" describes an eventual progression to daily use, single or multidrug intensive ingestion, and increasing time and money spent trying to acquire these substances. This is accompanied by a concomitant deterioration in social and emotional functioning. Stage 4, or "doing drugs to feel OK," describes substance abuse resulting in less euphoria. Drugs are used more for warding off dysphoria and psychosocial deterioration. He suggests that the diagnosis is best established by a drug use history on admission and that a behavioral inventory or a history of progressive behavioral change can more reliably determine the severity of abuse and indicate the proper level of treatment.

A second but similar scheme by Nowinski (1990) emphasized diagnostic criteria closer to DSM-III-R in terms of tolerance, loss of control, and continued use in spite of the resulting clear-cut negative consequences: using carefully structured interview skills. The author cited the following five stages, which correspond closely to Macdonald's (1984) stages:

1. Experimental (use motivated by curiosity and/or risk taking)
2. Social (event-related use)
3. Instrumental (seeking chemicals to manipulate emotions and behaviors for hedonistic purposes or compensatory to cope with stress and dysphoria)
4. Habitual (accommodation—the gray area that leads to dependence, in which using chemicals becomes a lifestyle for coping and recreation as former interests are dropped)
5. Compulsive (complete accommodation, preoccupation, and deterioration of global functioning)

These conceptual frameworks promote early screening, diagnosis, and treatment of adolescent substance abuse problems. Several problems arise, however, because again they do not clearly differentiate between abuse and dependence. This transition from abuse to dependence falls somewhere between Stages 3 and 4 in Macdonald's proposal, whereas Nowinski calls it the "habitual stage." This stage may better reflect the reality of the transition from abuse to dependence, but there is no research to validate this clinical impression. Furthermore, clinical experience suggests that a significant number of teenagers have probably found a particular chemical of choice and are physically dependent on it by the time they reach Stage 3 or 4. The later stages of each set of criteria include characteristics of both severe abuse and dependence, but they do not define the point at which abuse changes into dependence.

Adult Criteria: DSM-III-R Definitions

DSM-III-R attempted to solve some of these nosological dilemmas. It favors the flexibility needed to diagnose teenagers by defining *psychoactive substance dependence* according to the drugs being abused. It also lists "other features of psychoactive substance use disorders" to be considered in making a diagnosis, even though they are not formal criteria:

- route of administration
- duration of effects
- repeated intoxication
- personality and mood disturbances
- age of onset
- reduction in goal-directed behaviors
- social/occupational impairment
- course of illness
- predisposing factors, such as a specific psychiatric disorder and/or a positive family history for substance use disorders
- gender ratio
- differential diagnosis

Adolescents do not commonly display the most severe physical signs of tolerance or withdrawal. In addition, polysubstance dependence can be diagnosed when no single substance predominates and the criteria are met for at least three chemicals "as a group, but not for any specific substance" (American Psychiatric Association 1987, p. 185). A more conservative definition of dependence or addiction is restricted to use that is compulsive, occupies a significant portion of a person's time and energy, and displays physiological states of tolerance and/or withdrawal (Cambor and Millman 1991).

According to one pilot study, DSM-III-R can help identify substance use dependence and abuse in adolescents. Stowell and Estroff (1992) found that of 226 adolescents entering inpatient treatment for a primary substance abuse disorder, 81% were dependent on one or more substances, whereas 29% met criteria for a substance abuse disorder (the numbers were greater than 100% because multiple substances were abused). One or more organic mental disorders were found in 16% of this sample, including alcohol intoxication and/or withdrawal (10%), alcohol withdrawal requiring detoxification (5%), substance-induced delusions and/or hallucinosis (5%), and substance-induced dementia (11%). Alcohol, marijuana, LSD, and PCP, whether alone or in combination, were the primary substances associated with these organic disorders.

Adult Criteria: DSM-IV Definitions

DSM-IV and its text revision, DSM-IV-TR (American Psychiatric Association 2000) further defined the difference between substance abuse and dependence: substance abuse remains a residual diagnosis that can progress to dependence. In DSM-IV, abuse and dependence are most clearly differentiated by the amount of loss of control, that is, "a maladaptive pattern of substance use, leading to clinically significant impairment or distress,...occurring at any time in the same 12-month period" (p. 181). For substance abuse, only one item from the list of criteria is required to make the diagnosis, whereas substance dependence requires the presence of at least three listed items. Substance abuse criteria include use associated with physically hazardous situations, legal problems, and interpersonal problems. Failure to fulfill major role obligations is now a criterion for abuse, not dependence; it was moved from its former place in the dependence criteria of DSM-III-R.

A transition is assumed when abuse becomes dependence, although DSM-IV does not describe this transition stage explicitly. The substance-dependent patient has symptoms and signs concerning *physiology* and *loss of control* that are qualitatively different from abuse. The physiological signs of tolerance and withdrawal, as stated earlier, are less likely to be seen among adolescents. Loss of control is described as increased use or use beyond intended limits; a persistent desire or inability to cut down or control use; time spent in obtaining or using substances or recovering from their effects; reduction or surrender of important activities; and continued use despite physical or psychological problems. Duration of use is not directly addressed, except that at least three criteria must occur at any time in the same 12-month period.

Notably missing in DSM-IV is the diagnosis of polysubstance abuse, which would be helpful with regard to teenagers who fulfill the criteria for abuse of three or more chemicals. This diagnosis is now subsumed under the category of other (or unknown) substance use disorders, which also includes the use of unusual substances such as anabolic steroids, nitrite inhalants, nitrous oxide, catnip, betel nut, kava, antiparkinsonian agents, and antihistamines.

It is now possible under DSM-IV to add the diagnosis of *with physiological dependence* if withdrawal or tolerance is present. If not, the residual category *without physiological dependence* is more appropriate among teenagers. The difficulty of defining psychological dependence has been wholly avoided in DSM-IV.

In addition, course modifiers for dependence include more detail. Early remissions, which last less than 12 months, address the highest risk period for relapse. Sustained remissions must last at least 12 months. Recovery from dependence can also be defined as a partial or a full remission. A 1-month transition period is required before the patient is qualified for a remission diagnosis.

Another modifier is available for patients receiving agonist therapy who do not fit the criteria for dependence or abuse for 1 month. Examples are patients dependent on barbiturates who are being detoxified with a sedative hypnotic and cocaine-dependent patients who are being treated with bromocriptine. A final modifier describes patients who are dependent but are in a controlled environment that is highly supervised and are substance-free for at least 1 month.

A final significant change moved the psychoactive substance–induced organic mental disorders of DSM-III-R to the category of specific substance-related disorders in DSM-IV: the list of organically induced disorders expanded for every substance. For example, alcohol use disorders now consist of alcohol dependence, abuse, intoxication, withdrawal, delirium, persisting dementia, and sexual dysfunction. Disorders of amnesia, psychosis, mood, anxiety, and sleep are also listed.

Additional Adolescent Criteria

Halikas et al. (1984) noted clinical differences in the way that adolescents manifest alcohol abuse that make the DSM-III-R criteria less applicable.

They proposed that abuse should be based on adverse consequences occurring in multiple life areas. The life areas of adolescence in which substance abuse can present problems are biomedical complications, school problems, and psychosocial complications (Halikas et al. 1984). The authors modified adult criteria for substance abuse for use with a sample of juvenile offenders. A clear difference was found between abusers and users based on the existence of problems in these three areas.

This research pointed to the possibility of diagnostic subtypes. For example, teenagers who were dependent on alcohol and who used cigarettes and alcohol 1½ years earlier became intoxicated at an earlier age than a control group. Parents and siblings of these probands were respectively two and four times more likely to have an alcohol or drug problem.

Blum (1987) further refined the above criteria to include alcohol and other substance abuse. He also proposed an assessment instrument that focuses on the four areas:

- problem severity
- precipitating factors: signs, symptoms, consequences, patterns of substance use
- predisposing and perpetuating risk factors: genetic, sociodemographic, intrapersonal, interpersonal, environmental
- diagnostic criteria

His diagnostic criteria required at least one symptom from each of the three life areas. These criteria still need to be validated but are helpful guides in determining the existence of substance abuse. No attempt has been made to define the line at which substance abuse becomes dependence. In addition, these criteria do not specifically help the evaluator determine what level of care and type of treatment plans and interventions an adolescent requires.

Additional Diagnostic Issues

Genetics

From the above discussion, it appears that family genetics can play an important part in the development of substance abuse disorders. The risk of a child developing alcoholism is four times greater if one biological parent is also alcoholic. Many families exhibit large numbers of substance abuse disorders that persist across many generations (Goodwin 1985).

Drug of Choice

When adolescents finally become physically dependent on a drug, what accounts for their drug of choice? Many individuals will argue that it is a combination of a predisposing chemical vulnerability and the biochemical effects of the particular drug on that individual's brain chemistry. The situation is often likened to a lock and key. Many addicted teenagers will state that they tried a variety of drugs and were not in danger of becoming addicted until they tried their eventual drug of choice. They often state, "It was as though I finally found something that had been missing from my brain." Other individuals fall victim to various substances and are seemingly susceptible to any class of abusable drugs. The availability and price of abusable substances purchased in the marketplace or provided by peers may dictate choice in youngsters who do not have the economic freedom to choose.

Age and Vulnerability to Substance Abuse

The risk of drug abusers becoming addicted increases inversely with age. The younger the individual is when starting drug use and abuse, the more likely he or she is to become addicted. The age factor represents a vulnerability that is not applicable to adults. The adolescent brain is not fully mature and is thus more susceptible to insults of any kind (Cambor and Millman 1991). Thinking processes are also not fully mature. Judgment, which can be faulty even under the best circumstances, is further impaired under the influence of drugs. As the drug abuse or dependence progresses, social awareness and tact can progressively disappear to the point at which they are almost nonexistent. The end result is that substance abuse and dependence proceed much more rapidly among adolescents. Older, more mature individuals often take years, even decades, to become addicted, whereas adolescents can develop severe behavioral problems in the space of a few weeks or months (Estroff et al. 1989; Stowell and Estroff 1992).

Recommendations

Substance use disorders in an adolescent are not easily diagnosed by the clinician because of the patient's denial and minimization. No diagnostic scheme is perfect. Each has its own strengths and weaknesses. DSM-IV is currently the best for adults. Understanding the diagnostic criteria and other features of these disorders is relatively easy. Sensing the possibility that these disorders are present is more difficult. This sense can be defined as clinical intuition or having a "feel for a disease." Some individuals are more sensitive and better able to detect adolescent substance abuse. Because the major goal of this chapter is to increase a clinician's sensitivity to these disorders, several practical points can help identify and treat substance-abusing and -dependent youngsters.

The clinician should start with the DSM-IV criteria and its "other features" and complement the evaluation with the criteria proposed by Blum (1987) and Halikas et al. (1984) for adolescents. The latter criteria should be regarded as sensitive for substance abuse but not dependence. Criteria for dependence in adolescents are not as well defined as for abuse. When DSM-IV criteria do not indicate dependence, the diagnosis can be left to the discretion of the evaluator, based on his or her understanding of the natural history of the disorder. Factors such as a positive family history, patterns of use, or preoccupation with drugs may be more significant than DSM-IV or other diagnostic criteria.

The staging systems proposed by Macdonald (1984) and Nowinski (1990) are dimensional—i.e., they have greater utility as descriptions of the severity of substance use. These systems have value as a teaching tool and give mental health and chemical dependency counselors a way to base the treatment plan on the severity of the substance abuse. In contrast, DSM-IV is categorical because it uses absolute criteria that define a diagnosis regardless of severity of symptoms. Diagnosis alone does not readily translate into treatment planning.

Multiple sources of information are necessary for diagnosing these disorders. When there is uncertainty, consultation with an expert who has a greater feel for these disorders is important. Substance abuse disorders are primary disorders requiring specialized treatment. When planning treatment and choosing the intensity of level of care, the following rules of thumb should apply:

The treatment plan should focus on the substance abuse as a primary disorder when increased frequency and quantity of use, increased severity of behavior, a characteristic chronic pattern of use, an increase in the number of criteria above the minimum required to make a diagnosis, evidence of the patient's preoccupation with substance use, and a positive family history predominate.

A higher level of intensity of care is required as more criteria are met. Short-term hospitalization for detoxification and evaluation is often indicated. A controlled, chemical-free setting is needed to assess the patient's mental status and to consider the effect of drugs on his or her school and psychosocial life. Outpatient treatment failure or evidence of biomedical complications, such as worsening physical illness, would also indicate inpatient hospital care. Inpatient treatment failure requires residential care.

References

American Psychiatric Association: Diagnostic and Statistical Manual of Mental Disorders, 3rd Edition, Revised. Washington, DC, American Psychiatric Association, 1987

American Psychiatric Association: Diagnostic and Statistical Manual of Mental Disorders, 4th Edition. Washington, DC, American Psychiatric Association, 1994

American Psychiatric Association: Diagnostic and Statistical Manual of Mental Disorders, 4th Edition Text Revision. Washington, DC, American Psychiatric Association, 2000

Bailey GW: Current perspectives on substance abuse in youth. J Am Acad Child Adolesc Psychiatry 28:151–162, 1989

Blum RW: Adolescent substance abuse: diagnostic and treatment issues. Pediatr Clin North Am 34:523–537, 1987

Bukstein OG, Brent DA, Kaminer Y: Comorbidity of substance abuse and other psychiatric disorders in adolescents. Am J Psychiatry 146:1131–1141, 1989

Cambor R, Millman RB: Alcohol and drug abuse in adolescents, in Child and Adolescent Psychiatry. Edited by Lewis M. Baltimore, MD, Williams & Wilkins, 1991, pp 736–755

Estroff TW, Gold MS: Chronic medical complications of drug abuse. Psychiatr Med 3:267–286, 1985

Estroff TW, Schwartz RH, Hoffman NG: Adolescent cocaine abuse: addictive potential, behavioral and psychiatric effects among adolescent abusers. Clin Pediatr 28:550–555, 1989

Geller B, Cooper TB, Sun K, et al: Double-blind and placebo-controlled study of lithium for adolescent bipolar disorders with secondary substance dependency. J Am Acad Child Adolesc Psychiatry 37:171–178, 1998

Goodwin DW: Alcoholism and genetics: the sins of the fathers. Arch Gen Psychiatry 42:171–174, 1985

Halikas JA: Substance abuse in children and adolescents, in Psychiatric Disorders in Children and Adolescents. Edited by Garfinkel BD, Carlson GA, Weller EB. Philadelphia, PA, WB Saunders, 1990, pp 214–221

Halikas JA, Lyttle M, Morse C, et al: Proposed criteria for the diagnosis of alcohol abuse in adolescence. Compr Psychiatry 25:581–585, 1984

Johnson VE: I'll Quit Tomorrow. New York, Harper & Row, 1980

Macdonald DI: Drugs, drinking, and adolescence. Am J Dis Child 138:117–125, 1984

Nowinski J: Substance Abuse in Adolescents and Young Adults: A Guide to Treatment. New York, WW Norton, 1990, pp 38–65

Rinaldi RC, Steindler EM, Wilford BB, et al: Clarification and standardization of substance abuse terminology. JAMA 259:555–557, 1988

Stephenson JN, Moberg P, Daniels BJ, et al: Treating the intoxicated adolescent: a need for comprehensive services. JAMA 252:1884–1888, 1984

Stowell RJA, Estroff TW: Psychiatric disorders in substance-abusing adolescent inpatients: a pilot study. J Am Acad Child Adolesc Psychiatry 31:1036–1040, 1992

Williams AR, Feibelman ND, Moulder C: Events precipitating hospital treatment of adolescent drug abusers. J Am Acad Child Adolesc Psychiatry 28:70–73, 1989

Winters KC, Henly G: Assessing adolescents who abuse chemicals: the Chemical Dependency Adolescent Assessment Project, in Adolescent Drug Abuse: Analyses of Treatment Research (NIDA Res Monogr 77). Rockville, MD, National Institute on Drug Abuse, 1988, pp 4–18

5 Comorbidity and Adolescent Substance Abuse

Oscar G. Bukstein, M.D., M.P.H.

Substance use and abuse in adolescents can have a tragic impact on the lives of the adolescents and on their families. However, substance use disorders are but one of a group of many behavioral and emotional disorders that affect youth. Several surveys of children and adolescents in the general population have provided information on the prevalence of psychiatric disorders in young people. The results of these surveys indicate that at least 12% of children and adolescents have clinically significant psychiatric disorders that compromise their ability to function. At least half of these children are severely disordered with high levels of dysfunction.

The rate of co-occurrence or comorbidity between different psychiatric disorders in adolescents is high (Offord and Fleming 1991). Evidence of the coexistence or comorbidity of substance abuse disorders and other psychiatric disorders is well documented in adults. In the Epidemiologic Catchment Area Study, a large epidemiological study of adult mental health problems, 37% of adults reported having either an alcohol or other drug disorder and a comorbid or coexisting psychiatric disorder (Regier et al. 1990). Among adults with a psychiatric disorder, the risk of having some substance use disorder was 2.7 times greater than those without a psychiatric disorder and the lifetime prevalence of about 29%.

There are few community studies of the prevalence of coexisting psychiatric and substance use disorders in adolescents. The Oregon Adolescent Depression Project (OADP) (Lewinsohn et al. 1993) assessed the lifetime comorbidity of substance use disorders among 1,710 high school students and reported that 66.2% of adolescents with substance use disorders also had a lifetime psychiatric disorder, compared with 31.3% of adolescents who had a psychiatric disorder but did not have a substance use disorder. Adolescents with substance use disorders reported a lifetime prevalence of 25.4% for any disruptive behavior disorder, 49.4% for any mood disorder, and 16.2% for any anxiety disorder. In the Methods for the Epidemiology of Child and Adolescent Mental Disorders (MECA) study of mental disorders in the community (Kandel et al. 1999), adolescents ages 14–18 years old diagnosed with a current substance use disorder were 1.5 times more likely to be diagnosed with any anxiety disorder, 3.7 times more likely to be diagnosed with any mood disorder, and 20.3 times more likely to diagnosed with a disruptive behavior disorder than adolescents without current substance use disorders. Comparisons with adult samples such as the Epidemiologic Catchment Area Study and the National Comorbidity Survey (Kessler et al. 1997) suggest that comorbidity rates for adolescents are the same as those for adults. In the MECA study, 76% of adolescents with substance use disorders had at least one comorbid psychiatric disorder, whereas only 27.8% of adolescents without substance use disorders had a psychiatric disorder.

Existing research of adolescent comorbidity in clinical populations suffers from significant methodological problems that limit the ability to generalize these findings to other adolescent populations (Bukstein et al. 1989). Among these methodological problems are the lack of valid, reliable nosology; failure to articulate specific criteria for substance use disorders in adolescents; problems in assessment methods; and questions about the representativeness of the population assessed. Because the existing studies examine the occurrence of comorbidity of substance abuse and other psychiatric disorders, comorbidity may be a function of severity. Patients with comorbid disorders may be more severely impaired and thus likely to seek and enter treatment. Such a selection bias, also known as Berkson's bias (Berkson 1946), may lead to misleading associations between substance abuse and coexisting psychiatric disorders. However, we treat those who seek treatment or who are brought in by others (usually in the case of adolescents), therefore existing studies of clinical population are useful in describing the characteristics of our patients.

Relationships Between Coexisting Substance Abuse and Psychopathology

A number of possible casual relationships exist between substance abuse and psychopathology. Several specific relationships are suggested by Meyer (1986), including 1) psychiatric symptoms or disorders developing as a consequence of substance use or abuse, 2) psychiatric disorders altering the course of substance abuse, 3) substance abuse altering the course of psychiatric disorders, 4) psychopathology, both in the individuals and their families, as a risk factor for the development of substance abuse, and 5) substance abuse and psychopathology originating from a common vulnerability. Beyond documenting the prevalence of comorbidity among specific adolescent populations, much of the research involving comorbidity has attempted to elucidate these relationships.

The use of the primary-secondary paradigm (Winokur et al. 1970) or a hierarchical approach are two proposed solutions to classification of psychopathology and its relationship to addictions or substance use disorders. The primary-secondary classification refers to ordering the diagnoses according to their chronological appearance. The diagnosis for which specific signs and symptoms appeared first is considered primary and the later-appearing diagnoses are considered secondary. Although as originally conceived, this paradigm does not propose a direction of causality or an etiology, many clinicians often assume the primary disorder is the underlying problem. This is particularly true of substance abuse and other problems in adolescence.

However, some consider substance abuse the primary or most important or underlying problem relative to other coexisting problems regardless of chronology (MacDonald 1984). This position is plausible because of the conflicting evidence; although the onset of comorbid psychiatric disorders appears to usually precede rather than to follow the onset of substance use disorders (Boyle and Offord 1991; Deykin et al. 1987; Kessler et al. 1997), substantial numbers of adolescents display substance use disorder onset prior to the onset of psychiatric disorder (Brook et al. 1998; Rhode et al. 1991).

The influence of the coexisting disorders is often bidirectional—that is, substance use/abuse and psychiatric disorders can influence each other. The co-occurrence of both types of problems produces a third entity, often called *dual diagnosis*. This label may be a misnomer because many individuals with substance abuse disorders also have two or more psychiatric diagnoses. The term *multidiagnosed* may be a more accurate and appropriate descriptor for individuals with coexisting problems.

Common Comorbid Psychiatric Disorders

Disruptive Behavior Disorders

Disruptive behavior disorders, which include conduct disorder, oppositional defiant disorder, and attention-deficit/hyperactivity disorder (ADHD), are among the most common comorbid psychiatric disorders found in adolescents with substance use disorders (Bukstein et al. 1989). In studies of clinical populations of adolescents with substance use disorders, disruptive behaviors are found in most of the youths in these clinical programs. Prospective and retrospective studies have suggested that children with disruptive behavior disorders are at risk for the development of substance use disorders as adolescents and adults (Gittelman et al. 1985; Hechtman et al. 1984; Robins 1966).

In the MECA study, 68% of adolescents with a substance use disorder had comorbid disruptive behavior disorder (Kandel et al. 1999). Rates of disruptive behavior disorders in clinical populations of adolescents with substance use disorders range up to 80% (Bukstein et al. 1989; Hovens et al. 1994; Riggs et al. 1998). Investigators have observed that childhood antisocial behavior, including aggressiveness, predicts adult alcohol and drug problems (McCord and McCord 1960; Robins 1966). Deviant behavior and conduct disorder usually precede substance abuse (Elliot et al. 1985). Such factors as an earlier onset and greater variety of early conduct problems, aggressive behavior, and the presence of ADHD may increase not only the risk for later antisocial behavior but also that for later substance abuse (Loeber 1988). The early onset of conduct problems is associated with a higher frequency and greater variety of antisocial behavior, including substance abuse.

Loeber (1988) proposed three paths of development to explain differential outcomes among deviant children who have many symptoms or behaviors of disruptive behavior disorders. The first path, the aggressive versatile path, is characterized by an early onset of conduct problems, aggressive behavior, greater rates of ADHD, poor social skills and peer relations, male predominance, and a low remission rate. The aggressive versatile path is more likely to show an early onset of substance use and abuse. A nonaggressive antisocial path is described as having a later onset; few problems with attention, impulsivity, social skills, peer relations, and aggression; and a higher remission rate. Although nonaggressive deviant behaviors may be more predictive of later substance use or abuse, aggression may be a more robust predictor of polysubstance use. Aggression in adolescence, rather than in childhood, may be a better predictor of the stage of substance abuse or negative consequences of use (Brook et al. 1986). A third pathway, the exclusive substance abuse path, is manifested by the development of alcohol and/or other drug abuse in middle to late adolescence without significant antecedent deviant behavior. The onset of substance use and subsequent abuse is generally later than in the more deviant pathway groups.

Conduct disorder and substance use/abuse appear to have significant interactive effects. Among adolescents who have an early onset of substance use, there is an increased risk of continued substance use, continuation of antisocial behavior, and more substance abuse–related symptoms (Robins and Przybeck 1985).

ADHD is also a common comorbid disorder found in adolescents with substance use disorders (Bukstein et al. 1989; Wilens et al. 1994). Studies of clinical populations of adolescent substance abusers have found high rates of ADHD (Horner and Schiebe 1997). Several retrospective studies reported a greater frequency of childhood hyperactivity among adult substance abusers (Alterman et al. 1985; Tarter et al. 1977). Other studies observed an increased occurrence of drug abuse among adolescents with a history of ADHD (Blouin et al. 1978). Family studies have found high rates of alcoholism and antisocial personality disorder in the parents of hyperactive children (Cantwell 1972; Morrison and Stewart 1971). ADHD appears to be a significant risk factor for adult substance use disorders (Biederman et al. 1995). The increased prevalence of drug use by adolescents with a history of ADHD is reported by several prospective studies (Biederman et al. 1997; Gittleman et al. 1985; Weiss and Hechtman 1986). A number of additional studies have found an association between ADHD and early-onset substance use disorders (Wilens et al. 1997).

It has been suggested that the risk for subsequent substance use disorders among youths with ADHD may be mediated by the common comorbidity of ADHD with conduct disorder (Alterman and Tarter 1986; Barkley et al. 1990), which may place affected youth at higher risk for the development of substance use disorders than either disorder alone (Lahey et al. 1988; Loeber 1988). ADHD appears to make a substantial contribution to substance use problems and delinquency in adolescents (Thompson et al. 1996). The combination of ADHD and conduct disorder appears to be a more significant risk factor for later substance abuse than conduct disorder alone (Lahey et al. 1988).

The relation between conduct disorder, ADHD, and substance abuse may point to interesting interactional effects. Several possible mechanisms might be involved in explaining the possible role of ADHD in the development of substance abuse in children with conduct disorder. The added impulsivity observed in youths with ADHD may produce poorer social choices in the areas of both behavior and association with other deviant peers as well as poor problem solving. Substance use might serve as a form of self-medication for children with ADHD. Finally, ADHD may reflect a type of brain functioning with a high level of reinforcement from certain psychoactive agents. It has been suggested that the use of stimulants, the primary drug for the treatment of ADHD in children, may increase the risk for later substance abuse. There is currently no evidence associating the long-term use of stimulants to treat children with ADHD with higher rates of substance abuse (Barkley et al. 1990; Weiss and Hechtman 1986); in fact, emerging data suggest that current therapeutic stimulant use for adolescents with ADHD may result in reduced rates of substance use disorders (Biederman et al. 1999).

Aggression is a specific behavior that merits further discussion when considering the relationship of disruptive or deviant behavior with adolescent substance use/abuse. Aggressive behaviors are present in a large number of adolescents who have conduct problems or deviant behavior and who also abuse substances (Milan et al. 1991). Among the causes of aggression in substance-abusing adolescents are the direct pharmacological effects of the substances, disinhibition, and the presence of other coexisting psychopathology (e.g., bipolar disorder).

Conduct disorder or delinquency usually precedes substance use and the onset of substance use disorders (Clark et al. 1997a, 1997b; Loeber 1990). In such cases, aggressive behavior patterns can be noted early in males, with aggressiveness in the first grade being predictive of substance use 10 years later (Kellam et al. 1983). The more serious the interpersonal aggressive behavior is before drug use, the more serious the subsequent involvement with drugs will be (Johnston et al. 1978). Other findings indicate that early aggressive behavior leads to later increases in alcohol use and alcohol-related aggression but that levels of alcohol use are not related to later aggressive behavior (White et al. 1993). Whereas nonaggressive antisocial behavior appears to be predictive of later onset substance use or abuse, aggressive antisocial behavior is more predictive of polydrug abuse, especially in males (Loeber 1990). Childhood aggressive behavior appears to be a better predictor than antisocial personality disorder of increases in anger and aggression when drinking. Generally, the more serious the substance use is, the higher the likelihood is of more serious forms of delinquency (Bohman et al. 1983; Dishion and Loeber 1985).

Mood Disorders

Mood or affective disorders are perhaps the most studied psychiatric problems coexisting with substance abuse. The high prevalence of depressive disorders and depressive symptoms in adult substance abusers is well established (Regier et al. 1990; Schuckit 1986).

In the MECA study, 32% of adolescents with a substance use disorder also reported a current mood disorder (Kandel et al. 1999). Studies of various clinical adolescent populations have observed high rates of substance abuse and mood disorders. The percentages of depressed adolescents in clinical populations of adolescent substance abusers have ranged as high as 50% (Bukstein et al. 1992; Hovens et al. 1994; Riggs et al. 1997; Stowell 1991). Deykin et al. (1987) found that alcohol abuse was associated with major depression only, whereas drug abuse was associated with major depression as well as other diagnoses in a study of college freshmen. In another study of adolescents in residential drug and alcohol treatment, Deykin et al. (1992) observed a high rate of depression (24.7%), although only 8.1% had primary depression. Female adolescents with paternal psychopathology and a history of physical abuse were more likely to have major depression, especially primary depression. As in the adult literature, females were generally more likely to have primary depression and an earlier age of onset of depression. The existence of multiple comorbid diagnoses—usually substance abuse, conduct disorder, and depression—is also common (Bukstein et al. 1992; Riggs et al. 1997; Stowell 1991).

Major depressive disorder is the most common mood disorder noted in adolescents with substance use disorders whether in the clinic or the community (Bukstein et al. 1992; Lewinsohn et al. 1993; Riggs et al. 1997). Although bipolar disorder has a modest prevalence in adolescent populations with substance use disorders, there is evidence that adolescent or preadult onset of bipolar disorder is associated with a higher risk of subsequent substance use disorders in adolescence or adulthood (Biederman et al. 1997; Dunner and Feinman 1995; Wilens et al. 1999). Prominent mood liability and dyscontrol are noted in many adolescents with substance use disorders regardless of whether a substantial number of them have a definitive diagnosis of bipolar disorder (Wills et al. 1995; Young et al. 1995).

Few studies have examined the natural history or treatment response of adolescents with comorbid depression and substance abuse. Hovens et al. (1994) reported that among hospitalized adolescent substance abusers, the onset of psychopathology preceded or coincided with substance abuse except for major depression, which most commonly had a later onset than substance abuse. However, dysthymia preceded substance abuse in most of the patients. This finding suggests a prior vulnerability toward mood disorder. Bukstein et al. (1992) found that the primary-secondary distinction did not predict acute remission of depressive symptoms in a clinical population. In other words, it may not matter which came first in predicting the short-term course of depressive symptoms in adolescents. Riggs et al. (1996, 1997, 1998) also found an absence of remission in depressed adolescents with substance use disorders as well as more substance dependence diagnoses, more prevalent ADHD diagnoses, and earlier development of comorbid conduct disorder symptoms.

Suicide

Suicidal behavior is a critical complication of mood disorders. Increasing research in adolescent suicide reveals a relationship between substance abuse and suicidal behavior. Accumulating evidence suggests that much of the increase in the adolescent and young adult suicide rate since the 1960s may be related to substance use and abuse (Brent et al. 1987; Rich et al. 1986a, 1986b). Various studies support substance abuse as a risk factor for suicidal behavior, including ideation and attempted and completed suicide (Bukstein et al. 1993; Crumley 1990).

The association of adolescent substance abuse with other forms of psychopathology may also mediate both the acute and chronic effects noted above in suicidal behavior in this population. Substance abuse in adolescents is often evident concurrently with several other psychiatric disorders, including mood disorders, anxiety disorders, bulimia nervosa, schizophrenia, and conduct disorder (Bukstein et al. 1989; Greenbaum et al. 1991). Each of these disorders carries an increased risk of suicidal behavior (Brent and Kolko 1990) as well as an increased risk of substance abuse (Bukstein et al. 1989) in adolescents. However, comorbidity, especially mood disorders with other non-mood disorders including substance abuse, is one of several putative risk factors for completed suicide (Brent et al. 1988).

Although conduct disorder is also frequently comorbid with mood disorders (Ryan et al. 1987), many adolescents with substance abuse and conduct disorder can manifest suicidal behavior without the presence of a mood disorder (Apter et al. 1988). Aggression and impulsivity, both common in conduct disorders, may be important factors in the risk for suicidal behavior in substance-abusing adolescents (Apter et al. 1988).

Study of impulsivity and aggression as risk factors for suicidality may reflect underlying cognitive problem-solving styles or underlying neurobiology as true risk factors rather than discrete diagnoses. Adolescents with high rates of aggressive-type conduct disorder and ADHD are more likely to engage in substance abuse than are those with ADHD alone or nonaggressive conduct disorder (Bukstein 1994; Milan et al. 1991). Youths displaying explosive, aggressive outbursts appear to be at greatest risk for repetitive suicidal behavior (Pfeffer et al. 1988). Research on low serotonergic states with suicidal and aggressive behavior in substance-abusing adults (Roy and Linnoila 1986) indicates that impulsivity and aggression may be as critical as depression in the etiology of suicidal behavior. This is further evidenced by the fact that adolescents with conduct disorder have higher suicidality scores than those with major depression (Apter et al. 1988).

Anxiety Disorders

Until recently, anxiety disorders were underappreciated as a potential comorbid diagnosis for adolescents with substance use disorders (Clark et al. 1995). In the MECA study, 20% of adolescents with substance use disorders reported coexisting anxiety disorder (Kandel et al. 1999), whereas in the OADP project, 16.2% of adolescents with substance use disorders reported anxiety disorder diagnoses (Lewinsohn et al. 1993). Rohde et al. (1991) reported that anxiety disorders were associated with problematic alcohol use. Other clinical samples of adolescents with substance use disorders have shown high rates of comorbid anxiety disorder (Clark and Sayette 1993; Clark et al. 1997a, 1997b). Hovens et al. (1994) found a high prevalence of social phobia among adolescents with substance use disorders in an inpatient treatment program. In a comparison of young male alcoholic patients and subjects who did not use alcohol, Rydelius (1983) found that the heavy alcohol users were more likely than the nonusers to report anxiety symptoms and interpersonal difficulties due to shyness.

Posttraumatic stress disorder (PTSD) is also commonly noted in clinical populations, especially among females (Clark et al. 1997a, 1997b, 1998). Clark et al. (1994) found that anxiety disorders were common in an adolescent treatment population with early-onset alcoholism. Half of this sample had at least one lifetime anxiety disorder diagnosis, with PTSD as the most common diagnosis (25% of total sample). Substance-abusing adolescents without diagnoses of anxiety disorders still had higher anxiety levels than a normal control group. Adolescents with comorbid substance abuse, conduct disorder, and anxiety disorder had more depressive symptoms and suicidal behavior than normal control subjects, although the comorbid group did not differ on these variables from a group with comorbid substance abuse and conduct disorder but not anxiety disorder. The comorbid group with anxiety disorders was less impaired in terms of substance abuse behavior, school problems, peer relations, and overall problem density than the comorbid group without anxiety disorders.

For adolescents in the earlier stages of alcohol use, their reasons for use and continued abuse may hold clues as to the role of anxiety in eventually leading to anxiety disorders. Forty-one percent of high school seniors in the United States reported that they used drugs "to relax or relieve tension"; 64% of barbiturate users, 69% of tranquilizer users, and 40% and 41% of alcohol and marijuana users, respectively, mentioned tension reduction as a reason for their substance use (Johnston and O'Malley 1986). As with adults, many adolescents view alcohol and other substances as social lubricants that may allow them to be more social in the many anxiety-provoking social situations that occur during adolescence. In some individuals, the exacerbation of anxiety symptoms with alcohol use may raise anxiety symptoms to clinical levels. McKay et al. (1992) found that alcohol-abusing adolescents with high problem severity were more likely than those with low problem severity to report believing that alcohol enhances social behavior.

In clinical populations of adolescents with comorbid anxiety and alcohol abuse, Clark and Jacob (1992) found that a substantial proportion of adolescents (85%) had onset of anxiety disorder before onset of alcohol abuse. The order of appearance of comorbid disorders appears to be variable depending on the specific anxiety disorder. Social phobia and agoraphobia usually precede alcohol abuse, whereas panic disorder and generalized anxiety disorder tend to follow the onset of alcohol abuse (Kushner et al. 1990).

The pharmacologic effects of alcohol and other substances may explain much of the relationship between substance use and abuse and anxiety disorders. Although alcohol, for example, has direct anxiolytic properties, the expectation or belief that alcohol will reduce anxiety may often promote alcohol use despite the real effects of alcohol in actually reducing anxiety (Clark and Sayette 1993). Consistent with such theories of tension reduction or self-medication, the early onset of phobic disorders suggests attempts at self-medication. The later appearance of panic and generalized anxiety disorders may be due to preexisting excessive consumption and/or withdrawal states.

Eating Disorders

Eating disorders are another type of psychiatric disorder often associated with substance abuse. Studies point to a high incidence of substance abuse among bulimic patients as opposed to those with restrictive anorexia nervosa (Hatsukami et al. 1984; Pyle et al. 1981). Among women presenting for the treatment of alcoholism, there appears to be an increased risk of eating disorders, and several studies have reported high rates of substance abuse among relatives of bulimic women (Bulik 1987; Hudson et al. 1987).

Comorbidity and the Development of Substance Abuse in Adolescence

Specific psychiatric disorders likely influence the risk, onset, and course of substance abuse disorders in adolescents. This relationship between substance abuse and psychopathology is probably not a simple one, and it may be nonspecific in terms of how these additional problems add to other social stressors or risk factors for substance abuse. Whether they receive discrete psychiatric diagnoses or not, many substance-abusing adolescents appear to have higher levels of psychiatric symptoms including mood and anxiety symptoms (Bukstein et al. 1992). For example, adolescents with conduct disorder and substance abuse commonly have affect regulation problems manifesting as labile, irritable, and highly reactive mood states (Wills et al. 1995; Young et al. 1995).

In reviewing the psychological and biological characteristics associated with vulnerability to alcoholism, Tarter et al. (1985) suggested that vulnerability could be explained in terms of empirically established temperamental traits such as strength and speed of response and quality and lability of prevailing mood. Identification of temperamental traits in adolescents may be useful for identifying the characteristics that distinguish alcoholic patients or those at risk for alcoholism who have these traits from those who do not have these traits. Temperamental traits may be the basis for a common diathesis for substance use disorders, antisocial personality, and/or other psychiatric disorders (Tarter et al. 1994).

Cloninger (1987) proposed that clinical subgroups differing in patterns of abuse, personality traits, neurophysiological characteristics, and inheritance result from various response biases or neurogenetic adaptive mechanisms that mediate individuals' adaptation to experiences, including their responses to substance use. Cloninger's Type I and Type II alcoholic patients may reflect various combinations of these adaptive mechanisms that result in substance-seeking behavior and later dependence after initial or early exposure. As previously discussed, dimensional characteristics of adolescents, including aggression and behavioral disinhibition, may be even more important than categorical comorbid diagnoses in subtyping adolescent substance abusers according to natural history, prognosis, and treatment response. Mezzich et al. (1993) reported that alcohol-abusing adolescents from a clinical population formed two clusters: behavioral disinhibition and hypophoria characterized most of the adolescents, and negative affect characterized the rest. The first group had an earlier age of onset, more substance abuse involvement, and greater severity of psychiatric disorders and behavioral disturbance.

Substance use as self-medication of coexistent psychiatric symptoms is one hypothesis that attempts to explain comorbidity. On the basis of psychodynamic and other clinical findings, Khantzian (1985) suggested that the specific psychotropic effects of illicit drugs, especially cocaine and heroin, interact with psychiatric disturbances and painful affects to predispose to addictive disorder. Substance abusers' drug choices may be the result of an interaction between the psychopharmacologic properties of the drug and the primary feeling state experienced by the addict. Other investigators support the theory that adolescents use substances in response to distress and negative affective states. Kandel et al. (1978) found that psychological distress predicted the use of hard or illicit drugs other than marijuana. McKay et al. (1992) observed that alcohol-abusing adolescents with high problem severity reported a greater propensity of drinking in response to unpleasant emotions.

Self-medication of psychiatric symptoms may be the common denominator in explaining the relationship between various psychiatric disorders coexisting with pathologic substance use. Several studies have identified psychological distress as a contributing factor or explanation for relapse in alcoholic and opiate-dependent populations (Ludwig 1989). Consistent with classical conditioning models, negative affective states (e.g., depression or anger) appear to be able to directly trigger craving and possibly precipitate relapse (Childress et al. 1992).

Assessment and Comorbidity

The high prevalence of comorbity between substance use disorders and psychiatric disorders in adolescent clinical populations demands that clinicians develop skills in dealing with both mental health and substance abuse assessment and treatment issues. Screening and the subsequent comprehensive assessment of coexisting psychopathology are essential during each step of the assessment process for adolescents with suspected substance use disorders. Screening questions about depression, suicidal ideation and behavior, anxiety, aggressive behavior, and current and past mental health treatment should be a part of every evaluation. Questions should include whether the symptoms or behaviors are present during both substance use or intoxication and abstinence. Clinicians should attempt to establish the chronology of symptoms and behaviors relative to the onset of specific substance use behaviors, such as onset of first use, regular use, and pathologic use. It should also be determined if the symptoms or behaviors exist independently of substance use or intoxication and if they continue well into significant periods of abstinence.

A family history of psychiatric disorders can often provide clues to understanding a confusing set of symptoms and behaviors. The clinician should ask not only about past treatment history and established psychiatric diagnoses of family members, but also whether similar but undiagnosed comorbid symptoms or disorder patterns exist in other family members.

When choosing the level of inquiry into psychopathology, clinicians are usually guided by the setting and the purpose of the assessment. Several screening questions into depression, suicidality, aggression, psychosis, and treatment history may be sufficient to augment other information in determining where an adolescent should be referred for a more comprehensive psychiatric evaluation. In a comprehensive assessment of the adolescent with comorbid disorders, questions about psychiatric and behavioral problems should cover every major diagnostic group. Tarter et al. (1990) suggested a step-wise assessment procedure for adolescents, beginning with the screening of multiple domains of adolescent functioning (i.e., substance use, psychiatric/behavioral, family, school/vocational, recreational, peer, and medical). Positive responses in each domain are then followed by more detailed, focused assessment.

To augment the clinical interview, clinicians may wish to use one of several diagnostic instruments to assess the severity of psychopathology and to obtain psychiatric diagnoses. Such instruments include a highly structured diagnostic interview such as the Diagnostic Interview Schedule for Children (DISC) or the Diagnostic Interview Schedule for Children and Adolescents (DICA) or a semistructured interview format such as the Schedule for Affective Disorders and Schizophrenia for School-Age Children (K-SADS) for more experienced clinicians (Kaufman et al. 1997; Puig-Antich and Chambers 1978). Severity ratings can be obtained through the use of dimensional rating scales and other self-report or parent report instruments such as the Beck Depression Index (Beck et al. 1961) for depression, the Child Behavior Checklist (Achenbach and Edelbrock 1983) for general internalizing and externalizing problems, or the Iowa Conners Scale (Pelham et al. 1989) for ADHD. Such rating scales are often valuable to establish a baseline rating that can be compared with that of other adolescents to determine deviance from the norm and that can be use for repeated measures to assess response to treatment.

Conclusion: Clinical Implications of Comorbidity

It is essential that clinicians recognize the importance of comorbid psychiatric disorders in the assessment and treatment of adolescents with substance abuse disorders. In clinical settings, the risk of encountering coexisting problems is substantial. Comorbid psychiatric disorders influence the symptoms and behaviors displayed by adolescents, the course of the component disorders, and the approach and response to treatment.

Identification of subtypes of accompanying risk factors and more specific identification of populations at risk could be helpful in prevention, treatment, and follow-up. Because of the implications of additional diagnoses toward treatment and prognosis, evaluation of adolescents should be more thorough, whether the primary problem is identified as substance abuse or other psychopathology. Increased effort should be made in obtaining a thorough family history and chronology of symptom onset. Following such a complete evaluation and differentiation of individuals into subgroups, each subgroup could benefit from a specific individualized program or set of interventions (e.g., serotonin reuptake inhibitors for those in whom alcohol abuse was secondary to depressive symptoms). To ensure inclusion in the appropriate subgroup, evaluation of patient symptoms, behavior, and response to treatment should be ongoing.

Treatment-matching of adolescents with various levels of dysfunction, including comorbid psychopathology, offers much promise as one guide to appropriate treatment selection for this population. Results from treatment studies of substance-abusing adults indicate that psychiatric severity may be an important determinant of treatment success. In a published report of a patient treatment-matching study for adolescents, Friedman et al. (1993) reported that compared with short-term inpatient treatment, long-term outpatient treatment had a significantly greater effect in reducing substance use/abuse for patients who had relatively more severe social, family, and employment problems. This study also found a trend toward better outcome for adolescents with more severe psychiatric problems.

As improved treatment methods are developed for psychiatric disorders in adolescents, these improvements can be potentially modified and applied to the comorbid group of adolescents. A more comprehensive but flexible approach to the assessment and treatment of adolescents should produce better treatment outcomes.

References

Achenbach TM, Edelbrock C: Manual for the Child Behavior Checklist and Revised Child Behavior Profile. Burlington, VT, University of Vermont, 1983

Alterman AI, Tarter RE: An examination of selected topologies: hyperactivity, familial and antisocial alcoholism, in Recent Developments in Alcoholism, Vol 4. Edited by Galanter M. New York, Plenum, 1986, pp 169–189

Alterman AI, Tarter RB, Baughman TG, et al: Differentiation of alcoholics high and low in childhood hyperactivity. Drug Alcohol Depend 15:111–121, 1985

Apter A, Bleich A, Plutchik R, et al: Suicidal behavior, depression, and conduct disorder in hospitalized adolescents. J Am Acad Child Adolesc Psychiatry 27:696–699, 1988

Barkley RA, Fischer M, Edelbrock CS, et al: The adolescent outcome of hyperactive children diagnosed by research criteria, I: an 8-year prospective follow-up study. J Am Acad Child Adolesc Psychiatry 29:546–557, 1990

Beck AT, Ward CH, Mendelsohn M: An inventory for measuring depression. Arch Gen Psychiatry 42:667–675, 1961

Berkson J: Limitations of the application of four fold table analysis to hospital data. Biometry Bulletin 47–53, 1946

Biederman J, Wilens TE, Mick E, et al: Psychoactive substance use disorders in adults with attention-deficit/hyperactivity disorder (ADHD): effects of ADHD and psychiatric comorbidity. Am J Psychiatry 152:1652–1658, 1995

Biederman J, Wilens TE, Mick E, et al: Is ADHD a risk for psychoactive substance use disorders? Findings from a prospective follow-up study. J Am Acad Child Adolesc Psychiatry 36:21–29, 1997

Biederman J, Wilens T, Mick E, et al: Pharmacotherapy of attention-deficit/hyperactivity disorder reduces risk for substance use disorder. Pediatrics 104:e20, 1999

Blouin AG, Bornstein MA, Trites RL: Teenage alcohol abuse among hyperactive children: a five-year follow up study. J Pediatr Psychol 3:188–194, 1978

Bohman M, Cloninger R, Sigvardsson S, et al: Alcohol abuse and personality factors, using a personality inventory. Acta Psychiatr Scand 68:381–385, 1983

Boyle MH, Offord DR: Psychiatric disorder and substance use in adolescence. Can J Psychiatry 36:699–705, 1991

Brent DA, Kolko DJ: The assessment and treatment of children and adolescents at risk for suicide, in Suicide Over the Life Cycle. Edited by Blumenthal SJ, Kupfer DJ. Washington, DC, American Psychiatric Press, 1990, pp 253–302

Brent DA, Perper JA, Allman C: Alcohol, firearms and suicide among youth: temporal trends in Allegheny County, Pennsylvania, 1960 to 1983. JAMA 257:3369–3372, 1987

Brent DA, Perper JA, Goldstein CE, et al: Risk factors for adolescent suicide: a comparison of adolescent suicide victims with suicidal inpatients. Arch Gen Psychiatry 45:581–588, 1988

Brook JS, Gordon AS, Whiteman M, et al: Dynamics of childhood and adolescent personality traits and adolescent drug use. Dev Psychol 22:403–414, 1986

Brook JS, Cohen P, Brook DW: Longitudinal study of co-occurring psychiatric disorder and substance use. J Am Acad Child Adolesc Psychiatry 37:322–330, 1998

Bukstein OG: Substance abuse, in Handbook of Aggressive and Destructive Behavior in Psychiatric Patients. Edited by Hersen M, Ammerman RT, Sisson LA. New York, Plenum, 1994, pp 445–468

Bukstein OG, Brent DA, Kaminer Y: Comorbidity of substance abuse and other psychiatric disorders in adolescents. Am J Psychiatry 146:1131–1141, 1989

Bukstein OG, Glancy LJ, Kaminer Y: Patterns of affective comorbidity in a clinical population of dually diagnosed adolescent substance abusers. J Am Acad Child Adolesc Psychiatry 31:1041–1045, 1992

Bukstein OG, Brent DA, Perper JA, et al: Risk factors for completed suicide among adolescents with a lifetime history of substance abuse: a case-control study. Acta Psychiatr Scand 88:403–408, 1993

Bulik CM: Drug and alcohol abuse by bulimic women and their families. Am J Psychiatry 144:1604–1606, 1987

Cantwell D: Psychiatric illness in the families of hyperactive children. Arch Gen Psychiatry 27:414–417, 1972

Childress AR, Ehrman R, Rohsenow DJ, et al: Classical conditioned factor in drug dependence, in Substance Abuse: A Comprehensive Textbook. Edited by Lowinson JN, Ruiz P, Millman RB. Baltimore, MD, Williams & Wilkins, 1992, pp 56–69

Clark DB, Jacob RG: Anxiety disorders and alcoholism in adolescents: a preliminary report (abstract). Alcohol Clin Exp Res 16:371, 1992

Clark DB, Sayette M: Anxiety and the development of alcoholism: clinical and scientific issues. Am J Addict 2:59–76, 1993

Clark DB, Jacob RG, Mezzich A: Anxiety and conduct disorders in early onset alcoholism. Ann N Y Acad Sci 708:181–186, 1994

Clark DB, Bukstein OG, Smith MG, et al: Identifying anxiety disorders in adolescents hospitalized for alcohol abuse or dependence. Psychiatr Serv 46:618–620, 1995

Clark DB, Pollock N, Bukstein OG, et al: Gender and comorbid psychopathology in adolescents with alcohol dependence. J Am Acad Child Adolesc Psychiatry 36:1195–1203, 1997a

Clark DB, Lesnick L, Hegedus AM: Traumas and other adverse life events in adolescents with alcohol abuse and dependence. J Am Acad Child Adolesc Psychiatry 36:1744–1751, 1997b

Clark DB, Kirisci L, Tarter RE: Adolescent versus adult onset and the development of substance use disorders in males. Drug Alcohol Depend 49:115–121, 1998

Cloninger CR: Neurogenetic adaptive mechanisms in alcoholism. Science 236:410–416, 1987

Crumley FE: Substance abuse and adolescent suicidal behavior. JAMA 263:3051–3056, 1990

Deykin EY, Levy JC, Wells V: Adolescent depression, alcohol and drug abuse. Am J Public Health 77:178–182, 1987

Deykin EY, Buka SL, Zeena TH: Depressive Illness among chemically dependent adolescents. Am J Psychiatry 149:1341–1347, 1992

Dishion TJ, Loeber R: Adolescent marijuana and alcohol use: the role of parents and peers revisited. Am J Drug Alcohol Abuse 11:11–25, 1985

Donovan SJ, Susser ES, Nunes EV: Changes in marijuana use in teenagers with temper outbursts and irritable mood after successful treatment with open-label Depakote. Presentation at the 58th Annual Meeting of the College on Problems of Drug Dependence, San Juan, Puerto Rico, June 1996

Dunner DL, Feinman J: The effect of substance abuse on the course of bipolar disorder. Presentation at the American College of Neuropsychopharmacology, San Juan, Puerto Rico, December 1995

Elliot DS, Huizinga D, Ageton SS: Explaining Delinquency and Drug Use in Adolescents. Beverly Hills, CA, Sage Publications, 1985

Friedman AD, Granick S, Kreischer C, et al: Matching adolescents who abuse drugs to treatment. Am J Addict 2:232–237, 1993

Gittelman R, Mannuzza S, Shenker R, et al: Hyperactive boys almost grown up, I: psychiatric status. Arch Gen Psychiatry 42:937–947, 1985

Greenbaum PE, Prange ME, Friedman RM, et al: Substance abuse prevalence and comorbidity with other psychiatric disorders among adolescents with severe emotional disturbances. J Am Acad Child Adolesc Psychiatry 30:575–583, 1991

Hatsukami D, Eckert E, Mitchell J, et al: Affective disorder and substance abuse in women with bulimia. Psychol Med 14:701–704, 1984

Hechtman L, Weiss G, Perlman T: Hyperactive as young adults: past and current antisocial behavior and moral development. Am J Orthopsychiatry 54:415–425, 1984

Horner BR, Scheibe KE: Prevalence and implications of attention-deficit/hyperactivity disorder among adolescents in treatment for substance abuse. J Am Acad Child Adolesc Psychiatry 36:30–36, 1997

Hovens JG, Cantwell DP, Kiriakos R: Psychiatric comorbidity in hospitalized adolescent substance abusers. J Am Acad Child Adolesc Psychiatry 33:476–483, 1994

Hudson JI, Pope HG Jr, Jonas JM, et al: A controlled family history study of bulimia. Psychol Med 17:883–890, 1987

Johnston LD, O'Malley PM: Why do the nation's students use drugs and alcohol? Self-reported reasons from nine national surveys. Journal of Drug Issues 16:29–66, 1986

Johnston LD, O'Malley P, Eveland L: Drugs and delinquency: a search for causal connections, in Longitudinal Research on Drug Use: Empirical Findings and Methodological Issues. Edited by Kandel DB. Washington, DC, Hemisphere Wiley, 1978, pp 137–156

Kandel DB, Kessler RC, Margulies RZ: Antecedents of adolescent initiation into stages of drug use: a developmental analysis, in Longitudinal Research on Drug Use: Empirical Findings and Methodological Issues. Edited by Kandel DB. Washington, DC, Hemisphere Wiley, 1978, pp 73–99

Kandel DB, Johnson JG, Bird HR, et al: Psychiatric comorbidity among adolescents with substance use disorders: findings from the MECA Study. J Am Acad Child Adolesc Psychiatry 38:693–699, 1999

Kaufman J, Birmaher B, Brent D, et al: Schedule for Affective Disorders and Schizophrenia for School-Age Children—Present and Lifetime Version (K-SADS-PL): initial reliability and validity data. J Am Acad Child Adolesc Psychiatry 36:980–988, 1997

Kellam SG, Stevenson DL, Rubin BR: How specific are the early predictors of teenage drug use? in Problems of Drug Dependence 1983 (NIDA Res Monogr 49). Edited by Harris LS. Washington, DC, U.S. Government Printing Office, 1983, pp 329–334

Kessler RC, Nelson CB, Warner LA, et al: Lifetime co-occurrence of the DSM-III-R abuse and dependence with other psychiatric disorders in the National Comorbidity Survey. Arch Gen Psychiatry 54:313–321, 1997

Khantzian EJ: The self-medication hypothesis of addictive disorders: focus on heroin and cocaine dependence. J Stud Alcohol 46:329–356, 1985

Kushner MG, Sher KJ, Beitman BD: The relation between alcohol problems and anxiety disorders. Am J Psychiatry 147:685–695, 1990

Lahey BB, Piacentini JC, McBurnett K, et al: Psychopathology in the parents of children with conduct disorder and hyperactivity. J Am Acad Child Adolesc Psychiatry 27:163–170, 1988

Lewinsohn PM, Hopps H, Roberts RE, et al: Adolescent psychopathology I: prevalence and incidence of depression and other DSM-III-R disorders in high school students. J Abnorm Psychol 102:133–144, 1993

Loeber R: Natural histories of conduct problems, delinquency and associated substance use, in Advances in Clinical Child Psychology, Vol 11. Edited by Lahey BB, Kazdin AE. New York, Plenum, 1988, pp 73–124

Loeber R: Development and risk factors of juvenile antisocial behavior and delinquency. Clin Psychol Rev 10:1–41, 1990

Ludwig AM: The mystery of craving. Alcohol Health Res World 11:12–17, 1989

MacDonald DI: Drugs, drinking and adolescence. Am J Dis Child 138:117–125, 1984

McCord W, McCord J: Origins of Alcoholism. Stanford, CA, Stanford University Press, 1960

McKay JR, Murphy RT, Maisto SA, et al: Characteristics of adolescent psychiatric patients who engage in problematic behavior while intoxicated. J Am Acad Child Adolesc Psychiatry 311:1031–1035, 1992

Meyer RE: How to understand the relationship between psychopathology and addictive disorders: another example of the chicken and the egg, in Psychopathology and Addictive Disorder. Edited by Meyer RE. New York, Guilford, 1986, pp 284–291

Mezzich A, Tarter RE, Kirisci L, et al: Subtypes of early age onset alcoholism. Alcohol Clin Exp Res 17:767–770, 1993

Milan R, Halikas JA, Meller JE, et al: Psychopathology among substance abusing juvenile offenders. J Am Acad Child Adolesc Psychiatry 301:569–574, 1991

Morrison JR, Stewart MA: A family study of the hyperactive child syndrome. Biol Psychiatry 3:189–195, 1971

Offord DR, Fleming JE: Epidemiology, in Child and Adolescent Psychiatry: A Comprehensive Textbook. Edited by Lewis M. Baltimore, MD, Williams & Wilkins, 1991, pp 1156–1167

Pelham WE, Milich R, Murphy DA, et al: Normative data on the IOWA Connors Teacher's Rating Scale. J Clin Child Psychol 18:259–262, 1989

Pfeffer CR, Newcorn J, Kaplan G, et al: Suicidal behavior in adolescent psychiatric inpatients. J Am Acad Child Adolesc Psychiatry 271:357–361, 1988

Puig-Antich J, Chambers W: The Schedule for Affective Disorders and Schizophrenia for School-Aged Children (unpublished interview schedule). New York, New York State Psychiatric Institute, 1978

Pyle RL, Mitchell JE, Eckert ED: Bulimia: a report of 34 cases. J Clin Psychiatry 42:60–64, 1981

Regier DA, Farmer ME, Rae DS, et al: Comorbidity of mental disorders with alcohol and other drug abuse. JAMA 264:2511–2518, 1990

Rich CL, Young D, Fowler RC: San Diego Suicide Study, I: young vs. old subjects. Arch Gen Psychiatry 43:577–582, 1986a

Rich CL, Young D, Fowler RC: San Diego Suicide Study, II: substance abuse in young cases. Arch Gen Psychiatry 43:962–965, 1986b

Riggs PD, Thompson LL, Mikulich SK, et al: An open trial of pemoline in drug dependent delinquents with attention-deficit hyperactivity disorder. J Am Acad Child Adolesc Psychiatry 35:1018–1024, 1996

Riggs PD, Mikulich SK, Coffman LM, et al: Fluoxetine in drug-dependent delinquents with major depression: an open trial. J Child Adolesc Psychopharmacol 7:87–95, 1997

Riggs PD, Leon SL, Mikulich SK, et al: An open trial of bupropion for ADHD in adolescents with substance use disorders and conduct disorder. J Am Acad Child Adolesc Psychiatry 37:1271–1278, 1998

Robins L: Deviant Children Grown Up. Baltimore, MD, Williams & Wilkins, 1966

Robins LN, Przybeck TR: Age of onset of drug use as a risk factor in drug and other disorders, in Etiology of Drug Abuse: Implications for Prevention. NIDA Research Monograph No. 56. Edited by Jones CL, Battjes RJ. Rockville, MD, National Institute on Drug Abuse, 1985, pp 178–192

Rohde P, Lewinsohn PM, Seeley JR: Comorbidity of unipolar depression, II: comorbidity with other mental disorders in adolescents and adults. J Abnorm Psychol 100:214–222, 1991

Roy A, Linnoila M: Alcoholism and suicide. Suicide Life Threat Behav 16:244–273, 1986

Ryan N, Puig-Antich J, Ambrosini P, et al: The clinical picture of major depression in children and adolescents. Arch Gen Psychiatry 44:854–861, 1987

Rydelius P: Alcohol abusing teenage boys: testing a hypothesis on alcohol abuse and social background factors criminality and personality in teenage boys. Acta Psychiatr Scand 68:381–385, 1983

Schuckit MA: Genetic and clinical implications of alcoholism and affective disorder. Am J Psychiatry 143:140–147, 1986

Stowell RJA: Dual diagnosis issues. Psychiatr Ann 211:98–104, 1991

Tarter RE, McBride H, Buonpane N, et al: Differentiation of alcoholics: childhood history of minimal brain dysfunction, family history, and drinking pattern. Arch Gen Psychiatry 34:761–768, 1977

Tarter RE, Alterman AI, Edwards KL: Vulnerability to alcoholism in men: a behavior-genetic perspective. J Stud Alcohol 46:329–356, 1985

Tarter RE, Laird SB, Mostefa K, et al: Drug abuse severity in adolescents is associated with magnitude of deviation in temperamental traits. British Journal of Addiction 85:1501–1504, 1990

Tarter R, Kirisci L, Hegedus A, et al: Heterogeneity of adolescent alcoholism. Ann N Y Acad Sci 708:172–180, 1994

Thompson LL, Riggs PD, Milulich SK, et al: Contribution of ADHD symptoms to substance use problems and delinquency in conduct disordered adolescents. J Abnorm Child Psychol 24:325–347, 1996

Weiss G, Hechtman LT: Hyperactive Children Grown Up. New York, Guilford, 1986

White HR, Brick J, Hansell S: A longitudinal investigation of alcohol use and aggression in adolescence. J Stud Alcohol Suppl 11:62–77, 1993

Wilens TE, Biederman J, Spencer TJ, et al: Comorbidity of attention-deficit hyperactivity and psychoactive substance use disorders. Hospital and Community Psychiatry 45:412–435, 1994

Wilens TE, Biederman J, Abrantes AM, et al: Clinical characteristics of psychiatrically referred adolescent outpatients with substance use disorder. J Am Acad Child Adolesc Psychiatry 36:941–947, 1997

Wilens TE, Biederman J, Millstein RB, et al: Risk for substance use disorders in youths with child and adolescent-onset bipolar disorder. J Am Acad Child Adolesc Psychiatry 38:680–685, 1999

Wills TA, DuHamel L, Vaccaro D: Activity and mood temperament as predictors of adolescent substance abuse: test of a self-regulation model. J Pers Soc Psychol 68:901–916, 1995

Winokur G, Reichl T, Rimmer J, et al: Alcoholism, III: diagnosis and familial psychiatric illness in 259 alcoholic probands. Arch Gen Psychiatry 23:104–111, 1970

Young SE, Mikulich SK, Goodwin MB, et al: Treated delinquent boys' substance use: onset, pattern, relationship to conduct and mood disorders. Drug Alcohol Depend 37:149–162, 1995

6 Medical Evaluation of Substance-Abusing Adolescents

Anthony H. Dekker, D.O.
Todd Wilk Estroff, M.D.
Norman G. Hoffmann, Ph.D.

Unless they have specialized training in psychiatry and/or substance abuse treatment, physicians treating substance-abusing adolescents should initially limit their actions to identifying these patients and making an appropriate referral. Unfortunately, this does not happen for various reasons: Many physicians underestimate the extent of the adolescents' problems and consequently overestimate their own ability to treat the adolescents' addictions, and some physicians hang on to their patients, fearing that if they refer the patients they will not be able to continue to treat the adolescents' medical problems. This need not be the case if physicians cooperate with each other. When appropriate referrals are made and trusting relationships established, the referring physician and the specialist can function as equals in caring for the patients' needs. Failure to coordinate care in this manner can result from a general lack of training about substance abuse disorders in both medical school and residency training.

Lack of Training in All Specialties

Almost half of the pediatric residency programs in the United States reported they lacked the time, faculty, and curricula to teach anything about adolescent substance abuse (Faigel 1996; Werner and Adger 1995). There is a similar lack of training in many adult and child/adolescent psychiatric residencies (Wilens et al. 1997) as well as programs in emergency medicine; family medicine; internal medicine; obstetrics; gynecology; ear, nose, and throat; neurology; cardiology; orthopedics; and sports medicine (Arria et al. 1995; Dell 1996; Elias et al. 1994; Konings et al. 1995; Muramoto and Leshan 1993; Parrish 1994) despite the growing body of information about the interplay between medical problems and adolescent substance abuse (Kokotailo 1995). This connection is most apparent when teenagers with behavioral problems are seen in an emergency department or by psychiatrists, psychologists, and social workers (Barnett et al. 1998; Dell 1996; Gordon et al. 1996; Jenson et al. 1995; Spain et al. 1997; Wilens et al. 1997).

Identifying Adolescent Substance Abuse: Responsibility of Primary Care Physicians

General practitioners and pediatricians as primary care specialists are trained to keep an overall perspective of their patients treatment. As a result, they are often involved in adolescent substance abuse treatment in many different ways: 1) anticipatory guidance, 2) recognition of substance use and abuse, 3) treatment of urgent medical problems, 4) appropriate referral, 5) family support and reassurance, 6) education, and 7) community action (American Academy of Pediatrics 1988)

Importance of Suspecting Substance Abuse

Whenever a physician suspects substance abuse, he or she must investigate thoroughly. An adequate substance abuse history should be taken, the patient should be examined carefully for physical signs of substance abuse, and appropriate laboratory tests should be ordered, especially a sensitive urine drug screen. We believe testing should never be done deceptively or without informing both the adolescent and his or her parents. Testing should proceed only after the physician has carefully explained his or her concerns and the confirmatory tests to be ordered. Any refusal to allow testing must be carefully documented. This simple precaution can derail future malpractice suits over the failure to diagnose adolescent substance abuse.

Unfortunately, even when they suspect adolescent substance abuse, many physicians are uncomfortable questioning the truthfulness of their patients' histories, expressing their doubts, and asking direct questions about drug abuse. Physicians want to be perceived as allies, not adversaries, and as a result they tend to equivocate and avoid thinking about or addressing the topic altogether. Even if they do ask the correct questions, they tend to believe the adolescents' denials and decline to pursue the matter further.

Another reason that physicians avoid inquiring further into patients' substance abuse is that with the rise of managed care, physicians are under intense time and cost constraints. Stopping to ask more questions, order more tests, or ask for a second opinion takes more time and costs more money. Explaining what they are doing and why to the teenagers' parents or the managed care company takes even more time. The end result is that physicians infrequently order a urine drug screen or communicate their suspicions to the adolescents' parents.

Suspicion in Different Medical Settings

Substance abuse must be part of the differential diagnosis in a variety of medical settings. This is especially true in the emergency department in cases involving trauma (Barnett et al. 1998; Gordon et al. 1996; Loiselle et al. 1993; Spain et al. 1997). Each case of overdose, attempted suicide, unexplained unconscious states, unexplained fainting spells, or amnestic states should similarly prompt the taking of a drug and alcohol abuse history followed by a focused physical examination. Sexually transmitted diseases and pregnancy can also point to adolescent substance abuse.

Assessment of Suspected Substance Abuse

Whenever adolescent substance abuse is suspected, a complete evaluation should follow. As mentioned earlier, this assessment must include a thorough and focused history, review of systems, physical examination, and laboratory testing. Particular attention must be paid to various risk factors that indicate possible drug or alcohol abuse, including a family history of substance abuse, psychiatric disorders, sociopathic abuse or neglect, school problems or failure, association with dysfunctional peer groups, participation in high-risk activities, precocious or unprotected sexual activity, legal problems, and of course any history of substance abuse. Positive responses to any one of the following high-risk indicators should prompt an in-depth substance abuse evaluation:

- Involvement in gangs
- Previous arrests
- Incarceration
- Probation
- Running away from home
- Weapon possession or use
- Multiple sexual partners
- Lack of contraception
- Group sex
- Prostitution or posing for pornography
- Sexual abuse in childhood
- Sexual exploitation or abuse as an adolescent
- Pregnancy
- Sexually transmitted diseases
- HIV infections
- Physical abuse
- Substance abuse
- Suicide attempts
- Self-mutilation, including self-tattooing
- Physical examination

Physical Examination

The physical examination should focus on signs of substance abuse; in particular, attention should be focused on examining the skin for needle tracks. The nasal septum can reveal erythema and/or scabbing secondary to the intense vasoconstriction produced by intranasal cocaine abuse. A neurologic examination can reveal the impairment produced by volatile hydrocarbons. Hints of infectious diseases can also be found in icteric sclera, an enlarged or tender liver, or vaginal discharge. Unusual signs of trauma should also raise the possibility of a substance abuse etiology, especially if the circumstances or explanations do not make sense. A speculum examination is recommended for all female adolescents who are sexually active, have a history of a vaginal discharge or sexually transmitted disease, or have a history of prior sexual assault.

Laboratory Testing

When adolescent substance abuse is suspected, confirmatory laboratory testing is indicated. This testing includes but is not limited to a routine laboratory testing such as a complete blood count, a comprehensive blood chemistry profile, and a supervised comprehensive urine drug screen using a sensitive analytic technique. It is wise to order HIV testing and rapid plasma reagin as well. All females should have a pregnancy test and be screened for sexually transmitted diseases. Hair analysis is less useful and will reveal only whether drugs were used in the past month or two, not when they were used, how much, or how often. Further evaluation of behavioral abnormalities could be pursued if suspected, including thyroid function testing, an autoimmune evaluation, blood lead evaluation, electroencephalogram, electrocardiogram, and a PPD (purified protein derivative). Obviously any tests indicated for patients with other problems, such as chronic illness, should be pursued

Triage and Referral

Assessment can result in three scenarios: 1) there is no problem, 2) there might be a problem, and 3) there is a substance abuse problem. In the first case, it is acceptable to note the suspicions and follow-up with the adolescent to periodically reassess the situation. If these patients are followed long enough, time will resolve all lingering doubts. The problem will either get better, get worse, or stay the same.

In cases in which there might be a problem, it is important to obtain a second opinion even if the history and physical examination are negative. If the second opinion is still inconclusive and yet the suspicion of drug abuse remains, it is important to follow-up with the teenager over time and to order further confirmatory tests such as a weekly random supervised comprehensive urine drug screen. Ongoing regular contact with an adolescent substance abuse specialist is also important.

If any of these evaluations is either positive or inconclusive, the experienced clinician should refer the patient to a mental health specialist in adolescent substance abuse for day-to-day management. This is the position with the lowest risk. Physicians must avoid the idea that they can handle the problem all by themselves; the fact is that physicians do not have the time, ability, or skepticism necessary to treat these patients.

Medical Treatment of Substance-Abusing Adolescents

Despite their fear that they will be prevented from following up with or treating their patients, primary care and specialist physicians have an important role to play in the medical treatment of substance-abusing teenagers. They must to work in concert with an adolescent substance abuse specialist and provide long-term care after the initial phases of substance abuse treatment have been successfully accomplished. Physicians must be careful to always maintain a high index of suspicion and to question information that does not make sense. Most importantly, they must make a prominent note about the substance abuse disorders in the adolescents' charts to avoid prescribing potentially addicting medications. It is hoped that adolescents will automatically remind physicians about their substance abuse disorders and remind them not to prescribe an addicting substance; this does occur, but infrequently.

No Addicting Medications

Avoiding abusable medications is especially important if the teenager requests a controlled substance. If it is necessary to use a scheduled medication, consultation with an addiction medicine specialist or addiction psychiatrist is mandatory. These conversations should be prominently noted in the patient's chart before the medication is prescribed.

When such medications are prescribed, it should be under extremely carefully controlled circumstances and for a very limited time. For example, opiates can be used for pain relief in trauma or postoperatively but only for a few days and only when someone is administering the medication. These limitations should also be carefully described in the patients' records.

Communication

All specialists treating substance-abusing adolescents should maintain frequent communication with a specialist in adolescent addictions and with the individual patient's family to promote trust and understanding of what is being done and why treatment is occurring in such a manner. This communication helps avoid the many possible mistakes that can be made when treating these adolescents while maximizing their comfort and optimizing their medical treatment. Establishing communication also helps ensure that the adolescent is referred back when further medical care is necessary.

Summary

This chapter describes the basic role of physicians who are in contact with substance-abusing adolescents. Unless they have specialized training in substance abuse or psychiatry, physicians treating these patients should limit their actions primarily to identification and appropriate referral.

When adolescent substance abuse is suspected, confirmatory history, physical examination, and laboratory testing are indicated. If these investigations are inconclusive, a second opinion is indicated. If the second opinion is still inconclusive but the suspicion of drug abuse remains, it is important to follow the teenager over time and to order a weekly random supervised comprehensive urine drug screen.

If adolescent substance abuse is diagnosed, transfer to day-to-day management is strongly suggested. After diagnosis it is critical to avoid the prescription of abusable medications. The only exception to this rule is in specially circumscribed situations such as postoperatively or after trauma.

Primary care and specialist physicians have an important role to play in the medical treatment of substance-abusing adolescents. This is best accomplished by working in concert with the adolescent substance abuse treatment team and having as an ultimate goal the comprehensive care of the substance-abusing patient.

References

American Academy of Pediatrics: Substance Abuse: A Guide for Health Professionals. Elk Grove, IL, American Academy of Pediatrics, 1988

Arria AM, Dohey MA, Mezzich AC, et al: Self-reported health problems and physical symptomatology in adolescent alcohol abusers. J Adolesc Health 16:226–231, 1995

Barnett NP, Spirito A, Colby SM, et al: Detection of alcohol use in adolescent patients in the emergency department. Acad Emerg Med 5:607–612, 1998

Dell ML: Medical considerations in child and adolescent substance abuse. Child Adolesc Psychiatr Clin N Am 1:1–28, 1996

Elias MJ, Kress JS, Gager PJ, et al: Adolescent health promotion and risk reduction: cementing the social contract between pediatricians and the schools. Bull N Y Acad Med 71:87–110, 1994

Faigel HC: Primary care of the adolescent patient. Hosp Pract (Off Ed) 31:127–133, 137–138, 144–148, 1996

Gordon S, Toepper WC, Blackman SC: Toxicology screening in adolescent trauma. Pediatr Emerg Care 12:36–39, 1996

Jenson JM, Howard MO, Yaffe J: Treatment of adolescent substance abusers: issues for practice and research. Soc Work Health Care 21:1–18, 1995

Kokotailo P: Physical health problems associated with adolescent substance abuse, in Adolescent Drug Abuse: Clinical Assessment and Therapeutic Interventions (NIDA Res Monogr 156). Edited by Rahdert E, Czechowicz D. Washington, DC, U.S. Government Printing Office, 1995, pp 112–129

Konings E, Dubois-Arber F, Narring F, et al: Identifying adolescent drug users: results of a national survey on adolescent health in Switzerland. J Adolesc Health 16:240–247, 1995

Loiselle JM, Baker MD, Templeton JM, et al: Substance abuse in adolescent trauma. Ann Emerg Med 22:1530–1534, 1993

Muramoto ML, Leshan L: Adolescent substance abuse: recognition and early intervention. Prim Care 20:141–154, 1993

Parrish SK: Adolescent substance abuse: the challenge for clinicians. Alcohol 11:453–455, 1994

Spain DA, Boaz PW, Davidson DJ, et al: Risk-taking behaviors among adolescent trauma patients. J Trauma 43:423–426, 1997

Werner MJ, Adger H Jr: Early identification, screening, and brief intervention for adolescent alcohol use. Arch Pediatr Adolesc Med 149:1241–1248, 1995

Wilens TE, Biederman J, Abrantes AM, et al: Clinical characteristics of psychiatrically referred adolescent outpatients with substance use disorder. J Am Acad Child Adolesc Psychiatry 36:941–947, 1997

7 Psychiatric and Substance Abuse Evaluation of Adolescents

R. Jeremy A. Stowell, M.D.
Todd Wilk Estroff, M.D.

A basic tenet of modern medicine is that proper diagnosis is necessary before definitive treatment can begin. Symptoms of many psychiatric and substance use disorders are nonspecific and nondiagnostic (Estroff and Gold 1984). The clinical presentation of substance-abusing adolescents usually involves multiple symptoms, behaviors, and social problems, making it more difficult to identify central clinical issues. Because of this clinical complexity, careful evaluation is critical to determine which problems are primary to the initiation and perpetuation of adolescent substance abuse (Winters and Henley 1988a, 1988b). Additionally, substance-abusing adolescents are often dual-diagnosis patients who have at least one psychiatric diagnosis and also abuse multiple substances (Stowell 1991). Therefore, in the evaluation of adolescent substance abuse, it is critical to simultaneously evaluate both the substance abuse and psychiatric disorders.

No validated diagnostic system is specific for adolescent substance abuse and dependence. Applying the DSM-IV (American Psychiatric Association 1994) criteria for substance use disorders to adolescents may not be as useful as it is for adults (Stowell 1996). This is especially true for a subgroup of substance-abusing adolescents who have been called "diagnostic orphans": They may not meet the current criteria for dependence or abuse, but they have substantial alcohol and drug abuse problems (Pollock And Martin 1999). Lewinsohn et al. (1996) found that 13% of high school students fit this "diagnostic orphan" category.

Certain symptoms of drug abuse can be easily confused with psychiatric symptoms and vice versa. Drug-induced violence or related temper outbursts can easily be confused with and misdiagnosed as an intermittent explosive disorder. Attention-deficit/hyperactivity disorder (ADHD) symptoms can also mimic stimulant abuse or intoxication and withdrawal symptoms of several drugs. It is noteworthy also that only 10% of males with ADHD develop substance use disorders (Rapaport et al. 1993) and that using stimulants to treat adolescents with ADHD does not appear to significantly increase the risk of subsequent adolescent substance abuse problems (Disney et al. 1999). Marijuana-induced amotivational syndrome can imitate a major depressive episode and is often mistaken for major depression when drug testing is either not performed or is performed using insensitive techniques. Drug-induced psychotic disorders can occur with marijuana, cocaine, amphetamine, and hallucinogens. These drugs can also induce behavior that is indistinguishable from other classic psychiatric diagnoses, such as bipolar disorder and schizophrenia. When drug-induced psychiatric symptoms are diagnosed, it is wise for the treating physician to wait and see if the symptoms clear as the drugs are metabolized and excreted. Behavioral control is sometimes necessary, but treatment with psychotropic medications should be used only if absolutely necessary. If an incorrect diagnosis is made and the patient is treated with the wrong medication, his or her drug-induced psychiatric symptoms may be exacerbated (see case examples at the end of this chapter).

Conduct disorders frequently accompany substance use disorders. (Stowell and Estroff 1992). The presence of a conduct disorder appears to increase the risk of substance use and abuse among adolescents regardless of their gender (Disney et al. 1999). Bukstein et al. (1992) found conduct disorder to be the most common diagnosis in a clinical inpatient population of dually diagnosed adolescent substance abusers. In that study, 70.5% of patients met criteria for a conduct disorder. The percentage of males and females with conduct disorder was equal. In this study, a high percentage of adolescents (30.7%) had a comorbid diagnosis of major depression. The major depressive symptoms spontaneously improved in 19% of the males and 48% of the females 3 weeks after cessation of drug use and without medication. The conduct disturbance will also spontaneously subside over time and without medication in many individuals. For these reasons it is important to have the patient detoxified for a sufficient period of time before making any firm psychiatric diagnoses, especially on Axis II.

At the level of social, emotional, and personality development, a lag or arrest may be observed in the substance-abusing adolescent. This can appear as a personality disturbance as the individual's emotional age falls increasingly behind the chronological age. Such individuals often appear extremely immature, childish, demanding, and wanting immediate gratification of all their needs. Their ability to participate in treatment is often severely limited. The age of developmental arrest often is correlated chronologically with the age of onset of severe abuse of alcohol and drugs. If the personality disturbance persists, it tends have a particularly ominous outcome (Kasen et al. 1999).

A thorough and structured approach that evaluates all aspects of the substance-abusing adolescent's presentation is the one most likely to succeed. By identifying all of the problems to be addressed and defining their relative importance, decisions about the treatment plan can be made more accurately (Winters and Henley 1988a, 1988b). Excellent guidelines in the diagnostic process for adolescents and their parents have been developed (Young et al. 1990).

Diagnostic problems can result from overcommitment to a particular theoretical framework during the evaluation process. This can result in one disorder, either the substance abuse or the psychiatric problem, being minimized while the other disorder is overemphasized. Winters and Henley (1988a) called for better instruments that would increase the objectivity of client assessment, provide meaningful differentiation of the adolescents' stage of chemical involvement, identify different problems that accompany chemical abuse, and assign the adolescents to the appropriate treatment level and modality.

Developmental Issues

When evaluating the substance-abusing adolescent, it is important to note the developmental issues—i.e., biological, psychological, and sociological—

that the adolescent must resolve to successfully reach mature adulthood. Adolescent development is characterized by rapid growth and sexual maturation as well as changes in cognitive development that lead to the ability to think in abstract terms. A shift occurs from dependence on adults (parents in particular) to a strong identification with the peer group. Values and lifestyles are explored. The developmental tasks include

1. Adapting to physical growth and hormonal changes
2. Separating and individuating from parents
3. Attaining adult cognitive development and abstraction
4. Developing a sexual identity and achieving aspects of intimacy; developing sexual relationships
5. Developing moral and ethical values
6. Preparing for further educational and vocational goals

Abuse of drugs on a regular basis may produce a delay, disruption, or even arrest of these developmental tasks in adolescents. This developmental perspective is critical in the overall evaluation of the substance-abusing adolescent.

Outpatient Evaluation

The first and one of the most difficult decisions of the outpatient evaluation is whether the evaluation can continue in an outpatient setting or whether the severity of clinical problems requires inpatient or partial hospitalization. A screening clinical interview with the parents and the adolescent is needed to answer this basic question. Potential patients are usually identified by their parents, school, or legal system as possibly having a substance abuse problem. They are then referred for an initial evaluation that usually occurs in an outpatient setting. The evaluator is then charged with making an assessment of the extent and severity of the substance use and the potential psychiatric diagnoses and making appropriate treatment recommendations. To make the initial treatment placement decision, the question must be answered: Is there a drug abuse problem, and how severe is it? Sometimes the problem is minor. The patient has become intoxicated as a result of experimentation or is abusing substances as a way of dealing with emotional or social stress. Referral for substance abuse education can be useful in the experimental drug-use phase. Psychotherapy or counseling for the individual and family can be useful for adolescents who abuse substances to deal with their internal stresses. In more severe cases in which a definitive substance use disorder exists, intensive treatment is indicated. The treatment decision then becomes whether to continue the evaluation on an outpatient basis or to refer to a more intensive level of treatment. The least restrictive and most appropriate level of care is the one to recommend initially. We have found it useful to have criteria that can be clearly conveyed to the patient, the parents, and the third-party payor. The reasoning behind the decision can be especially clear if the American Society of Addiction Medicine (ASAM) criteria are used.

The Cleveland Criteria was the first multilevel criteria set for assigning adolescents to treatment. It was developed for treatment providers in Ohio (Hoffmann et al. 1987). These initial criteria formed the foundation for a special task force of both the ASAM and the National Association of Addiction Treatment Providers (NAATP). The combined criteria produced from these efforts resulted in the initial ASAM Patient Placement Criteria (Hoffmann et al. 1991). Subsequently, ASAM revised these criteria to develop the ASAM Patient Placement Criteria 2 (American Society of Addiction Medicine 1996).

Interview with the Parents

As part of the evaluation, the parents of the adolescent are interviewed. They can provide important information about the adolescent's premorbid functioning and personality as well as behavioral issues. They can best address symptoms of preexisting psychiatric disorders. Structured data collection in the following areas is essential:

1. Developmental history
2. Medical history
3. Social and educational history
4. Substance use history
5. Family history, including parental use of substances and extended family data on substance use and psychiatric disorders
6. Emotional, physical, and sexual abuse

Parents may be able to provide some limited information about which drugs are being abused by their adolescent. They may have found drug paraphernalia or other signs of drug use. However, parents are usually unable to give information about specific drugs and the amounts used. This is partly because adolescent drug abuse is a covert illness based on denial and lies and partly because the drugs sold to adolescents may actually be different from what they thought they were purchasing. It is also possible that the drug they have purchased has been "cut" with other unidentified psychoactive substances.

It is useful to question the parents about behavioral symptoms such as violence, temper tantrums, oppositional behavior, severe mood swings, psychotic symptoms, suicidal statements, suicidal behavior, and possible suicide attempts. When an interview with the parents discloses imminent danger to the adolescent or others, inpatient treatment must be strongly considered.

A sensitive area of exploration is the matter of the parents' personal substance abuse and their own possible need for treatment. This can be such a delicate matter and the parental denial can be so powerful that the parents become frightened and pull both the adolescent and themselves out of the evaluation and treatment process. It sometimes may be necessary to delay obtaining complete information until the adolescent is engaged in treatment and the parents are under less stress. The importance of understanding whether there has been alcohol and drug abuse in the family is underscored by findings that families in which a parent is alcoholic are generally less successful in establishing a well-planned, stable, and meaningful family life style than are families where neither parent is abusing alcohol or other drugs. The lack of a healthy family environment is reflected in significantly greater problems in the adolescent's cognitive and emotional spheres (Bennett et al. 1988).

When interviewing the parents, the clinician must be sensitive to certain information that may signal a substance abuse problem in the adolescent. Behavioral manifestations can include poor grades, delinquent behavior, having few friends or a change in friends, having overt aggression toward other siblings or peers, withdrawing from peers, and having somatic symptoms such as stomachaches or headaches.

The substance-abusing adolescent has a number of other signs and symptoms that indicate probable substance abuse problems, including staggering, smelling of alcohol or marijuana, nausea or vomiting, glassy or bloodshot eyes, problems with coordination, speech that is slurred, or notable changes in physical appearance. With depressant drugs such as alcohol, barbiturates, and sedative hypnotics symptoms such as staggering, slurred speech, dilation of pupils, problems with concentration, and falling asleep at inappropriate moments often occur. With marijuana, users may have red eyes, time distortion, a change in appetite, memory impairment (especially recent), chronic coughing, chest pain, fatigue, sleep disturbance, menstrual irregularities, diminished hygiene, and a general decline of performance in most areas. Stimulant abuse such as cocaine and amphetamine abuse often presents as an excessively active adolescent who may be overexcited, euphoric, hyperverbal, argumentative, or paranoid. On a physical level these drugs can cause pupillary dilatation, decreased appetite, and increased blood pressure and pulse rate.

Hallucinogens such as lysergic acid diethylamide (LSD) and phencyclidine hydrochloride (PCP) can cause an increase in blood pressure and heart rate as well as irregular breathing, sweating, and tremulousness of the hands. There may be notable changes in hearing, touching, smelling, tasting, and vision. Inhalants can produce physical changes such as the odor of the inhalant, nasal secretion, watering of the eyes, difficulties with balance, sedation, slurred speech, and altered cognitive perceptions and abilities.

Marked behavioral changes also usually occur in the chemically abusive adolescent including disruptive behaviors such as refusal to follow rules and guidelines, disciplinary problems in school, outbursts of abusive language, irresponsibility in relationships and home and school areas, fighting, negative attention seeking, and an increase in negative mood states such as anger and depression. These adolescents usually change from a family orientation to an orientation toward drug-using peers, and they are much more secretive and dishonest.

It is important to explore the parents' own history of psychiatric disorders and treatment and to determine if they have any current psychiatric problems or treatment needs. The extended family history should determine whether familial alcoholism, drug abuse, or psychiatric disorders exist that could predispose the adolescent to substance abuse and/or psychiatric disturbances. Other questions during the family interview should address the adolescent's legal problems, including arrests, convictions, and probation status. This information may provide potent sources of leverage that can be useful in keeping substance-abusing adolescents in treatment, especially if they are resistant. It is also useful to ask the parents if they have told their adolescent that he or she may not live at home unless he or she accepts treatment and complies with specific rules and guidelines. Such strong family support of the treatment program, the staff, and the primary clinicians makes a successful outcome more likely (Peircy and Frankel 1989).

Interview with the Adolescent

In the adolescent diagnostic interview it is important to try to establish some rapport and to initiate a relationship. It is useful to allow part of this interview to be unstructured to enable the adolescent to express personal concerns or issues. This should be followed by a review of the important areas of the adolescent's life, and then the interview should turn to more specific areas of concern such as substance abuse.

Specific material should be obtained about each family member—the relationship of the adolescent to each parent, stepparent, sibling, and any other person living in the home. Information should be gathered about the adolescent's friends and athletic, social, and leisure activities. Problem behaviors such as stealing, running away, and any contact with the courts should be explored. Information should also be gathered about the emotional life of the adolescent, including feelings that can figure prominently in the present illness such as anger, depression, anxiety, and other painful emotions. It is important to obtain data about physical, emotional, or sexual abuse. Developmental areas need to be traced carefully, including the physical, emotional, cognitive, and sexual development of the adolescent. Details of any counseling or psychotherapy, including any efforts at substance abuse treatment, should be obtained, and the adolescent should be asked to share his or her perceptions of these experiences. Evaluation of peer associations and influences deserves special attention because a strong relationship exists between ongoing alcohol abuse and association with peers who use alcohol (Oetting et al. 1989).

This phase of the interview is followed by a psychiatric and mental status examination and the taking of the adolescent's substance use history. There are various formal instruments for this type of evaluation currently in use; these are reviewed in Chapter 6.

Each clinician and substance abuse program should have a systematic way of approaching substance use disorders in adolescents. If the patient is forthcoming about the substance abuse, it is important to determine the particular drugs of choice and place the substance abuse problem into a coherent program of recovery (see case examples at the end of this chapter).

Disclosing to the parents what the adolescent has said about his or her substance use can present problems of confidentiality. There are various approaches. We have found it best to help adolescents tell their parents about their personal substance use. Occasionally, life-threatening conditions require informing parents and breaking confidentiality. Even then, the adolescent should be given the choice of telling the parents before the clinician does this independently. Other disclosures of privileged clinical material should be made only if the adolescent is aware and agrees to it. Documentation of the adolescent's consent should be prominently noted and maintained in his or her chart. Confirmation of what the adolescent has stated needs to be corroborated by other sources of information, including but not limited to his or her parents, school, friends, other relatives, and the legal system.

Spiritual Evaluation of the Patient and Family

Spiritual evaluation can be one of the most important aspects of the evaluation and subsequent treatment at any level of care. Although there appears to be no exact methodology for the spiritual evaluation in peer-reviewed literature, we recommend inquiry into the adolescents' and families' beliefs in a higher power or the god of their understanding. It is useful to obtain details of their beliefs, attitudes, experiences, and current practices in the religious and/or spiritual areas. It is also necessary to determine whether the adolescent and family are willing to involve themselves in the spiritual dimension of recovery work (e.g., 12-step program). During the spiritual evaluation it is useful to bear in mind the degree to which the family and adolescent may have been harmed by years of psychological pain and dysfunction.

Look for Leverage

Because adolescents who are abusing substances are often not motivated toward treatment, it is important to find as many possible routes for producing leverage as possible. Through direct questioning it is possible to find out whether the parents are going to stand firmly behind the evaluation process or will enable the adolescent to sabotage treatment. Parents may tell their adolescent that he or she must participate in the evaluation and treatment or significant consequences will occur. Some parents have told their adolescent that if he or she resists treatment, he or she will have to live in an alternative setting. Parents can sometimes turn to the juvenile court or family court system for help with resistant adolescents. It is useful in the interview to look for possible motivators such as severely painful emotions (i.e., suicidal feelings), school failure, a bad LSD trip, social ostracism, and parental and peer support. Being able to live at home or to use a vehicle may be important motivators for adolescents to participate in their own recovery. Several other motivators for the recovery process exist, including the therapeutic rapport between the therapist and adolescent as well as treatment approaches employed to help adolescents in the recovery process. For example, Kaminer et al. (1992) found that inpatient substance-abusing adolescents who completed treatment placed a high value on individual treatment contracting, therapeutic community meeting, and educational counseling.

The drug involvement may have become so severe that the patient has resorted to selling drugs, stealing, or prostitution. Income from these sources may not be sufficient to cover the expenses of a heavy drug habit, and these patients may owe significant amounts of money to other drug suppliers. Sometimes one of the reasons that an adolescent agrees to enter the evaluation and treatment process is because of threats from drug dealers or unhappy customers. These threats can also be a powerful motivator for the initiation and continuance of the recovery process. When the choice is between going to jail and getting treatment, most substance-abusing adolescents choose treatment. A judicial order can be another incentive for the adolescent to comply with treatment; under certain circumstances in which the adolescent may be in danger of self-harm or harm to others or is not cooperative with treatment, a judge may order him or her to complete treatment as a hospital inpatient or, if still uncooperative, to a detention facility.

Physical Examination

After the interview process is complete, a physical examination by a physician is the next step in the diagnostic work up. This examination can help identify potentially severe medical complications due to substance abuse. Further details of the physical examination are addressed in Chapter 6.

One of the questions that remains controversial is whether to test the substance-abusing adolescent for HIV/AIDS during the evaluation. A number of physicians feel that only individuals who are intravenous drug users or who are active sexually should be tested for this disease. As is emphasized in this chapter and throughout this book, substance abuse is a disease marked by denial and deceit. Therefore, it is best not to fully trust the substance abuser's denials of intravenous drug abuse or sexual activity. It is recommended that most substance-abusing adolescents be tested for both hepatitis B exposure and HIV/AIDS. It should be pointed out that many of the previously described behavioral symptoms may also be the first sign of AIDS encephalopathy.

Laboratory Testing

A complete blood count, rapid plasma reagin test, hepatitis B profile, and blood chemistry may be necessary in the course of outpatient evaluation. All females should be tested for pregnancy. Supervised urine drug screens should be performed. AIDS testing may also be advisable; if done, informed consent must be obtained from and an appropriate explanation given to the adolescent and his or her parents.

The Imaginary Urine Test

Occasionally it is not necessary to perform a urine drug screen on the adolescent. Sometimes the mere suggestion that the physician is going to request a supervised urine test is enough to produce a strongly negative response from the patient. This particular response is highly suggestive that the patient is abusing drugs. If the patient continues to refuse urine testing, it is reasonable to speculate, to the parents and the adolescent, that drug abuse is indeed occurring.

The Actual Urine Test

An important step in the evaluation of the substance-abusing adolescent is to order a supervised urine specimen, which is tested using precise assay techniques. The particular technique used for the analysis can be of great importance. Significant advances have been made during the past 10–20 years in the testing of urine samples for drugs of abuse. Immunoassay techniques (enzyme immunoassay, radioimmunoassay, enzyme-linked immunosorbent assay) use a sensitive cutoff point such as 300 ng/mL for many drugs. Cannabinoids are usually detected at a 20 ng/mL cutoff using this technique. Gas chromatography/mass spectrometry (GC/MS) cutoff levels are usually lower. These are approximately 100 ng/mL for most drugs, whereas it is even more sensitive for cocaine at 50 ng/mL and for cannabinoids at 10 ng/mL. Drug detection after last use is usually in the range of 1–3 days, but with marijuana, it can be anywhere from 2 to 40 days depending on the severity and chronicity.

Urine collection must be accomplished with direct observation of the adolescent patient (Dackis et al. 1982). Observers must actually see the urine emerging out of the patient's body. Modesty and deference to the patient's wishes must be secondary to making certain that the liquid obtained is actually urine and not apple juice, tap water, or someone else's urine. Other ways to confirm the integrity of the specimen are to measure the specific gravity of the urine and/or to measure the urine temperature immediately and compare it to the core body temperature (Ehrenkranz J, personal communication, 1987).

Urine testing may provide additional useful information. For instance, the adolescent may be telling the truth about which drugs he or she thinks he or she has purchased and abused, but other substances may appear in the urine as well. A good example of this is PCP, which is often added to weak marijuana preparations to make them seem more powerful.

Some other drugs are not picked up by urine test because either they are not commonly abused or they are active in such small quantities that they are difficult to assay. LSD is not readily detectable in the urine but can be identified in blood samples. This is also true for anabolic steroids. Certain sedative hypnotics that were abused more frequently in the past, such as glutethimide (Doriden), ethchlorvynol (Placidyl), and meprobamate (Miltown), may be detected using urine drug screens but are more easily picked up in serum samples if these samples are ordered.

Inhalants are also not picked up in the urine drug screen because they are principally excreted by the lungs. Inhalant abuse is usually diagnosed by the patient's own history. Broken vials of amyl nitrate, empty tubes of glue, and bottles of solvents or paint are physical evidence of inhalant abuse. Similarly, observing a youngster obtaining Freon from an air conditioner can confirm this diagnosis. A blood test for inhalants does exist, but it is uncommonly used and must be specifically ordered when inhalant abuse is suspected.

Contracting for Outpatient Treatment

If it is decided that outpatient work is the appropriate level of care, it is useful to suggest to the parent and adolescent that a written contract be drawn up and signed. Elements of the contract should include

- Total abstinence from any alcohol or mind-altering drugs
- Supervised urine drug screening once or twice per week on an unannounced basis
- Attendance and active participation at the outpatient treatment sessions for both individual and family therapy unless there is an emergency
- Attendance at 12-step recovery meetings (Alcoholics Anonymous, Narcotics Anonymous, Cocaine Anonymous) at a frequency recommended by the clinician
- Setting of a curfew and other reasonable guidelines agreed to by the adolescent and parent in the evaluation

The patient and parents agree to immediate intervention, increased frequency of treatment, or hospital-based treatment if any of the above conditions are not complied with or if drugs are detected in a urine test. (Please see case examples at the end of this chapter.)

Limits of Outpatient Evaluation

There can be significant limitations in the outpatient evaluation and treatment of substance-abusing adolescents. Problems can arise when the parents and adolescent are told in a summation diagnostic conference that adolescent substance abuse has been diagnosed. A strong negative reaction can occur when either the parent or the patient refuses to deal with the substance abuse diagnosis. Fear and anger may exacerbate the clinical situation and the adolescent may act out with further substance abuse. The parents may persist in their denial and resistance to treatment. As outlined previously, if the guidelines for the contract cannot be complied with, then outpatient treatment is unlikely to work and a partial hospital program or inpatient treatment must be considered. Many parents and patients are not ready to accept a more restrictive recommendation. If the risks of *not* following through with the contract are carefully explained, then the more restrictive intervention often becomes acceptable. Sometimes a second opinion consultation is useful along with the recommendation that they return after this has occurred.

It should be emphasized again that among substance-abusing adolescents, no evaluation is complete unless the patient has been reexamined for associated psychiatric disorders in a fully detoxified and drug-free state. Ideally, this psychiatric evaluation will be performed by a psychiatrist who specializes in treating children and adolescents and who is knowledgeable in addiction medicine.

Guidelines for Selecting Day Hospital or Inpatient Treatment

Day Treatment

Day treatment should be considered when the risk of relapse is severe and/or there is a treatment failure at a less intensive level of care. This level of treatment also should be considered when family pathology exists, including physical, emotional, or sexual abuse, that precludes safe treatment on an outpatient level of care and/or prevents recovery. Many times, for other reasons, the parents or legal guardians are unable to provide the consistency or participation necessary to support a less intensive level of care. In such cases residential placement should be considered.

Other criteria for the day hospital program may include 1) need for non-intensive medical monitoring, 2) suicidal ideation but no plan, 3) moderate emotional lability and poor impulse control, 4) moderate to severe educational and social deterioration, 5) moderate to severe denial and minimization of the substance abuse problem, and 6) inability to stay drug and alcohol abstinent without daily intensive treatment and moderate risk of withdrawal. Most adolescent inpatient hospital admission criteria include the risk of a withdrawal syndrome, extreme depression with suicidal risk, violence, and/or homicidal risk. At the neuropsychiatric level, severe confusion, delirium, coma, hallucinations, toxic psychosis, extreme emotionality, volatility, and a history of recent seizures will justify an admission. Inpatient treatment should also be considered if there are conditions and complications of addiction requiring medical management or if the patient is in immediate danger of self-harm.

Suicide

Suicide in a substance-abusing adolescent is a distinct possibility, especially if the patient has a history of suicide attempts. It is important to understand that a suicide attempt among substance-abusing adolescents is much more likely to result in death than it would for adolescents with a purely psychiatric disorder such as depression or mania (Fowler et al. 1986; Kaminer 1992). Loss of control over drug use is often a precipitant for a suicide attempt (Crumley 1979). Therefore we recommend careful evaluation of suicide risk in this population and use of the day hospital or inpatient treatment when indicated.

Possible Withdrawal

Many physicians believe that adolescents will not have a significant withdrawal syndrome. Although this may be true of most, a small number of adolescents exhibit full withdrawal syndromes from alcohol, opiates, or sedative hypnotics. If a withdrawal syndrome is likely, inpatient treatment is advisable at least until the danger of withdrawal complications has passed.

Other Conditions

There are times when adolescents exhibit acute psychotic symptoms secondary to drug abuse. These adolescents need to be in the hospital. Hospitalization is also strongly indicated if there is active family alcoholism or drug use or if the environment is dangerous to the adolescent. In the event that inpatient treatment is selected, the adolescent and his or her parents should be given a detailed explanation about plans for further evaluation, stabilization, and treatment. Even after the parents agree to hospitalization, significant problems may occur. Many times the adolescent is resistant to treatment. One or both parents and the clinician may be needed to help convince the patient to enter the hospital. In more extreme cases, parents may be forced to consider obtaining a court order for the safety and welfare of their teenager. In such a case, it is important to remember that strong measures to achieve hospitalization may be lifesaving.

Inpatient Evaluation

Inpatient evaluation must also be accomplished in a comprehensive and systematic manner. Evaluation at this level of care should provide the most complete diagnostic profile possible. Although much information may have already been gathered from the parents during the initial outpatient evaluation, it is important to review all of the data again in detail. Many times, under the stress of the initial evaluation the parents will leave out clues to the substance abuse or gloss over significant facts. A careful, systematic medical and psychiatric review may turn up psychiatric symptoms that preceded the substance abuse.

School

Information from the adolescent's school can be useful in pointing out behavioral disturbances, unexplained absences, and declines in the patient's grades. Often the grades may decline so profoundly that they are placed in special classes for emotionally handicapped or for learning disabled students. Sometimes these changes in the student's behavior are incorrectly assessed by the school system as a specific learning disability. Adolescents sometimes use drugs to self-medicate painful feelings about their ADHD or learning disabilities. School-based treatment teams need to address both the educational and substance abuse issues.

Inpatient Urine Testing

Inpatient urine testing is usually performed by the same laboratories that do the outpatient urine testing. The first void in the morning is more apt to be concentrated and more likely to produce a positive result. Inpatient urine drug samples are more easily obtained than outpatient samples. Urine drug screens should be obtained routinely on all adolescents entering inpatient treatment and should also be obtained after therapeutic passes. During the actual hospitalization, if an adolescent's behavior or mood changes without known reasons, it is important to again test the urine for drugs of abuse brought into the hospital.

Environmental Control

When an adolescent is hospitalized, environmental controls prevent drugs from flowing into the hospital and getting into the hands of the patient. These controls also prevent the patient from leaving the hospital to obtain drugs (Gold and Estroff 1985). However, drugs can flow into an open or closed hospital through various means, and it is important to place the patient in a locked inpatient unit with limited visitors. No visitor should be allowed to visit the patient unsupervised if the patient is a substance abuser. All packages and mail that arrive at the hospital for the patient must be inspected. United States mail may not be opened by hospital staff before it is received by the patient, but staff may observe the patient opening any mail and inspect all contents for drugs. There should be a high index of suspicion for packages and envelopes that arrive on the unit but are not part of the mail.

Environmental control is important in the maintenance of behavioral control when resistant patients exhibit dangerous and/or disruptive behaviors and need added structure. It is recommended that a behavioral modification system using positive reinforcement as well as a point system be instituted. This should be accompanied by the possibility of a progression through a series of privileges and responsibilities. On some units there may be a level system, starting with an orientation or entry level and progressing to more advanced levels. This progress reflects treatment compliance and gains.

How Long After Detoxification Should a Psychiatric Diagnosis Be Made?

One of the many questions that arise in the treatment of substance-abusing adolescents is how long after detoxification the treating physician should wait before making a psychiatric diagnosis. A psychiatric disorder is usually present if 1) psychiatric symptoms persist after detoxification, 2) clear psychiatric symptoms preceded the substance abuse, 3) severe psychiatric symptoms exist beyond what would normally be expected, or 4) there is a strong family history of certain psychiatric disorders in first-degree relatives. It is clear that many individuals have a highly fluctuating course of psychiatric symptoms. Some individuals may enter treatment severely depressed but eventually develop manic symptoms when fully detoxified. Similarly, other individuals who have presented with normal affect or even hypomanic symptoms can become significantly depressed after detoxification (see case examples at the end of this chapter).

Making a psychiatric diagnosis depends mainly on the point of view of the treating physician and his or her understanding of psychiatric disorders. We believe that in the detoxification phase it is a mistake to make more than a provisional psychiatric diagnosis. In certain instances, adolescents may require even longer periods of detoxification; cannabinoid metabolites are released from fat stores for up to 4 weeks after detoxification starts (Dackis et al. 1982). Certain psychiatric diagnoses such as depression often persist after detoxification. For instance, Deykin et al. (1992) showed that depressive illness among chemically dependent adolescents is about three times greater than among adolescents not referred for medical treatment. Unlike some psychiatrists who insist on waiting months before diagnosing an affective disorder, we believe that this lengthy wait may lead to needless suffering for the patient. Untreated depression can contribute to relapse if the appropriate treatment is postponed.

Above all, clinical judgment is paramount in deciding when to institute psychotropic medications for the treatment of psychiatric disorders. Severe or persistent symptoms may force the treating physician's hand earlier in the course of treatment. However, more subtle and variable symptoms may lead to longer periods of observation to ensure that the diagnosis and proposed treatment are correct. It is always useful when there is diagnostic uncertainty to go to other data sources to assist in determining the timing and order of appearance of psychiatric and substance abuse symptoms.

A strong family history of affective disorder, including major depression and bipolar disorders, can provide powerful clues to the diagnosis and treatment of these disorders among substance-abusing adolescents. Psychiatric symptoms may remit spontaneously when they have developed after substance abuse has started (Lewis et al. 1982). However, psychiatric symptoms may persist long after the cessation of drug and alcohol abuse. Strong evidence argues for the simultaneous evaluation of both substance use and psychiatric disorders in this type of adolescent population (Stowell and Estroff 1992).

Conclusion

A thorough and structured approach is required in the evaluation of substance-abusing adolescents. Multiple comorbid psychiatric and/or medical disorders usually exist in both the adolescent and his or her family members. Determining the appropriate level of care for the substance-abusing adolescent is part of the evaluation process, and each practitioner needs to be aware of the clinical criteria for each level of care. The details of the evaluation process outlined in this chapter form the basis for treatment recommendations.

Case Examples

Case 1

Patient A was a 17-year-old white male in the eleventh grade. He had had behavior problems since kindergarten and was diagnosed as hyperactive while in the fourth grade. He was being reevaluated in the eleventh grade because he was depressed and had become increasingly withdrawn, sad, and tired. He exhibited decreased motivation and his grades were so poor that he had failed his freshman year in high school and had to go to summer school for both the tenth and eleventh grades. He was also having increased temper outbursts and was becoming increasingly irritable. He adamantly denied taking any drugs.

The patient started counseling 1 year prior to being seen by the addictions professional. Four months prior to being seen, he was identified in school as a possible drug abuser and forced to submit to a urine test, the results of which were positive for marijuana. The school pressed charges, and the patient was mandated to go to an adolescent outpatient drug program for evaluation. While in this program, he admitted to abuse of cocaine in addition to marijuana. His treatment in the program failed, and he was sent to an adolescent residential treatment center. He was not seen by a psychiatrist until he attempted to hang himself. The pressure of the program had caused him to reveal, under intense peer pressure, that he had been homosexually raped by an older boy when he was 7 or 8 years old.

After his attempted suicide, the patient was seen by a psychiatrist who recommended immediate discharge from the residential program. The patient returned to the outpatient program in which he had previously failed treatment. He was again pushed beyond his limits and became violent, which led to a complete diagnostic reevaluation.

At the time of his presentation, the patient was attending Alcoholics Anonymous meetings daily, but he suffered prominent symptoms of guilt, loneliness, boredom, decreased sleep, and depression. He was neither suicidal nor homicidal. He admitted to having used cocaine (up to 1 gram a day on a regular basis), crack, marijuana, PCP, mescaline, hashish, stimulants, quaaludes, LSD, and mushrooms. He denied using heroin.

Initial diagnosis was

- Axis Ia, Major Depression
- Axis Ib, Conduct Disorder
- Axis Ic, Attention-Deficit/Hyperactivity Disorder
- Axis Id, Polysubstance Abuse and Dependence (alcohol, cocaine, marijuana)

- Axis Ie, Posttraumatic Stress Disorder (secondary to being a victim of sexual abuse at age 7–8 years)
- Axis II, Oppositional Traits
- Axis III, Rule Out Partial Complex Seizures

The patient was encouraged to continue attending Alcoholics Anonymous groups. He also had weekly supervised urine testing and psychotherapy. Antidepressants were prescribed to treat his depressive symptoms, which persisted despite the fact that he had been abstinent for several months. A computed tomography scan and 24-hour electroencephalogram were negative.

The patient responded well to gentle but firm encouragement in Alcoholics Anonymous meetings as well as in his own individual psychotherapy. Family sessions were helpful in allowing him to ventilate his feelings and develop a closer relationship with his family members.

Comment

Clearly, this patient would never have responded to treatment in either a pure psychiatric setting or a pure substance abuse setting. It was only by addressing simultaneously both his substance abuse and his psychiatric problems that this patient was able to make a prolonged sustained recovery.

Case 2

Patient B was a 14-year-old white male in the eighth grade. He presented with the chief complaints of trouble sleeping and depression. The patient had been an ideal child until the previous year, when his mother noted a gross personality change. Symptoms gradually worsened over a 6-month period until everyone around him noted that he was depressed. He had difficulty falling asleep because thoughts kept running through his head; he would not fall asleep until 2 A.M. and would awaken by 7:30 A.M. He was tired all the time; had no energy; felt depressed most of the time; was sad and blue; felt helpless, hopeless, worthless, and bored; and experienced no pleasure out of life. He did not participate in any hobbies, stayed away from his friends, and was increasingly isolated. His sex drive, while not disappearing totally, had markedly decreased. He wanted many times to disappear, and he had some suicidal ideation but no concrete plans.

He had temper outbursts and was increasingly irritable. He would punch walls in his room, bang his head against boards, and constantly argue with family and friends. He could not remember what he had read from newspaper articles or books. His appetite was voracious—he could eat three "Big Macs," french fries, and a milkshake and state that he was hungry 1 hour later. He denied any history of substance use or abuse.

His evaluation by an experienced child psychiatrist revealed a DSM-IV diagnosis of

- Axis I, Major Depressive Episode
- Axis II, No Diagnosis
- Axis III, No Diagnosis

A urine test was not obtained. He was started immediately on antidepressant medication and weekly psychotherapy. The patient showed a dramatic response in his depressive symptoms, to the point of almost total recovery. He then reached a plateau from which he did not improve. Most notable of all was his continued academic failure, even after 1 year of antidepressant therapy. He was successfully tapered off the medication and did not become depressed. After 3 years of treatment, he was arrested for alcohol intoxication and was later discovered to be smoking marijuana in school. He was later arrested in a drug raid for possession of cocaine and marijuana.

Comment

The treating psychiatrist totally missed the diagnosis of substance abuse. Major errors were made in not checking the patient's urine on initial evaluation and on a regular basis when the patient did not continue to improve. Treatment of the psychiatric disorder alone was not sufficient and led to the patient's continued abuse of drugs and alcohol and his relapse.

Case 3

Patient C was a 15-year-old white female in the tenth grade. She was brought to psychiatric attention for possible substance abuse after she got into a fight with her mother that had resulted in the police being called. Her grades had been poor to failing, and she was going to repeat algebra in summer school. The patient was reported as having increasing irritability, including fighting with her mother over curfew restrictions and her ability to date older boys. There were no signs of depression or psychosis. Her psychiatric history was negative. Her parents were afraid that she was abusing drugs. Mental status examination was within normal limits. Initial diagnostic impression was

- Axis Ia, Possible Polysubstance Abuse
- Axis Ib, Parent–Child Problem
- Axis II, No Diagnosis
- Axis III, Rule Out Partial Complex Seizures

The patient was given a complete diagnostic workup including a urine drug screen; the results of these tests were negative. She was started in weekly individual and family psychotherapy and observed for signs of depression and drug abuse, none of which appeared. The patient made significant progress and was released from treatment after 6 months. She was greatly improved. Her urine drug screens were consistently negative throughout the course of treatment and her parents felt that she was more open and honest with them.

Comment

This is obviously one of the most difficult cases to diagnose and treat, one in which substance abuse is suspected and yet cannot be confirmed. In cases such as these the judicious course is to assume that the possibility exists and to observe the patient over a period of time. In this case, 6 months was chosen as the observation period. When no signs of drug abuse were found during and at the end of this period, the diagnosis was dropped. The patient was released from treatment with the proviso that if things deteriorated again, she would be brought back for reevaluation and treatment.

Case 4

Patient D was a 14-year-old white male who lived with his mother and stepfather. He was repeating the seventh grade for the third time. His behavioral problems included running away, alcohol abuse, possible cannabis abuse, school failure and truancy, fighting, and verbally abusing his school's vice principal. He had been suspended from school and had been told that he could not return to school until he had received treatment.

The patient gave a history of being depressed 60%–75% of the time for almost 1 year. He stated that he did not feel like being around anybody and had decreased interest in pleasurable activities. He had been very irritable and was fighting at school. He denied suicidal and homicidal ideation. He had lost weight, going from 165 pounds to 148 pounds during the previous 2 months, but still stated that he was fat. He had been in psychotherapy for several months without success. The patient would not admit to any drug abuse other than Dexatrim (phenylpropanolamine) daily for at least 3 weeks prior to admission. The mental status examination revealed a nonpsychotic depression. His urine drug screen was negative. The initial diagnostic impression was

- Axis Ia, Rule Out Major Depression
- Axis Ib, Conduct Disorder
- Axis Ic, Rule Out Polysubstance Dependence
- Axis IIa, Mixed Personality Disorder Traits
- Axis IIb, Rule Out Specific Developmental Disorder
- Axis III, No Diagnosis

The patient stuck to his story that he was depressed and did not abuse drugs over the next 3½ weeks of treatment. In the meantime, his mood improved tremendously, so much so that the therapist insisted that something more than simple depression was occurring. As a result of his therapist's pressure, he revealed that he had been smoking marijuana multiple times per day over the past 2 years. He and his therapist considered the marijuana abuse to be a major factor in both his conduct disorder and major depressive symptoms. Following this realization, the patient agreed to be treated for substance abuse disorder. His final DSM-IV diagnosis was

- Axis Ia, Cannabis Dependence
- Axis Ib, Substance (cannabis) Induced Mood Disorder (Depressed)
- Axis II, No Diagnosis
- Axis III, No Diagnosis

Comment

This patient was a particularly difficult and resistant patient who initially would not admit his substance abuse for reasons that remain unclear. The major factor that was instrumental in making the proper diagnosis was the clinician's understanding of both substance-induced psychiatric symptoms and the behavioral disorders that go along with them.

As the patient rapidly and steadily became less depressed without any medication, his insistence that he was not abusing any substances became less and less credible. He was confronted with this on a daily basis. After he admitted his marijuana abuse, he stated that he never would have revealed the true nature of his disorder unless there had been constant day-in and day-out pressure on him to tell the truth. It is unusual to find a patient who can hold out for this length of time. The usual period of denial in the face of overwhelming evidence to the contrary is 10 days to 2 weeks. This patient was stronger, more resistant, and able to hold out for a longer period of time.

Case 5

Patient E was a 15-year-old white male who had failed the eighth grade and was failing summer school. He had been ordered into psychiatric evaluation by the courts. His mother stated that he had been very depressed, angry, and hostile and had had dramatic mood swings from being calm to screaming and yelling. The patient had reportedly thrown a brick through the window and beat up the mailbox at their house. He often stated that he was stupid and not worth anything. He had a very poor relationship with his father.

His parents first noticed that something was wrong 1 year prior to evaluation, when they started receiving complaints about him from the school system. He was reported to be hyperactive with decreased attention span, inappropriately touching female students, pushing, and talking out of turn. He was treated with weekly psychotherapy for 2–3 months, the results of which were reported to be unhelpful. His behavior continued to deteriorate and became so far out of control that he started striking his parents' truck and boat, saying "I'll just kill myself," and threatening to kill both of his parents.

One year previously a general practitioner had treated the patient with Ritalin (methylphenidate) for presumed hyperactivity. The patient's grades did improve, but he did not like the way the medication made him feel and he threw it away.

Mental status examination revealed a thin, white male. Affect was extremely flat. Mood was depressed and thoughts were within normal limits. Urine drug screening was negative. His electroencephalogram was normal. Initial diagnosis was

- Axis Ia, Rule Out Major Depression
- Axis Ib, Rule Out Attention-Deficit/Hyperactivity Disorder (doubt)
- Axis Ic, Rule Out Polysubstance Dependence or Abuse
- Axis Id, Parent–Child Problem
- Axis Ie, Rule Out Eating Disorder Not Otherwise Specified
- Axis II, No Diagnosis
- Axis III, Rule Out Partial Complex Seizures

The patient's affect brightened somewhat in the hospital, and he was no longer suicidal. As an outpatient he continued to deny any drug abuse until he made an attachment with one of the substance abuse therapists. Approximately 6 weeks into treatment he confessed to daily use of marijuana, frequent use of LSD, and use of copious amounts of alcohol. The focus of his treatment was then shifted to emphasize his substance abuse and how it affected his behavior and mood.

Final diagnosis was

- Axis Ia, Substance (cannabis) Induced Mood Disorder (Depressed)
- Axis Ib, Cannabis Dependence
- Axis Ic, Hallucinogen Abuse (LSD)
- Axis Id, Alcohol Abuse
- Axis II, No Diagnosis
- Axis III, No Diagnosis

While in treatment, the patient did well. His depression remitted spontaneously, and he did not require treatment with medication.

Comment

This patient represents the normal course of events in an adolescent with behavioral disorders who is admitted to the hospital, denies drug abuse initially, and has an initial urine drug screen that does not confirm drug abuse. His experiences also demonstrate that substance abuse and psychiatric disorders can interact with each other to produce nonspecific but highly disturbed behavior. It is important to avoid a rush to diagnosis and medication. The diagnoses usually become more clear over time.

Case 6

Patient F was a 15-year-old white male who had been receiving outpatient psychotherapy with a therapist for 3 years. He was originally brought in for consultation because of oppositional behavior toward his parents and because of declining grades. The therapist treated the patient for the next 3 years without any marked change in his progress. He remained oppositional and defiant at home and at school and continued to have failing grades at school despite having been a straight-A student in the fifth grade. Much confusion surrounded the care and treatment of this patient because the oppositional and defiant behavior was not hostile in nature. It took the form of passive-aggressive behavior and lack of cooperation.

When the therapist finally decided that the patient was not getting better and should be reevaluated, there was much resistance to hospitalization because the patient did not clearly meet the admission criteria for being dangerous to himself, dangerous to others, or having behavior that was out of control. On this basis it was decided that the patient should be seen first on an outpatient visit to determine what was the most appropriate treatment setting for him.

When the patient arrived, it was impossible to complete the interview. He constantly interrupted and contradicted everything his mother tried to say. It was finally necessary to ask the patient to leave the office because of his interruptions and his inability to remain silent while his mother was speaking. She related that she was at her wit's end and could not get her son's cooperation. He was the opposite of his older brother, who was well behaved. It became clear that the patient could not be treated as an outpatient. Inpatient admission was approved due to failure to respond to outpatient therapy for 3 years and the patient's extreme lack of cooperation.

Although calm during his mental status examination it was unusual because this affect which was inappropriate and distant with a constricted range. His mood was slightly depressed, his thought content was decreased in production, and he was somewhat circumstantial and tangential. During a physical examination, when asked if he had a heart murmur, he stated, "my heart is like milk." He elaborated that blood and milk were thicker than water and that was why he had a heart murmur. The next day he admitted that he had been using LSD and marijuana on an every-other-day basis with alcohol for approximately 3 years. His story changed frequently. His medical and neurologic workup was entirely normal.

As the patient remained in treatment and was observed drug-free, he became more clearly psychotic and a clear thought disorder emerged. At that point it was evident that he could not be treated for his substance abuse disorder until the psychosis cleared because he was too fragile to withstand substance abuse treatment. Initial diagnosis was

- Axis Ia, Substance (marijuana, LSD, alcohol) Induced Mood Disorder (Bipolar Psychotic)
- Axis Ib, Cannabis Abuse
- Axis Ic, LSD Abuse
- Axis Id, Alcohol Abuse
- Axis II, Schizoid versus Schizotypal Personality Disorder Traits
- Axis III, No Diagnosis

Comment

There are several features to note in this case. First, the fact that this patient never saw a psychiatrist during 3 years of psychotherapy is somewhat startling, especially in view of his lack of progress. However, his behavior was not out of control, and he was thought to be simply oppositional. An error probably occurred when the therapist failed to arrange for sensitive drug testing. This might have picked up the disorder early on. Second, the decision to hospitalize when it was unclear whether or not the patient should be treated as an inpatient or outpatient was resolved by having an outpatient psychiatric evaluation performed. When it became clear that inpatient hospitalization was indicated because the patient could not and would not cooperate as an outpatient, his admission became much less controversial and hospitalization was justified.

An important part of the diagnostic work up was to observe the patient under drug-free conditions. Although there were early signs of psychosis, the attending psychiatrist did not rush in with antipsychotic medications. As the drugs washed out of the patient's system he became more clearly psychotic, and the diagnostic picture became more clear. It was necessary to treat the patient with antipsychotic medications because his psychosis continued to intensify. The patient became more fragile and unable to withstand any confrontation. It was also clear that the patient was inappropriate for substance abuse treatment *at that time* because he was too disturbed and disruptive and his ego was too weak to withstand the intense confrontation and introspection that frequently occur during such treatment.

When similar patients are stabilized on neuroleptic medication they usually develop enough ego strengths to allow substance abuse treatment to proceed. In this patient's case the patient did not stabilize sufficiently and it was necessary to treat the drug abuse component of his illness in the context of his psychiatric symptoms by emphasizing that the risk of relapse into psychosis was extreme if he ever again used drugs or alcohol. This became a primary component of his therapy along with traditional substance abuse 12-step programs. Additionally, the risk of relapse was emphasized both to the parents and to the therapist treating the patient.

Case 7

Patient G was a 17-year-old female. She had a 2-year-old daughter, and they were both living with the patient's parents. The patient had been previously admitted to the hospital because of a suicide attempt. She had had a 1-month history of mild depression after high school graduation caused by concerns about what she was going to do after graduation. She had become more depressed and had attempted to kill herself by overdosing on medication. The patient was then admitted to a local hospital intensive care unit. A psychiatrist had released her from the hospital because he felt that she was not suicidal and had referred her to a local psychologist who had treated her with psychotherapy for 6 weeks. She was given no medications and did not see a psychiatrist. She reportedly functioned well during this period of time but developed depression with constant suicidal ideation 1 week prior to her current admission. She also related that she had had periods of time during which she did not know her own name or where she was driving on at least six occasions previously.

Her mental status examination and medical and substance abuse work ups were unremarkable. All of her laboratory test results were normal. The initial diagnosis was

- Axis Ia, Major Depressive Disorder
- Axis Ib, Rule Out Panic Disorder
- Axis Ic, Possible Dissociative Disorder
- Axis II, No Diagnosis
- Axis III, Rule Out Partial Complex Seizures

At first, the patient maintained that she had no substance abuse problem except for smoking marijuana once and occasional drinks of alcohol but not to excess. She demonstrated symptoms of severe depression and was started on antidepressants. The patient was initially started on a normal dosage of an antidepressant, but she had a great deal of difficulty tolerating even minimal dosages due to side effects. Her dosage had to be reduced to one-quarter of the normal dosage and was later slowly increased to the normal adult dosage.

After several weeks of treatment, the patient admitted to heavy use of marijuana and ecstasy. She stated that her symptoms had not started until she began using these drugs. As treatment progressed, she admitted to more antisocial abnormal behavior, including ignoring her daughter and going out with friends to do drugs and attend parties. She demonstrated additional pathology in treatment that focused on her overinvolvement with male patients. This was successfully confronted and treated.

The final diagnosis was

- Axis Ia, Polysubstance Abuse (marijuana, alcohol, and ecstasy)
- Axis Ib, Major Depressive Disorder
- Axis II, No Diagnosis
- Axis III, Rule Out Partial Complex Seizures

Comment

In retrospect, it is evident that the patient should have received psychiatric or psychological counseling from the time her pregnancy became known. The fact that she had become pregnant should have raised concern that she was experiencing other problems in addition to early sexual activity, including possible substance abuse. The second point at which she could have been helped was when she made her first suicide attempt. She should not have been released from the hospital intensive care unit without outpatient therapy.

Her antidepressant intolerance is interesting; this is usually found only among patients with panic disorders. Therefore, it is interesting to note that this patient developed panic disorder–like symptoms after she started abusing drugs and that these symptoms became progressively worse. This may indicate a biological vulnerability to panic disorder. The most striking thing about this case is that substance abuse was not initially diagnosed because the patient had initially presented with clear depressive symptoms, had made a suicide attempt, and had produced a negative urine drug screen. It was only after the passage of time and the start of psychotherapy that she admitted that she had used drugs and that the drugs had probably caused most of her symptoms. This case demonstrates that it is very important not to make snap judgments or diagnoses when treating adolescent psychiatric patients because they may be substance abusers denying their illness. It is better to wait and pursue a thorough evaluation as outlined in this book to prevent similar diagnostic errors.

References

American Psychiatric Association: Diagnostic and Statistical Manual of Mental Disorders, 4th Edition. Washington, DC, American Psychiatric Association, 1994

American Society of Addiction Medicine: Patient Placement Criteria for the Treatment of Substance-Related Disorders, Second Edition. Chevy Chase, MD, American Society of Addiction Medicine, 1996

Bennett LA, Wolin SJ, Reiss DA: Cognitive, behavioral, and emotional problems among school age children of alcoholic parents. Am J Psychiatry 145:185–190, 1988

Bukstein OG, Glancy LJ, Kaminer Y: Patterns of affective comorbidity in a clinical population dually diagnosed adolescent substance abusers. J Am Acad Child and Adolescent Psychiatry 31:1041–1045, 1992

Crumley FE: Adolescent suicide attempts. JAMA 241:2404–2407, 1979

Dackis CA, Pottash AL, Annitto W, et al: Persistence of urinary marijuana levels after supervised abstinence. Am J Psychiatry 139:1196–1198, 1982

Deykin EY, Buka SL, Leena BS: Depressive illness among chemically dependent adolescents. Am J Psychiatry 149:1341–1347, 1992

Disney ER, Elkins IJ, McGue M, et al: Effects of ADHD, conduct disorder, and gender on substance use and abuse in adolescence. Am J Psychiatry 156:1515–1521, 1999

Estroff TW, Gold MS: Psychiatric misdiagnosis, in Advances in Psychopharmacology: Predicting and Improving Treatment Response. Edited by Gold MS, Lydiard RB, Carman JS. Boca Raton, FL, CRC Press, 1984, pp 34–66

Fowler RC, Rich CL, Young D, et al: Suicide Study II: substance abuse in young cases. Arch Gen Psychiatry 43:962–965, 1986

Gold MS, Estroff TW: The comprehensive evaluation of cocaine and opiate abusers, in The Handbook of Psychiatric Diagnostic Procedures. Edited by Hall CW, Beresford TP. New York, Spectrum Publications, 1985, pp 213–223

Hoffmann NG, Halikas JA, Mee-Lee D: The Cleveland Admission Discharge and Transfer Criteria. Cleveland, OH, Greater Cleveland Hospital Association, 1987

Hoffmann NG, Halikas JA, Mee-Lee D, et al: Patient Placement Criteria for the Treatment of Psychoactive Substance Use Disorders. Washington, DC, American Society of Addiction Medicine, 1991

Kaminer Y: Psychoactive substance abuse and dependence as a risk factor in adolescent attempted and completed suicide. Am J Addict 1:21–29, 1992

Kaminer Y, Tarter R, Bukstein O, et al: Treatment completers and noncompleters: perceptions of the value of treatment variables. Am J Addict 1:115–120, 1992

Kasen S, Cohen P, Skodol AS, et al: Influence of child and adolescent psychiatric disorders on young adult personality disorders. Am J Psychiatry 155:1529–1535, 1999

Lewinsohn PM, Rohde P, Seeley JR: Alcohol consumption in high school adolescents: frequency of use and dimensional structure of associated problems. Addiction 91:375–390, 1996

Lewis DO, Shanok SS, Pincus JH: A comparison of the neuropsychiatric status of female and male incarcerated delinquents: some evidence of sex and race bias. Journal of the American Academy of Child Psychiatry 21:190–196, 1982

Oetting ER, Swaim RC, Edwards RW, et al: Links from emotional distress to adolescent drug use: a path model. J Consult Clin Psychol 57:227–231, 1989

Peircy FP, Frankel BR: The evolution of an integrative family therapy for substance abusing adolescents. Journal of Family Psychology 3:3–17, 1989

Pollock N, Martin C: Diagnostic orphans: adolescents with alcohol symptoms who do not qualify for DSM-IV abuse or dependence diagnoses. Am J Psychiatry 156:897–901, 1999

Rapaport MH, Tipp JE, Schuckit MA: A comparison of ICD-10 and DSM-III-R criteria for substance abuse and dependence. Am J Drug Alcohol Abuse 19:143–151, 1993

Stowell RJA: Dual diagnosis issues. Psychiatr Ann 21:98–104, 1991

Stowell RJA: Evaluation and treatment of the substance abusing adolescent, in The Hatherleigh Guide to Child and Adolescent Therapy. Edited By Lonsdale J. New York, Hatherleigh Press, 1996, pp 227–249

Stowell RJA, Estroff TW: Psychiatric disorders in substance abusing adolescent inpatients: a pilot study. J Am Acad Child Adolesc Psychiatry 31:1036–1040, 1992

Winters KC, Henley G: Assessing adolescents who abuse chemicals: the Chemical Dependency Adolescent Assessment Project, in Adolescent Drug Abuse Analyses of Treatment Research (NIDA Res Monogr 77). Washington, DC, U.S. Government Printing Office, 1988a, pp 4–18

Winters KC, Henley G: Personal Experience Inventory Test and Manual. Los Angeles, CA, Western Psychological Services, 1988b

Young JG, Leven L, Ludman W, et al: Interviewing children and adolescents, in Psychiatric Disorders in Children and Adolescents. Edited by Garfinkel BD, Carlson GA, Weller E. Philadelphia, PA, WB Saunders, 1990, pp 443–468

8 Treatment Planning and Case Management

Linda Semlitz, M.D.

Substance abuse programs proliferated during the 1980s. This was followed by a period of decline during which many programs either closed their doors entirely or redefined their structures and purposes. This evolution occurred largely as a consequence of managed care, which sharply curtailed the generous funding of the earlier decade. Despite a growing body of literature documenting the general efficacy of addictions treatment and the financial returns of the treatment investment, policymakers and much of the research community have remained skeptical of treatment benefits. Many researchers discount the naturalistic studies that have been done because the research did not involve the randomized clinical trial design that is more appropriate to medication research. In addition, when experimental studies using the treatment randomization technique were used, they often were too narrowly focused and did not provide generalizable findings. This lack of consensus about treatment results between the clinical and research communities led policymakers to severely cut funding for addictions treatment.

Treatment providers contributed to the decline by underestimating the impact of managed care and failing to adapt their treatment models to accommodate clinical innovations and economic reality. Matching appropriate treatment with the patient's substance, social, and psychological problems remains largely based on the biases of the evaluator and on financial resources (McLellan et al. 1997). Adolescent treatment resources and sound treatment outcome research are alarmingly scarce (Bruner and Fishman 1998).

In this context, this chapter reviews the current literature on treatment planning (Godley et al. 1994; Semlitz 1996), the role of assessment outcome research, and contracting as an integral part of treatment planning for substance-abusing adolescents. The chapter also discusses appropriate documentation of the treatment plan, treatment matching, and utilization review.

Assessment as the First Step in Treatment Planning

Treatment planning does not mean just choosing the appropriate treatment program. It is a continuously evolving process resulting in a continuously evolving document: the treatment plan. Both the process and the document must be reevaluated over time.

Effective interventions are predicated on a valid and clinically relevant assessment (American Academy of Child and Adolescent Psychiatry 1998; Bruner and Fishman 1998; Bukstein 1997; Tarter 1990; Weinberg et al. 1998). Nonetheless, most adolescent substance treatment facilities employ locally developed (and idiosyncratic) assessment methods or use procedures developed for adults (Owen and Nyberg 1983). Factors that influence treatment planning include 1) patterns of substance abuse; 2) behavior patterns such as running away, delinquency, and legal problems; 3) medical problems such HIV risk and pregnancy; 4) the presence of comorbid psychiatric disorders; 5) developmental status, including level of social skills; 6) the family system, level of pathology, denial, and substance abuse among family members; 7) school behavior, attendance, academic progress, and coexisting learning disabilities; 8) vocational skills; 9) peer relationships; 10) leisure/recreational interests; 11) cultural factors; and 12) risk of relapse. It is the function of the treatment plan to target special interventions with specific areas of disturbance identified by diagnostic assessment. Thus, the needs of a 15-year-old male high school dropout who uses cocaine and is involved in a gang differ vastly from those of a 15-year-old female with possible bipolar disorder who deteriorates into episodic marijuana and alcohol use.

Treatment planning responds to the specific problem identified during screening and comprehensive assessment. Once a problem is identified using the outline previously described, it is possible to specify the presence, type, and severity of the areas of dysfunction that require intervention. Thus, every treatment plan is individualized to the patient and requires a multimodal response.

Tarter (1990) has developed a decision tree method for systematic evaluation and treatment of adolescent substance abuse. His model integrates assessment with intervention, allowing for both thorough evaluation of the adolescent and for quantitative monitoring of treatment progress and outcome. This elegant model will be described here in some detail.

Tarter's model employs a multiphase decision tree format. The Drug Use Screening Inventory (DUSI) is used to systematically screen for problems related to drug use in 10 domains. The adolescent's scores on the DUSI document each problem's density or severity. Results of the initial screening influence the direction of subsequent comprehensive diagnostic evaluations using the same 10 problem domains identified by the DUSI. These domains include 1) substance use, 2) behavior patterns, 3) health status, 4) psychiatric disorder, 5) social skills, 6) family system, 7) school adjustment, 8) work, 9) peer relationships, and 10) leisure/recreation. This process results in a diagnostic summary identifying and integrating all of the patient's treatment needs.

The DUSI is intended to identify the medical and psychiatric disturbances and psychosocial maladjustment that are frequently concomitant to substance use in adolescents. Tarter (1990) recommended several specific instruments for more thorough diagnostic assessment in the specific domains tapped by the DUSI. For example, the Achenbach Child Behavior Checklist (CBCL; Achenbach and Edelbrock 1983) is used to delineate behavior patterns, and the Schedule for Affective Disorders and Schizophrenia for School-Age Children (K-SADS; Puig-Antich 1982) is used to identify comorbid Axis I psychiatric disorders. The final step involves the preparation of a treatment plan that targets interventions to specific areas of disturbance based on evaluation findings.

Patient Placement Criteria

Determining acceptable treatment options is frequently influenced as much by those programs that are reimbursable as by clinical need. In an attempt to resolve the reimbursement crisis facing inpatient programs, the American Society of Addiction Medicine (ASAM) developed criteria for determining what level of care a patient needs (American Society of Addiction Medicine 1996; Hoffmann et al. 1991). These criteria assist clinicians in deciding whether a patient needs inpatient treatment or some level of outpatient treatment.

The ASAM patient placement criteria were developed in response to several concerns. Treatment providers charged that managed care treatment reviewers deny coverage based on criteria that the reviewers frequently will not disclose. At the same time, treatment providers acknowledged that they were open to criticism given the frequent use of fixed protocols, such as 28-day hospitalizations, independent of patient need. ASAM responded by proposing criteria for four levels of care: outpatient, intensive outpatient/partial hospitalization, medically monitored intensive inpatient, and medically managed intensive inpatient. Length of stay was determined by an individual's clinical appropriateness for transfer to a less restrictive level of care. Criteria were delineated for both adults and adolescents (American Society of Addiction Medicine 1996; Hoffmann et al. 1991). These criteria were later revised to provide additional differentiation within the base levels of care (American Society of Addiction Medicine 1996).

Outcome as a Factor in Treatment Planning

Many adolescents experiment with drugs and alcohol or become involved with regular episodic use, yet most do not develop significant negative consequences. Most adolescents demonstrate spontaneous cessation of substance use after a period of experimenting (Jessor 1977; Kandel 1978a, 1978b; Kandel and Logan 1984). Despite several longitudinal studies, more is known about the antecedents of initiation to drug use than about the consequences in adolescence or young adulthood (Kandel et al. 1986). Knowledge of the consequences of use ought to influence decisions about treatment planning, especially in an atmosphere of limited resources.

Kandel et al. (1986) identified four major consequences of substance use on the lives of young people who use cigarettes, alcohol, or illicit drugs. Use of a particular drug class between adolescence and adulthood most strongly predicted the continued use of the same class of drugs in young adulthood. Use of a particular substance directly reinforced further use of that same substance. Illicit drugs have an adverse effect on employment and marriage and enhance the effect of delinquency as well as predict negative reports of health. The consequences of substance use seem to be related to cumulative use. Age of onset is highly related to continued and thus greater cumulative use (Kandel and Logan 1984). The consequences of substance use affect every aspect of young people's lives.

Substance Abuse as a Continuum

Substance abuse can be viewed as a continuum ranging from nonuse to experimental use, casual use, and compulsive use (Bailey 1989). Substance abuse is often described as a developmental process in which adolescents pass through a sequence of stages, with each prior drug state acting as a potential gateway to the next stage (Dupont 1987; Kandel 1978a, 1978b; MacDonald and Newton 1981).

Clear temporal developmental stages emerge from the data on the use of substances by adolescents, and these result in a progression of substance use from adolescence through young adulthood, when the period of risk for initiation into substance use essentially ends (Yamaguchi and Kandel 1984a, 1984b). The sequence of involvement with substances progresses from the use of at least one legal (for adults) substance such as alcohol and/or cigarettes to the use of marijuana and then on to other illicit and/or prescribed psychoactive drugs. A direct progression from nonuse to illicit drug use is very rare. Some suggest that a stage of problem drinking follows marijuana use but occurs before other illicit drug use (Donovan and Jessor 1983). Once initiation of substance use has occurred, continued use is best explained by the self-reinforcing effects of a particular substance (Kandel and Logan 1984).

Clayton (1986) confirmed this consistent and predictable pattern of progression despite differences in sociodemographics. Alcohol and cigarettes are thus "gateway drugs": their use predicts later use of illicit drugs. Nonetheless, multiple drug use is the rule, not the exception, for most substance-using adolescents (Clayton 1986).

During the earliest stages of substance use, experimenters or casual drug users who go on to develop a substance-related disorder are indistinguishable from their drug-using peers with respect to the type and frequency of drug use. Adolescents at high risk for substance abuse or dependence show signs of preoccupation with drugs and/or alcohol. Regular use of the gateway drugs (alcohol and marijuana) increases along with more frequent episodes of intoxication and concurrent use of other psychoactive drugs (Christie-Burke et al. 1990; Dupont 1987). These adolescents tend to gravitate toward their drug-using peers and to spend more time in drug-related activities. They begin to demonstrate difficulties with academic performance and peer and family relationships and show signs and symptoms of conduct disturbance. They may obtain increased experience with drugs whose use carries greater potential for drug dependence and may develop both a drug of choice and a preference for a specific route of administration. Substance-related disorders may affect their affective stability, cognitive functioning, and psychosocial development.

Levels of Use

Critical to the field of adolescent substance abuse treatment is the concept of levels of use. This construct can be very useful for the practitioner who must determine what, if any, treatment is appropriate for a substance-using adolescent. However, this concept is descriptive only and has not been validated by research. See Simpkin (1992) for a review of the literature on levels of use.

Although no DSM-IV (American Psychiatric Association 1994) criteria specifically define substance abuse and dependence in adolecents, the adult criteria are fully applied without exception to adolescents. However, it has been argued that the adult criteria are incomplete for attempting to diagnose adolescent substance abuse. Zoccolillo et al. (1999) recently examined the issue of problem drug and alcohol use in a Quebec community sample. Drug use in this sample, once it passed a threshold of using drugs more than five times (two-thirds of those who had ever used an illegal drug), suggested that these teens were not just experimenting. Almost 45% of boys and 42% of girls were using drugs in the morning, suggesting that a significant number of adolescents spend a part of the day intoxicated. Drug use appears to be incorporated into at least two major daily activities—sports and school. Therefore, the authors concluded, "normative" use of drugs really means normative use. The authors defined *normative use* as using several times per week, attending school and sports while intoxicated, and using in the morning. These findings raise questions about the diagnosis of drug use in adolescence. Teenagers who attend school intoxicated, play sports while intoxicated, and use drugs several times per week may still not meet DSM-IV criteria for substance abuse with regard to "substance related absences, suspensions, or expulsions from school." (DSM-IV, p. 184). Nevertheless, this pattern of use is clearly problematic from a developmental perspective. Thus, meeting DSM-IV criteria for substance abuse may artificially delay treatment for teenagers engaging in problem drug use. Unfortunately, as Zoccolillo et al. pointed out, the absence of a diagnosis is often equated with the absence of a problem or disorder.

Psychoactive substance dependence can be grouped into three aspects that fit the criteria for alcoholism as defined by the National Council on Alcoholism. These criteria are continued use despite adverse consequences, preoccupation, and loss of control. Neither tolerance nor withdrawal is necessary to diagnose dependence or addiction. The definition of *addiction* (which includes preoccupation, compulsive use in spite of adverse consequences, and a pattern of relapse or inability to cut down despite adverse consequences) is strikingly similar to that of alcoholism. In sum, the dividing line between psychoactive substance abuse disorders and psychoactive substance dependence usually involves the loss of control. DSM-IV-TR (American Psychiatric Association 2000) criteria for substance dependence and substance abuse appear in Table 8–1 and Table 8–2, respectively. A few guides exist that help to determine the level of use based on the elements that define addiction.

Schaefer (1987) defined *substance use*, or the first level of use, as a point in normal development when the adolescent discovers that alcohol or drugs of abuse can produce a pleasant mood swing. The adolescent seeks the drug or drugs because he or she is curious and associates the use of the substance with the thrill of using a "forbidden" substance. Nowinski (1990) called this the *experimental stage*. Situational drug use (e.g., parties) may occur when the adolescent's motivation is social acceptance by peers. Nowinski calls this the *social stage*.

The second level of use as defined by Schaefer (1987) is called *substance misuse*. Both Schaefer and Nowinski (1990) described this level as "seeking a mood swing." Nowinski refers to this level as *instrumental use*. He subdivides this level into *hedonistic use* and *compensatory use*. Hedonistic use implies seeking out a pleasurable or euphoric state induced by a substance. Compensatory use implies seeking out a drug to inhibit or suppress emotions (e.g., feel less sad, less angry, less lonely). During this second level, indicators that the adolescent is in serious trouble are minimal. Grades may be only slightly erratic, and the adolescent may have only occasional blackouts or hangovers that are not noticeable to anyone else.

The third level as defined by Schaefer (1987) is referred to as *substance abuse*. Nowinski (1990) denotes the difference between use and misuse by the chronicity of the problem. He refers to this chronicity as the *habitual stage*. Adolescents at this stage habitually seek out the mood swing, and their lifestyles change to accommodate their use. Their peer groups change from nonusers to users. To experience a greater high, they may be high for days at a time, and the toll this takes is dramatic. Their grades fall, their absenteeism increases, and they are more moody and irritable. Physical effects such as

Table 8–1. DSM-IV-TR Criteria for Substance Dependence

A maladaptive pattern of substance use, leading to clinically significant impairment or distress, as manifested by three (or more) of the following, occurring at any time in the same 12-month period:

(1) tolerance, as defined by either of the following:
  (a) a need for markedly increased amounts of the substance to achieve intoxication or desired effect
  (b) markedly diminished effect with continued use of the same amount of the substance

(2) withdrawal, as manifested by either of the following:
  (a) the characteristic withdrawal syndrome for the substance (refer to Criteria A and B of the criteria sets for Withdrawal from the specific substances)
  (b) the same (or a closely related) substance is taken to relieve or avoid withdrawal symptoms

(3) the substance is often taken in larger amounts or over a longer period than was intended

(4) there is a persistent desire or unsuccessful efforts to cut down or control substance use

(5) a great deal of time is spent in activities necessary to obtain the substance (e.g., visiting multiple doctors or driving long distances), use the substance (e.g., chain-smoking), or recover from its effects

(6) important social, occupational, or recreational activities are given up or reduced because of substance use

(7) the substance use is continued despite knowledge of having a persistent or recurrent physical or psychological problem that is likely to have been caused or exacerbated by the substance (e.g., current cocaine use despite recognition of cocaine-induced depression, or continued drinking despite recognition that an ulcer was made worse by alcohol consumption)

Specify if:

With Physiological Dependence: evidence of tolerance or withdrawal (i.e., either Item 1 or 2 is present)

Without Physiological Dependence: no evidence of tolerance or withdrawal (i.e., neither Item 1 nor 2 is present)

Course specifiers (see text for definitions):

Early Full Remission

Early Partial Remission

Sustained Full Remission

Sustained Partial Remission

On Agonist Therapy

In a Controlled Environment

Source. American Psychiatric Association 2000, p. 197.

Table 8–2. DSM-IV-TR Criteria for Substance Abuse

A. A maladaptive pattern of substance use leading to clinically significant impairment or distress, as manifested by one (or more) of the following, occurring within a 12-month period:

(1) recurrent substance use resulting in a failure to fulfill major role obligations at work, school, or home (e.g., repeated absences or poor work performance related to substance use; substance-related absences, suspensions, or expulsions from school; neglect of children or household)

(2) recurrent substance use in situations in which it is physically hazardous (e.g., driving an automobile or operating a machine when impaired by substance use)

(3) recurrent substance-related legal problems (e.g., arrests for substance-related disorderly conduct)

(4) continued substance use despite having persistent or recurrent social or interpersonal problems caused or exacerbated by the effects of the substance (e.g., arguments with spouse about consequences of intoxication, physical fights)

B. The symptoms have never met the criteria for Substance Dependence for this class of substance.

Source. American Psychiatric Association 2000, p. 199.

weight loss begin to occur, and the adolescents may have their first bout with the law. During this time, they continue to use despite these adverse consequences, thus fulfilling the criteria for diagnosis of psychoactive substance abuse found in DSM-IV. Tolerance may develop faster than in adults. The frequency of use, types of drugs used, and quantity used may increase until the adolescents may occupy much of their time using or anticipating how, when, and where they will use next. This second important element, preoccupation, satisfies the second requirement of addiction and psychoactive substance abuse.

According to both Schaefer (1987) and Nowinski (1990), only when adolescents have met the third requirement for addiction, loss of control, can they be diagnosed with psychoactive substance dependence. This loss of control denotes inability to abstain, regulate, or cut back from substance use. Schaefer refers to this loss of control as level IV, or *addiction*. Nowinski refers to this stage as the *compulsion stage*. The adolescents go to greater extremes to obtain drugs. This behavior can be used to measure the severity of their dependence on the substances. Substance-abusing adolescents may engage in unlawful behavior; they may resort to selling drugs or prostitution to obtain money for drugs or may offer sex in exchange for drugs. They may also begin stealing and selling their stolen goods to obtain money to buy drugs.

Their home lives are chaotic, and they may have little emotional support. This lack of support, combined with their increasingly low self-esteem and the effects of their drug use, may cause the adolescents to feel increasingly depressed and suicidal. They may also start using one substance to increase the effects of another drug or to let them down easily after using another drug. They may experience withdrawal. As noted earlier, neither tolerance nor withdrawal is required to meet the criteria for diagnosing psychoactive substance dependence.

Use of Contracting

Diagnostic assessment, treatment intervention, and treatment planning begin with the first contact a family makes with their family doctor or mental health professional. Despite performing multiple interviews, administering rating scales, and organizing collateral data, the practitioner may still be left with an ambiguous situation and/or an ambivalent family. This is especially true when an adolescent presents in the earlier phases of substance abuse or with a style of abuse characterized by episodic dyscontrol and negative consequences. In addition, families can be in significant denial about their adolescent's difficulties and can be unprepared to endorse and follow through with specific treatment recommendations. The use of serial contracting and follow-up with the adolescent over time serve multiple functions. They can be powerful diagnostic tools in assisting the practitioner to obtain additional measures of the adolescent's functioning, to assist in alliance building with families, and to begin to provide parents with the appropriate tools with which to intervene with their acting-out adolescent.

Schaefer (1987) describes the use of serial contracting in terms families can readily use. Contracting involves the suspension and monitoring of target behaviors at home, at school, and in the community. Both the target behaviors as defined by the contract as well as the consequences for breaking the contract are clearly established with both the adolescent and the parents. The adolescent's ability to abide by the contract assists in determining both the level of use and the level of intervention required.

Thus, when an adolescent and/or family presents an ambiguous situation or seems to minimize the severity of substance use, the practitioner can establish a "no use contract" and then reevaluate the adolescent at a later date. The "no use" rule includes prohibition against drinking, possession or use of illegal drugs, and illegal actions related to drug or alcohol use. To make a no use rule effective, it must have consequences. Consequences may include enforcement of local school rules (e.g., prohibition from participation in school activities if caught using drugs/alcohol) or spending a night in juvenile detention if arrested for possession or driving under the influence. Other logical consequences may include curtailed telephone or driving privileges or attendance at an information group about substance dependence. If the adolescent is able to abide by the no use rule, there is a probability that substance use is not out of control. If the adolescent continues to use despite the rule, the therapist and family can assume the need for both additional confrontation and the next level of intervention as exemplified by a simple contract.

The simple contract should include basic nonnegotiable rules: no alcohol or drug use, no physical or verbal aggression, and no skipping of classes (or, when appropriate, drug and alcohol education group sessions). It addresses misuse of drugs most likely resulting in school or legal consequences. Consequences for breaking this contract include the choice of an evaluation in either an outpatient substance dependence treatment setting or an inpatient setting and placement on a contract. An adolescent at this level (abuse) is preoccupied with drugs or alcohol.

An additional contract is usually needed that includes all the rules of the simple contract and outlines the specific behaviors required to earn privileges at home or school. Target behaviors may include improved school performance, keeping to curfew, and doing chores. Consequences for breaking this contract include the choice between treatment in an outpatient or inpatient setting and placement on a final contract. At this level, substance use has become compulsive.

Each contract must spell out, in writing, the specific behaviors required for the teenager to retain the privileges of living at home and staying in school. Consequences for breaking this contract include the choice between two available and reputable inpatient treatment centers.

Patient Treatment Matching

> The outsider seeking to assess various treatment programs in any particular geographic area may find himself or herself enmeshed in local territorial disputes, local jargon or code words, local personality conflicts among elders of the treatment community, and local philosophic monopolies, all of which thwart objective assessment adequacy in ways not seen in medicine since the 1930s. Indeed, the closest analogy to this current state of treatment perspectives is found historically in that era's various treatment approaches used for the management of polio patients. (Hoffmann et al. 1987, p. 450)

McLellan and Alterman (1991) reviewed the conceptual and methodological issues with respect to matching adult patients to drug and alcohol treatments. What follows summarizes much of their thinking.

The idea of patient matching has become increasingly attractive along with the increase in treatment options and the political and economic pressures to reduce health care cost. In addition, it is a widely held belief that certain kinds of treatments are optimal for certain kinds of patients. McLellan and Alterman (1991) concluded that the limited scientific literature demonstrates very little evidence that a matching strategy can be practical or worthwhile in most clinical settings (Bruner and Fishman 1998; McLellan et al. 1997). There are numerous methodological and conceptual problems with patient matching research (American Academy of Child and Adolescent Psychiatry 1998; Bruner and Fishman 1998; Bukstein 1997; McLellan et al. 1997; Weinberg et al. 1998). Matching is viable only in a treatment network in which each program is both different and effective. In addition, it is not possible to demonstrate the superiority of a specific program for a specific type of individual if the program is generally poorly administered and only minimally effective. If it cannot be specified that a treatment was delivered in the intended manner by adequately trained individuals and in sufficient quantity and intensity to effect the desired change, then the results of treatment matching will remain inconclusive.

There are at least four levels of treatment intensity that have been studied with regard to matching. These include advice or self-help, brief interventions (less than five therapist visits lasting about 1 week), outpatient or partial hospitalization, and inpatient care. The patient factors that are predictive of treatment outcome at a reduced level of treatment intensity (i.e., no treatment or brief treatment) usually continue to be predictive even at more structured or intensive levels of treatment. The level of social support has been reliably associated with posttreatment outcome at all levels of treatment intensity (Hoffmann et al. 1987; N.G. Hoffmann, personal communication, 1998).

Matching can also take place at the treatment component level. There is a fairly discrete set of treatment components available to most substance-abusing patients in treatment. These include group therapy (usually focusing on need for treatment and denial), interpersonal therapy, substance abuse treatment, education, 12-step self-help groups, and social service assistance. Matching at the treatment component level is important, as similarity among treatment programs may account for the failure to find evidence of matching between programs.

Friedman et al. (1993) published a study in which they matched substance-abusing adolescents and various inpatient and outpatient treatments. Unfortunately, this study is limited by inadequate matching of inpatients and outpatients to the severity of their substance abuse and their demographics. Another problem is that the time between initial and follow-up assessments varied significantly. Compared with short-term inpatient treatment, long-term outpatient treatment was shown to have significantly greater effect in reducing substance use/abuse. This was particularly true for patients who had relatively more severe social lifestyle problems, family problems, and employment problems. Outpatient treatment also showed a trend toward a significantly better outcome for patients with more severe psychiatric problems. The authors of the study speculated that the longer course of outpatient treatment explained the advantages of this mode of treatment.

The work to date on patient treatment matching has thus far suggested three conclusions: 1) Patient factors have been more predictive of outcome than treatment process factors. Treatment process or methods have been virtually unstudied. 2) Patients with better social and economic supports and fewer psychiatric problems do well in most treatments and seem to benefit equally from inpatient or outpatient treatments. Patients with lower socioeconomic status and/or greater psychiatric morbidity do particularly poorly in outpatient care. Patient factors, such as severity of drug dependence, family history of substance abuse, and especially the presence of antisocial personality disorder, have been generally predictive of poor outcomes from all treatments but not differentially predictive of response to specific treatments. 3) There are no clear predictors from any specific treatment components secondary to a paucity of studies.

Treatment Plan Documentation

An excellent guide to treatment plan documentation can be found in Kennedy's *Fundamentals of Psychiatric Treatment Planning* (1992). The treatment plan reduces the many assessments and evaluations into a coherent statement of the patient's diagnosis, deficits, and assets and establishes a series of treatment goals. It outlines the treatment program, including the specific treatment methods to be employed, the clinician(s) responsible for segments of treatment, the time frames for reaching specific treatment objectives, and discharge criteria. The treatment plan begins the process of first review and concurrent review by utilization management (American Psychiatric Association Committee on Managed Care 1992).

Special attention must be paid to the documentation of the treatment plan for various reasons. The patient record serves as a legal record of delivered services. It assists in the development of clear, observable treatment guidelines that generate successful patient outcomes. The record is increasingly used to support or deny third-party reimbursement. Significant external influences are pressuring providers to change not only how they deliver services but also how they document them (Joint Committee on the Accreditation of Health Care Organizations 1992).

Treatment planning has, for the most part, emerged from the concerns of accreditors, not clinicians. Accreditors want the record to reflect what is happening to the patient (Siegel and Fisher 1981). Providers of substance abuse treatment are being held to increasing levels of clinical accountability by those receiving treatment, the public, third-party payors, other fiscal intermediaries, and occasionally by the judicial system (Joint Committee on the Accreditation of Health Care Organizations 1992). Diagnostic summaries, problem statements, and treatment plans should clearly portray the individuality of the patient in observable behavioral terms.

Common Problems with Documentation

Treatment planning emerges from assessments and multidisciplinary treatment team meetings. It includes lists of problems, goals, objectives, and interventions. Although accreditation is a necessary goal, clinicians must not lose sight of the fact that a good treatment plan greatly contributes to high-quality clinical care and outcome. Most high-caliber substance abuse treatment requires the participation of a multidisciplinary team that formulates a multidisciplinary assessment. There are many potential problems in developing high-quality treatment plans. A good treatment plan must articulate clinical problems that communicate across disciplines. The use of jargon or vague clinical statements is unacceptable. It is not uncommon for documentation to be ignored in favor of providing treatment for the patient in the competition for professional time. With the provision of multidisciplinary care, the joint responsibility for a treatment plan, coordination, and accountability can become vague. Many patients have multiple diagnoses including multiple substance abuse diagnoses, psychiatric diagnoses, and medical diagnoses. Every problem identified must generate a list of goals, objectives, interventions, and progress notes. Thus, there may be a disincentive to identify problems. Concentration on diagnoses can lead to an emphasis on biological interventions at the expense of psychosocial treatments. Managed health care providers and many other third party payors do not consider the standard 21- or 28-day treatment program to be individualized care. Treating substance use issues alone without attending to comorbid psychiatric, educational, family, and medical problems is no longer considered an acceptable community standard of care. The sole use of patient self-rating forms does not make up an adequate psychosocial intervention. Documentation of assessment and treatment should enhance clinical care and outcome as well as assist in efforts to maintain organizational efficiency and cost containment on inpatient units. Treatment plans are very difficult to complete today, given the short patient stays of 2–4 days. Sometimes a problem list is the only thing that can be accomplished.

Components of the Treatment Plan

Treatment plans are continuously evolving documents intended to guide treatment intervention and trace patient progress. Consistency must be established between assessment, development of a master treatment plan and tracking patient progress via progress notes, and treatment plan updates.

The Diagnostic Summary

A biopsychosocial diagnostic summary is based on the integration of salient medical and clinical information from the assessments and individual disciplines. Its goal is to define the placement and treatment of patients in addition to summarizing multiaxial diagnoses. The diagnostic formulation will naturally lead to a problem list and definition of specific treatment goals. Skilled addiction professionals realize the need for multimodal treatment to target complicated multidimensional biopsychosocial problems.

The greater the level of dysfunction, the more intensive the level of care required and the greater the likelihood that length of stay within a continuum will be prolonged. Treatment in the least restrictive modality is chosen for both ethical and financial reasons. As a patient's condition changes, recommendations should also be made for either a more-intensive or a less-intensive level of care.

The Problem List

Treatment planning interacts with all aspects of the clinical process. There is a critical connection between thorough multidisciplinary assessments and the development of a master treatment plan, beginning with a problem list.

As stated earlier, use of jargon cannot capture the individuality of a patient. Problem statements must be written precisely and specifically, defining the targeted problem behaviors. They should include the patient's strengths and problems documented with a comprehensive biopsychosocial history interpreted specifically for the patient. Unless this is done first, it is impossible to determine the appropriate level of care and the necessary treatment (Joint Committee on the Accreditation of Health Care Organizations 1992).

A clinical problem should be documented as soon as it is identified during any phase of treatment. If treatment of a particular identified problem is to be deferred, clinical justification must also be documented. The problem list should contain all significant clinical problems as well as clinical factors requiring treatment (e.g., pregnancy, criminal charges). Historical factors that have continued clinical significance should also be included (e.g., history of suicide attempt). Generally, a review of the problem list can serve as the most efficient manner by which a professional can obtain an overview of a particular patient's individual care.

A master problem list can help capture the dynamic nature of the treatment plan. New problems must be listed whenever they are identified. A treatment plan should document treatment progress as well as the need for change in interventions when the desired results are not achieved. The problem list should indicate the date each problem was established as well as the date of onset of each problem. The date established serves the purpose of marking how far back in the chart one must search in order to review the documentation of a specific problem. The date of onset indicates, as best as possible, the time a particular set of symptoms began. Finally, problem resolution must also be dated in the treatment plan.

Kennedy (1992) devised a classification system to simplify problem identification and treatment planning. He devised Axis V subscales from the DSM-III-R (American Psychiatric Association 1987) because of its focus on adaptive function, problematic behavior, and outcome. These Axis V subscales divide the symptoms and behaviors into five problem areas: psychological impairment, social skills, dangerousness, activities of daily living and occupational skills, and substance abuse. Kennedy added two additional categories: medical problems and ancillary problems (i.e., placement problems, legal problems, financial problems).

Treatment Objectives

A treatment *objective* is a desired behavior that is related to the ultimate achievement of a clinical goal. It is probably one of the least understood and misused concepts in treatment planning. Objectives are usually written using action verbs that reflect the desired behavioral change, for example, "The patient is to recognize that he/she has an alcohol problem."

Kennedy recommended the use of short-term goals and long-term goals to measure outcome. He maintained that the concept of *objectives* was confusing and required special training, whereas long- and short-term goals fit well along a continuum. As a rule of thumb, Kennedy suggested that long-term goals mean essentially the same thing as *goals* and short-term goals mean the same as *objectives*. All outcome measures must be both observable and measurable.

Treatment Goals

Treatment *goals* can most clearly be defined as targeted, measurable behavioral changes that occur in the patient. Goal statements should document the desired behaviors that will demonstrate resolution of the identified problem(s). For example, "The patient will learn to apply the skills necessary for abstinence." The goal statement should be logically and directly linked to the problem statement (Joint Committee on the Accreditation of Health Care Organizations 1992). The primary goal of substance abuse treatment is achieving and maintaining abstinence from all illicit substances and/or alcohol.

Treatment Goals Versus Treatment Modalities

Kennedy (1992) discussed the need to differentiate treatment goals and treatment modalities. Treatment modalities are defined as actions that staff members take by which a patient is assisted in reaching targeted, measurable change. Treatment modalities often have effects across several problem areas such as medications or group therapy. It is recommended that the treatment modality be limited to being listed only in one or two primary problem areas to which it is being targeted.

How comprehensive should the treatment plan be? The anticipated length of treatment greatly influences the breadth and complexity of a treatment plan. An acute 8–10-day inpatient stay requires a substantially different treatment plan than a long-term residential placement.

Utilization Review

The Committee on Managed Care of the American Psychiatric Association provided guidelines for the process of utilization management. *Utilization management* is a set of techniques used by or on behalf of purchasers of health care benefits to manage health care costs through case-by-case assessments of the care prior to and during its provision (Institute of Medicine 1989). *Prior review* (i.e., prior authorization, precertification) is the process by which a determination is made whether medical services proposed for a specific patient are consistent with the health plan for medical necessity.

Typically, prior review authorizes the initial procedures and initial amount, duration, and scope of services required to form a sufficient evaluation and to create a treatment plan. Submission of an initial treatment plan is required to follow quickly, and additional requests for service are subject to concurrent review. Prior review is used most frequently for inpatient care but is increasingly requested by managed care providers for outpatient care. Information requested for prior review usually includes the following: precipitants for seeking treatment, provisional multiaxial DSM-IV diagnoses, history, goals of treatment, length of treatment anticipated to meet goals, mechanisms used to measure patient progress, levels of treatment that will allow patients to best reach treatment goals, services used to achieve treatment goals, an initial discharge plan, risk assessment (including homicidal and suicidal potential), medical complications, patient score on the Axis V Global Assessment of Functioning Scale for DSM-IV, and a mental status examination.

Concurrent review assesses the clinical justification, the appropriateness of the treatment plan, the extent to which services provided correlate with treatment goals, and progress toward discharge planning. Concurrent reviews occur at regularly specified intervals in response to requests for continued inpatient stay or additional outpatient visits. Reviewers frequently request written modified treatment plans, progress notes, and treatment summaries as well as telephone contact with the treatment provider. Information frequently required for concurrent review includes any changes in diagnosis, evidence of patient progression or regression, medical/neurological problems requiring treatment, current mental status and behavioral functioning, special treatments such as suicide precautions or seclusion, and any adverse behavioral episodes such as self-injury or assault. In addition, the progress toward completion of each goal in the treatment plan and the time frame for meeting remaining goals are reviewed. Special attention is paid to progress in meeting goals toward discharge. Reviewers may request information about psychotherapy progress including the duration and frequency of sessions, the presence of family therapy and educational activities, progress in group and milieu therapies, and an explanation of the current medication progress including optimal dosing, serum levels, and side effects.

Utilization management makes decisions about requests for treatment based on a determination of medical necessity. To be deemed "necessary" a service must be

- adequate and essential for the evaluation and/or treatment of a disease, condition, or illness, as defined by standard diagnostic nomenclatures;

- reasonably expected to improve an individual's condition or level of functioning; and
- in keeping with national standards of psychiatric practice as defined by standard clinical references, valid empirical experience for efficacy, and national professional standards promulgated by medical associations and federal agencies using professional consensus development and scientific data.

Utilization management may add the requirement that treatment be provided at the most cost-effective level of care. The need for precise information and clear language for authorization of service based on medical necessity cannot be overestimated. Not all utilization management companies are willing to reveal their criteria for service. It is frequently considered proprietary. If the provider disagrees with the medical necessity criteria of the utilization management entity, appeal and/or provision of care without third party payment may be necessary. It is the moral, ethical, and legal obligation of the treating physician to provide medically necessary care, stabilization, and transfer of arrangements for additional care independent of utilization review.

Treatment Options and Approaches

The heterogeneity among treatment programs cannot be underestimated. Two philosophical controversies in the treatment field deserve comment (Wheeler and Malmquist 1987). Despite the general acceptance of substance abuse and dependency as valid clinical entities, there remains a belief among many psychodynamic psychiatrists that severe psychiatric pathology must antedate and contribute to substance abuse. Programs favoring this view are found in the mental health setting, especially among inpatient psychiatric units. Substance abuse is seldom the central focus in these psychiatric settings. It is often believed that by treating the underlying psychiatric condition, the substance abuse will abate.

The second philosophic model has to do with the definition of substance dependence. Although a diagnosis of substance dependence can be made without the presence of tolerance or withdrawal, many clinicians feel adolescents never meet criteria. Most treatment programs are designed for the chemically dependent adolescent, and referral for treatment primarily occurs among the most acute and severe cases, which demonstrates both the progression of chemical use as well as clearly related life consequences.

Intervention as Primary Treatment

An intervention is a highly organized, well-planned, and thoroughly practiced procedure using a trained facilitator. The goal is to help the adolescent see how substances have had an impact on his or her life and on the lives of those who care for him or her and to initiate treatment. Family members and concerned persons prepare for the intervention by listing in writing the harmful events in the life of the adolescent that can be directly or indirectly attributed to substance abuse. Judgmental attitudes, guilt, and shame are avoided; instead, the events are reported in a factual and empathic manner. Each confronter then tells the substance abuser what he or she is prepared to do to stop enabling the continued substance abuse and to inform the adolescent about plans for treatment.

The Spectrum of Treatment Options

A broad continuum of treatment options is available, although practically, local practitioners must often rely on limited local resources or those resources on contract to specific managed health care organizations. There has been a shift, largely because of fiscal concerns, away from traditional 21–28 day treatment programs to brief (1–2 weeks) residential treatment followed by a continuum of less restrictive outpatient alternatives. This generally includes day treatment (or partial hospitalization) followed by intensive outpatient treatment and weekly or biweekly "aftercare" for a total length of 6 months to 1 year of treatment. Therapeutic communities (e.g., Daytop Village in New York City), which provide long-term intensive residential care for individuals with significant conduct disturbances or who have been refractory to prior treatment, also still have a role.

In the past, practitioners were not kept informed about their referred patient's progress and were not involved in the treatment planning process. Practitioners suddenly found themselves reacquainted with their patient when he or she "graduated" from a program or was given a medical discharge secondary to treatment noncompliance. This situation is changing with the development of dual diagnosis programs, biopsychosocial treatment philosophies, and the recognition that the mental health practitioner may have a role throughout treatment.

At the less intensive end of the treatment spectrum are community-based programs, such as drug and alcohol assessment teams, that contract with the juvenile justice system or the school system, in-school drug and alcohol education and recovery support groups, and 12-step programs such as Alcoholics Anonymous (AA), Narcotics Anonymous (NA), and Cocaine

Anonymous (CA). Other treatment options include halfway houses, emancipation programs, treatment within the judicial system, and wilderness experiences (e.g., Outward Bound).

Many treatment programs have similar components. Abstinence and lifestyle changes are seen as necessary to facilitate recovery. There is a general assumption that self-disclosure, individually or in groups, about one's life and one's problems helps to provide patients with perspective and insight into their own use of substances. Group therapy is a mainstay of treatment. Patients who are farther along in treatment act as role models for abstinence and recovery. Drug and alcohol treatment counseling staff may include individuals in long-term recovery.

The ultimate goal of most treatment programs is long-term abstinence from all psychoactive substances. The use of self-help or 12-step groups as an adjunct to treatment is almost always recommended. Prescription medication is avoided whenever it is not indicated, although more enlightened treatment programs tolerate the judicious use of specific medications for various comorbid psychiatric disorders. (It is still assumed by many substance abuse professionals that there are "good medicines," such as lithium and tricyclic antidepressants, and "bad medicines, " such as Xanax). Most treatment programs endorse the disease concept of substance abuse disorders and see treatment as ongoing control rather than curative. Family education and family therapy are generally encouraged and often requested. Psychiatric services vary from program to program.

Choosing an appropriate level of care involves more than a determination of the level of substance abuse. Just as in any psychiatric evaluation, the following clinical factors will influence program choice: level of family support and/or pathology, existence of high-risk behaviors, psychiatric comorbidity, and degree of both family and individual motivation and cooperation. Finally, prior treatment failure in equal or less-intensive treatment programs should be considered. As previously described, treatment choice is also influenced by local availability of treatment programs (both public and private) as well as the bureaucratic demands of public agencies and private payors. Hospitalization should be considered under the following circumstances:

1. Drug overdose that cannot be safely treated in an outpatient or emergency room setting
2. Patients at risk for severe or complicated withdrawal
3. Patients with complicated medical conditions affecting detoxification
4. Patients with a documented history of inability to cooperate or benefit from less-restrictive treatment

5. Patients with marked psychiatric comorbidity (e.g., suicidality, psychosis)
6. Patients who pose an imminent danger to themselves or others

Residential treatment is indicated primarily for patients whose lives and social interactions have come to focus exclusively around drug use and who lack sufficient social and vocational skills and drug-free supports to remain abstinent in an outpatient setting.

The American Association of Partial Hospitalization Child and Adolescent Special Interest Group has developed its own standards and guidelines for the use of partial hospitalization, an increasingly prevalent form of treatment (Block et al. 1991). Under these guidelines, partial hospitalization is indicated if

1. The patient is at risk for exclusion from normative community activities or residence.
2. The patient exhibits psychiatric symptoms, chemical dependency, behavioral problems, and/or developmental delays of severity sufficient to bring about significant or profound impairment in day-to-day educational, social, vocational, and/or interpersonal functioning.
   A. The patient has failed to make sufficient clinical gains within a traditional outpatient setting or has not attempted such outpatient treatment, and the severity of presenting symptoms is such that success of traditional outpatient treatment is doubtful.
   B. The patient is ready for release from an inpatient setting but is judged to be in continued need of ongoing intensive therapeutic intervention to make the appropriate transition toward full community activities.
3. The patient's family, guardian, or custodian
   A. is able and willing to provide the support and monitoring of the patient, enabling adequate control over behaviors; and
   B. is involved in treatment.
4. The patient has the capacity to benefit from the therapeutic interventions provided.

A clinician's ability to clearly and concisely document the need for specific levels of care by referring back to the multidimensional assessment of an individual will increase the likelihood of appropriate treatment matching and reimbursement by third parties. Despite the similarities of many programs, their clinical sophistication, availability of well-trained multidisciplinary staff members, and flexibility to formulate logical, defensible, individualized treatment plans vary widely. The availability of full psychiatric assessment with or without the ability for ongoing concurrent psychiatric care also varies from program to program. Many programs profess to perform a full psychological assessment on each patient when in reality they are completing the Child Behavior Checklist (Achenbach and Edelbrock 1983) or performing the Minnesota Multiphasic Personality Inventory (MMPI; Hathaway and McKinley 1982). Programs that are advertised as providing dual diagnosis care may or may not have fully integrated substance abuse and psychiatric treatments. Finally, family education, as opposed to family therapy, tends to be the norm among many programs.

Outpatient treatment requires a comprehensive approach using a variety of cognitive, behavioral, and psychotherapeutic techniques. Behavioral monitoring at home, school, and in the community is combined with family therapy, and participation in a 12-step program is usually recommended. Better outcome is generally associated with longer treatment. Essential features of outpatient therapy include the development of a therapeutic alliance, vigilance toward the development of drug craving and drug use, providing a relapse plan, and psychoeducation about the patient's illness, prognosis, and treatment. The patient is urged to set realistic and tangible goals for treatment and is encouraged to seek new experiences and roles consistent with a drug-free existence. Functioning interpersonally in family and peer situations as well as academic/vocational progress is also monitored.

It is the responsibility of the referring clinician to research the components of local treatment programs before making a referral. I recommend that the referring mental health professional obtain the intake assessments of individual programs and require that the rationale for specific treatment modalities be clearly defined.

Summary

Treatment planning and case management of the substance-abusing adolescent (Godley et al. 1994) must reflect both the increasingly available (but still sparse) research on adolescent substance abuse as well as external pressures facing the United States health care system as a whole. In the current climate of managed health care, the use of precise and carefully documented treatment planning is a requirement for reimbursement. Well-organized and coordinated treatment planning and case management can help select the most appropriate level of care at various stages of treatment, help reduce the overall cost for care of the adolescent substance abuser, and increase the likelihood of reimbursement. Outcome and treatment matching studies are greatly needed and will shape existing practices of treatment.

References

Achenbach TM, Edelbrock C: Manual for the Child Behavior Checklist and Revised Child Behavior Profile. Burlington, University of Vermont, 1983

American Academy of Child and Adolescent Psychiatry: Summary of the practice parameters for the assessment and treatment of children and adolescents with substance use disorders. J Am Acad Child Adolesc Psychiatry 37:122–126, 1998

American Psychiatric Association: Diagnostic and Statistical Manual of Mental Disorders, 3rd Edition Revised. Washington, DC, American Psychiatric Association, 1987

American Psychiatric Association: Diagnostic and Statistical Manual of Mental Disorders, 4th Edition. Washington, DC, American Psychiatric Association, 1994

American Psychiatric Association: Diagnostic and Statistical Manual of Mental Disorders, 4th Edition Text Revision. Washington, DC, American Psychiatric Association, 2000

American Psychiatric Association Committee on Managed Care: Utilization Management: A Handbook for Psychiatrists. Washington, DC, American Psychiatric Association, 1992

American Society of Addiction Medicine: Patient Placement Criteria for the Treatment of Substance-Related Disorders, Second Edition. Chevy Chase, MD, American Society of Addiction Medicine, 1996

Bailey G: Current perspectives on substance abuse in youth. J Am Acad Child Adolesc Psychiatry 28:51–162, 1989

Block BM, Arney K, Campbell D, et al: American Association for Partial Hospitalization Child and Adolescent Special Interest Group: standards for child and adolescent partial hospitalization programs. International Journal of Partial Hospitalization 7:13–21, 1991

Bruner AE, Fishman M: Adolescents and illicit drug use. JAMA 280:597–598, 1998

Bukstein O: Practice parameters for the assessment and treatment of children and adolescents with substance use disorders. American Academy of Child and Adolescent Psychiatry. J Am Acad Child Adolesc Psychiatry 36(10, suppl):140S–156S, 1997

Christie-Burke K, Burke JD, Regier DE, et al: Age at onset of selected mental disorders in five community populations. Arch Gen Psychiatry 47:511–518, 1990

Clayton RR: Multiple drug use. Recent Dev Alcohol 4:7–38, 1986

Donovan JD, Jesser R: Problem drinking and the dimension of involvement with drugs: a Guttman Scalogram analysis. Am J Public Health 73:468–472, 1983

Dupont RL: Prevention of adolescent chemical dependency. Pediatr Clin North Am 34:495–505, 1987

Friedman A, Granick S, Krelsher C, et al: Matching adolescents who abuse drugs to treatment. Am J Addict 2:232–237, 1993

Godley SH, Godley MD, Pratt A, et al: Case management services for adolescent substance abusers: a program description. J Subst Abuse Treat 11:309–317, 1994

Hathaway SR, McKinley JC: Minnesota Multiphasic Personality Inventory. Minneapolis, MN, University of Minnesota Press, 1982

Hoffmann N, Sonis WA, Halikas J, et al: Issues in the evaluation of chemical dependency treatment programs for adolescents. Pediatr Clin North Am 39:947–959, 1987

Hoffmann NG, Halikas JA, Mee-Lee D, et al: Patient Placement Criteria for the Treatment of Psychoactive Substance Use Disorders. Washington, DC, American Society of Addiction Medicine, 1991

Institute of Medicine: Controlling Costs and Changing Patient Care: The Role of Utilization Management. Washington, DC, National Academy Press, 1989

Jessor R: Problem Behavior and Psychosocial Development: A Longitudinal Study of Youth. Orlando, FL, Academic, 1977

Joint Committee on the Accreditation of Health Care Organizations: Patient Records in Addiction Treatment: Documenting the Quality of Care. Oakbrook Terrace, IL, Joint Committee on the Accreditation of Health Care Organizations, 1992

Kandel D: Adolescent initiation into stages of drug use, in Longitudinal Research on Drug Use: Empirical Findings and Methodological Issues. Edited by Kandel DB. Washington, DC, Hemisphere-Wiley, 1978a, pp 75–100

Kandel DB: Longitudinal Research on Drug Use: Empirical Findings and Methodological Issues. Washington, DC, Hemisphere-Wiley, 1978b

Kandel D, Logan NA: Patterns of drug use from adolescence to young adulthood, I: periods of risk for initiation, continued use, and discontinuation. Am J Public Health 74:660–666, 1984

Kandel D, Davies M, Karus D, et al: The consequences in young adulthood of adolescent drug involvement. Arch Gen Psychiatry 43:746–754, 1986

Kennedy JA: Fundamentals of Psychiatric Treatment Planning. Washington, DC, American Psychiatric Press, 1992

MacDonald DI, Newton M: The clinical syndrome of adolescent drug use. Adv Pediatr 28:1–25, 1981

McLellan T, Alterman A: Patient treatment matching: a conceptual and methodological review, with suggestions for further research, in Improving Drug Abuse Treatment (DHHS Publ No ADM 91-1754; NIDA Res Monogr 106). Washington, DC, U.S. Government Printing Office, 1991, pp 114–135

McLellan AT, Grissom GR, Zanis D, et al: Problem-service "matching" in addiction treatment: a prospective study in 4 programs. Arch Gen Psychiatry 54:730–735, 1997

Nowinski J: Substance Abuse in Adolescents and Young Adults: A Guide to Treatment. New York, WW Norton, 1990

Owen P, Nyberg L: Assessing alcohol and drug problems among adolescents: current practices. J Drug Educ 13:247-254, 1983

Puig-Antich J: Major depression and conduct disorder in prepuberty. Journal of the American Academy of Child Psychiatry 21:118–128, 1982

Schaefer D: Choices and Consequences. Minneapolis, MN, Johnson Institute Books, 1987

Semlitz L: Adolescent substance abuse treatment and managed care, in Adolescent Substance Abuse and Dual Disorders. Child Adolesc Psychiatr Clin N Am 5:221–241, 1996

Siegel D, Fisher S (eds): Psychiatric Records in Mental Health Care. New York, Brunner/Mazel, 1981

Simpkin D: Levels of substance abuse. Presentation in the Clinical Practicum on Substance Abuse, Annual Meeting of the American Academy of Child and Adolescent Psychiatry, October 20, 1992

Tarter RE: Evaluation and treatment of adolescent substance abuse: a decision tree method. Am J Drug Alcohol Abuse 16:1–46, 1990

Weinberg NZ, Rahdert E, Colliver JD, et al: Adolescent substance abuse: a review of the past 10 years. J Am Acad Child Adolesc Psychiatry 37:252–261, 1998

Wheeler K, Malmquist J: Treatment approaches in adolescent chemical dependency. Pediatr Clin North Am 34:437–447, 1987

Yamaguchi K, Kandel DB: Patterns of drug use from adolescence to young adulthood, II: sequences of progression. Am J Public Health 74:668–672, 1984a

Yamaguchi K, Kandel DB: Patterns of drug use from adolescence to adulthood, III: predictors of progression. Am J Public Health 74:673–681, 1984b

Zoccolillo M, Vitaro F, Tremblay R: Problem drug use in a community sample of adolescents. J Am Acad Child Adolesc Psychiatry 38:900–907, 1999

9 Outpatient Treatment

Todd Wilk Estroff, M.D.

Greater demands are being made on adolescent outpatient substance abuse treatment because permission for inpatient hospitalization is often denied. When authorization is granted, the lengths of stay are usually much shorter. Acute stabilization is often the most that can be accomplished before discharge to the outpatient program. Substance-abusing adolescents must be treated as outpatients when they are denied inpatient treatment. As a consequence, outpatient treatment has expanded to accommodate these more severely impaired teens.

When substance-abusing adolescents enter outpatient treatment, they are sicker, have more severe behavioral problems, are less stable, and have a higher risk of relapse than in previous years. The result is that outpatient treatment programs currently must increase the intensity of treatment to be effective. There are at least five major paths through which these adolescents enter outpatient treatment.

From an Outpatient Evaluation

The first path to outpatient treatment is directly from an outpatient evaluation. The evaluation must determine that the adolescent has a substance abuse problem and that the problem is not life threatening. The procedures for a thorough outpatient evaluation are outlined in Chapter 8 and in the treatment guidelines published by the American Academy of Child and Adolescent Psychiatry (1998; Bruner and Fishman 1998; Bukstein 1997; Weinberg et al. 1998).

From Primary Care Physicians and Other Mental Health Professionals

The second route is from other health care professionals. One of the most frequent contacts substance-abusing adolescents have with physicians is in the emergency department. This occurs when their substance abuse has led to a traumatic injury or overdose or when they become comatose for any reason (Barnett et al. 1998; Dell 1996; Gordon et al. 1996; Loiselle et al. 1993). Emergency department doctors often do not consider the additional diagnosis of substance abuse because they are focused on the immediate problem and are under pressure to get the patients seen and referred out as quickly and inexpensively as possible. Ordering drug or alcohol testing takes time, delays getting the patient out of the department, and is considerably more costly. Even if the emergency department physician orders appropriate toxicologic screening tests, parents and other emergency department personnel who do not believe that drug abuse is a major problem in traumatic injuries often vigorously resist such testing. Emergency department physicians are also vulnerable to criticism because the quality of their care is often judged based on the time the patient spent in the emergency department rather than on a determination of whether additional appropriate diagnostic testing was ordered (Casalino 1999).

Pediatricians, general practitioners, and family physicians also have frequent contact with substance-abusing adolescents. Unfortunately, these professionals often have little or no training in *adult* substance abuse, let alone *adolescent* substance abuse (Loiselle et al. 1993; Parrish 1994; Werner and Adger 1995). They often do not even ask the screening questions that might reveal ongoing abuse for fear of offending the adolescent or his or her parents or guardians. There is a great deal of debate among physicians as to whether all adolescents should have regular drug testing as a part of their annual physical examination.

Other mental health professionals often refer adolescents to outpatient substance abuse treatment when they discover that the teenager's behavioral problems are related to or caused primarily by drug or alcohol abuse. Unfortunately, many social workers and psychologists also get little to no training in the diagnosis and treatment of adolescent substance abuse. The question of when any of the primary care physicians or other mental health workers should seek outside evaluation is complex and controversial. However, I believe that early referral is best and should be made when there is any suspicion of drug abuse.

From Higher Levels of Care

The third route by which adolescents can enter outpatient treatment is through transfer from a higher level of care such as inpatient or residential treatment programs. This transition constitutes a step down in the intensity of treatment and implies that the adolescent has made enough progress to enter outpatient treatment. These adolescents are referred for ongoing treatment to consolidate their therapeutic gains and to promote further progress. If the transition is carried out carefully and all relevant information is passed on and understood by the accepting outpatient program, relapse can be prevented. It is important also to select the most appropriate level of intensity of outpatient treatment for the individual substance-abusing adolescent. Options may include outpatient day hospital treatment, intensive after-school treatment, or aftercare. Enrollment in educational programs alone, when the adolescent has moved down from this level of severity, is generally contraindicated.

From the Courts and Juvenile Justice System

The fourth route of entry into outpatient treatment is from the courts. Once adolescents have been identified by the juvenile justice system, the chances of discovering their substance abuse rise. Often juvenile probation officers and juvenile judges, as a condition of probation or parole, mandate periodic drug testing. This is true even if the adolescents are not on probation for a drug-related offense. This testing often picks up drug abuse that was previously unknown to the parents, probation officer, or judge. Once detected, the adolescents are often sent for treatment at a local mental health center. They are usually mandated to once-a-week drug abuse treatment meetings for an 8–12-week period. Unfortunately, this approach is often ineffective because this intensity of treatment is usually too low for these teens. Frequently, the adolescents do not attend the meetings regularly and the probation officers do little to ensure their attendance even when informed of the teenagers' noncooperation. Other adolescents cooperate, attend the meetings, superficially participate, and bide their time until their mandated treatment is over. Rarely if ever do any of these adolescents voluntarily extend their treatment even if it is clearly indicated. If outpatient treatment fails under these conditions, further juvenile justice consequences, rather than adequate treatment, are likely to be imposed. Substance-abusing adolescents can be sent to a variety of different and progressively more restrictive settings. These programs are usually residential in nature, progressively more punitive, and less therapeutic and include group homes, outdoor therapeutic programs, boot camp, juvenile detention facilities, and the adult criminal justice system.

After Relapse

The fifth route is through a return to outpatient treatment after a mild to moderate relapse. If the relapse is severe, inpatient treatment is probably indicated. The entire issue of relapse—how to identify it and how to treat it—is dealt with in Chapter 15. It is sufficient to say that there are various degrees of relapse, and those that are not severe are best dealt with by further treatment in the outpatient setting.

Treatment Matching

Once the decision is made to treat the substance-abusing adolescent as an outpatient, the intensity of treatment must be selected. This can vary widely depending on the severity of abuse and the actual drugs abused. Multiple attempts have been made to match substance-abusing adolescents to a particular form of therapy. There has been little to no success in predicting who will remain in treatment or who will remain abstinent for long periods of time. Matching treatment to the severity of the substance abuse is an idealized goal that is not verified by research. Because of managed care's insistence that this idea is possible, many substance-abusing adolescents receive treatment at intensities that are neither effective nor realistic.

Levels of Outpatient Treatment

Drug Abuse Education

If the adolescent's substance abuse is found to be minor and is diagnosed at the experimental stage, then attendance at a drug abuse education program once a week may be sufficient treatment (Bailey 1996). This level of treatment is for substance experimenters whose problem is mild and who are having little to no dysfunction in their lives. The treatment provided is basically a series of lectures and group discussions about the dangers of various drugs and their addictive potentials. Most adolescents referred to outpatient drug education need no further intervention and have no further contact with drug abuse treatment providers.

Intensive Treatment After School

The next, more-intensive level is for adolescents who have a substance abuse problem. To be treated at this level, adolescents must be able to successfully attend school and to respond to daily treatment after school. There is a great advantage to these programs because they make certain that the substance-abusing adolescents are supervised after school and before dinner. This is the period of time during which adolescents are most likely to be unsupervised at home and to engage in risky behaviors such as drug abuse and/or sexual activities.

Day Hospital

Adolescents who cannot function at school because of behavioral problems, continued contact with substance-abusing acquaintances, or a previous relapse at a lower level of treatment should be treated in a day hospital setting. This means that they spend their entire day in a treatment setting where they attend school as well as receive treatment. They usually go home at night to their parents and return the next morning. These adolescents are more likely to include dual diagnosis patients and to have a more complicated long-term course.

Residential and Partial Residential Care

Residential care is best viewed as a mixture of inpatient and outpatient treatment. As they make progress, adolescents may go to regular school but must spend the night at the residential treatment center. Effective treatment is intensive, usually in individual, group, and family settings, and occurs after schoolwork and homework are completed. Group homes can also provide this level of care, but it is rare.

Aftercare

As the adolescents continue to make progress, all outpatient treatment merges into a final common pathway designed to maintain lifelong abstinence.

The objective of aftercare is to help the adolescent achieve a stable, pragmatic recovery plan that promotes abstinence. It is appropriate only after the substance-abusing adolescent has made significant progress. Aftercare usually begins when the adolescents have progressed beyond step 5. At this point they realize that they do indeed have a substance abuse disorder, accept the need for treatment, and make a commitment to further introspection and treatment. Few if any adolescent substance abusers should be guided onto this path directly from an initial evaluation. It is much more frequently selected either after a great deal of progress has occurred in an outpatient or an inpatient setting or if the adolescent has finished treatment and has had a minor relapse.

One of the greatest problems is maintaining the continuity of care between each level of treatment and effectively communicating information about the adolescent's history from one treatment provider to the next. Too often, a historical amnesia occurs at the moment of transfer. This is especially true if different agencies are involved and no unified charting and documentation plan is in place. Another problem is that even if the information is well thought out and well documented, clinicians in the receiving program frequently do not bother to read carefully the written information they have been given.

Failure to Respond to Outpatient Treatment

If a teenager fails to respond to or relapses in outpatient treatment, then a relapse evaluation is critical. This is described in further detail in Chapter 15. When this thorough failure analysis is completed, the adolescent can be redirected back into the most appropriate level of outpatient or even inpatient treatment.

If the failure is caused by ill will, such as not attending treatment, failure to take medications, or failure to participate in 12-step meetings, then it is important to determine whether the adolescents are in the wrong system and whether they more appropriately belong in the criminal justice system. This decision should not to be taken lightly because it implies that the adolescent and the substance abuse are essentially untreatable. Before this decision is made, it is important to explain to the adolescent in detail the repercussions of not committing to abstinence. Uncooperative adolescents most often wind up in the criminal justice system.

The courts can provide important leverage, through probation officers and threat of further restraint, to make sure that the adolescent stays in treatment, at least superficially cooperates, and conforms to substance abuse treatment expectations. In addition, the courts may provide the only way to have the adolescent's urine drug screened. Much depends on how enlightened the probation officer is and how sensitive he or she is to issues relating to the causes and treatment of both substance abuse and psychiatric disorders.

Long-Term Treatment Options in the Juvenile Justice System

Outdoor Therapeutic Programs

Although technically not an inpatient institutional treatment, outdoor therapeutic programs or wilderness programs are not as flexible as more classical outpatient treatments. The adolescents are neither voluntary participants nor able to leave as they choose. They are supposed to derive much of their treatment from group interaction and teamwork, which builds competence in caring for themselves and confidence in their ability to be successful. Drug treatment may be a part of an overall focus on decreasing antisocial behaviors. In some settings medications are acceptable and in others they are not.

Boot Camps

In many areas of the United States, juvenile judges send adolescents who are uncooperative or who have relapsed to boot camps. This placement can last for 3 months or longer. It is believed in the juvenile justice system that all teenagers need is a little discipline and that with this discipline they will straighten out. Unfortunately, these boot camps may be more punitive than therapeutic. In my experience very few teens exposed to boot camp implement significant changes in their lives or their lifestyles. They basically bide their time, do the minimum amount of work, and await their eventual release.

In the boot camps there is often little to no appreciation of either the psychiatric or the substance abuse issues that influence the adolescent's behavior. Psychotropic medications are sometimes dispensed, but rarely do these teenagers see a psychiatrist or an addiction medicine specialist. In some states the U.S. Department of Justice has stated that the juvenile justice system not only does not treat the adolescents in its charge but that it actually makes them worse (B.L. Lee, U.S. Department of Justice Civil Rights Division: "Findings of Investigation of State Juvenile Justice Facilities." Written communication to the Honorable Zell Miller, Governor Of Georgia, February 13, 1998; Georgia Mental Health Association, personal communication 1999; National Mental Health Association, personal communication, 1999; "U.S. Sues Louisiana in Move to Reform Its Juvenile Prisons" 1998).

If the adolescent still does not respond, there are three possible options. The first is to repeat the outpatient treatment, possibly at a higher intensity of care, and to demand proof that he or she is attending and cooperating. If this does not happen, then the teenager will be placed in a juvenile detention facility prior to further placement. The second option is to repeat the boot camp experience, but this is even less likely to be helpful than the first time. Third, the adolescent can be incarcerated.

Role of Drug Testing

Regular random supervised drug testing can play another important role in promoting adolescent abstinence. Testing often provides adolescents with an acceptable excuse not to use when other adolescents offer them drugs. They can truthfully respond that they cannot use any drugs because they are being tested and that if they test positive severe consequences will follow. For some teenagers this excuse is much more acceptable than saying that they are sober, working a recovery program, and do not want to relapse. Some adolescents ask to have drug testing continue even when it is no longer clinically necessary because it provides this acceptable rationale for refusing to use drugs.

Essential Therapies

One of the greatest problems with outpatient treatment is that it can be focused too narrowly. By concentrating on one or two issues, treatment may ignore the whole picture. This overly focused approach can preclude consideration of other important factors that actually lead the adolescent to relapse. If outpatient treatment programs are to be successful, they must provide the entire spectrum of therapies needed to treat the substance-abusing adolescent, including but not limited to 12-step treatment, individual psychotherapy, family therapy, group therapy, drug education, educational remediation, socialization, peer selection, and judicious use of medications. These therapies are described in greater detail elsewhere in this book. In all of these settings 12-step treatment plays a central role.

Summary

Financial and policy decisions have placed greater demands on outpatient programs to treat sicker substance-abusing adolescents. There are five possible pathways into outpatient treatment: 1) from outpatient evaluation, 2) from primary care physicians and other mental health professionals, 3) from higher levels of care, 4) from the juvenile justice system, and 5) after minor relapses. Treatment intensity must be carefully chosen to best meet the individual adolescent's needs. Outpatient treatment options include education, intensive after-school treatment, day hospitalization, and aftercare. Treatment matching remains unproven, although it should be attempted. Those individuals who fail to remain abstinent require a thorough relapse evaluation followed by further inpatient or outpatient treatment or referral back to the criminal justice system if they are determined to be untreatable. Urine drug screening and a wide spectrum of treatments that support 12-step treatment programs are more likely to be successful.

References

American Academy of Child and Adolescent Psychiatry: Summary of the practice parameters for the assessment and treatment of children and adolescents with substance use disorders. J Am Acad Child Adolesc Psychiatry 37:122–126, 1998

Bailey GW: Helping the resistant adolescent enter substance abuse treatment. Child Adolesc Psychiatr Clin N Am 5:149–164, 1996

Barnett NP, Spirito A, Colby SM, et al: Detection of alcohol use in adolescent patients in the emergency department. Acad Emerg Med 5:607–612, 1998

Bruner AE, Fishman M: Adolescents and illicit drug use. JAMA 280:597–598, 1998

Bukstein O: Practice parameters for the assessment and treatment of children and adolescents with substance use disorders. American Academy of Child and Adolescent Psychiatry. J Am Acad Child Adolesc Psychiatry 36 (10, suppl):140S–156S, 1997

Casalino LP: The unintended consequences of measuring quality on the quality of medical care. N Engl J Med 341:1147–1150, 1999

Dell ML: Medical considerations in child and adolescent substance abuse. Child Adolesc Psychiatr Clin N Am 5:123–147, 1996

Gordon S, Toepper WC, Blackman SC: Toxicology screening in adolescent trauma. Pediatr Emerg Care 12:36–39, 1996

Loiselle JM, Baker MD, Templeton JM, et al: Substance abuse in adolescent trauma. Ann Emerg Med 22:1530–1534, 1993

Parrish SK: Adolescent substance abuse: the challenge for clinicians. Alcohol 11:453–455, 1994

U.S. Sues Louisiana in move to reform its juvenile prisons. Orange County Register 6 November 1998

Weinberg NZ, Rahdert E, Colliver JD, et al: Adolescent substance abuse: a review of the past 10 years. J Am Acad Child Adolesc Psychiatry 37:252–261, 1998

Werner MJ, Adger H Jr: Early identification, screening, and brief intervention for adolescent alcohol use. Arch Pediatr Adolesc Med 49:1241–1248, 1995

10 Inpatient Programs

R. Jeremy A. Stowell, M.D.
Todd Wilk Estroff, M.D.

The success of the inpatient treatment of substance-abusing adolescents is measured by ongoing abstinence after completion of treatment and how functional and productive these adolescents are once they become drug free (Dobkin et al. 1998). This chapter addresses the treatment of adolescents whose addiction and/or comorbid psychiatric conditions require inpatient treatment as defined under level IV of the American Society of Addiction Medicine (ASAM) patient placement criteria (American Society of Addiction Medicine 1996; Hoffmann et al. 1987, 1991). Given the complexity of the issues that must be addressed in the typical adolescent requiring inpatient treatment, a specialized evaluation and treatment program capable of providing comprehensive treatment is required. This chapter focuses on the details of establishing and operating an inpatient treatment unit designed to treat this severe population. The following is an idealized description of a program designed to provide optimal care for these adolescents. We try to ignore managed care pressures and other financial constraints that would compromise the efficacy of the program until the last section of the chapter, in which we explain how even the best-run treatment program is modified in a managed care environment.

Setting Up an Inpatient Substance Abuse Unit

When an inpatient substance abuse program for adolescents is set up, the treatment philosophy should be clearly stated. These programs characteristically embrace a dual diagnosis approach in which psychiatric and substance use disorders are treated concurrently. They are more correctly classified as multiple-problem programs because the typical adolescent in these intensive programs has multiple problems including substance abuse/dependence, a range of psychiatric conditions, medical complications, developmental delays, educational deficits, poor or improper socialization, and a lack of effective coping abilities. Many of these adolescents are victims of repeated physical, sexual, and emotional abuse. Because many of these adolescents come from families in which multiple generations have exhibited significant alcohol or other drug abuse, the program must also be prepared to deal with the adolescent's dysfunctional family. Generally, the adolescents served in these programs are 13–18 years of age.

Although adolescents characteristically fall within a spectrum of substance abuse ranging from isolated experimentation to abuse and on to full-blown dependence, most of the severely afflicted adolescents treated in inpatient programs have alcohol and drug use patterns comparable with those of many adults. For these adolescents, experimentation with alcohol and drugs may have begun as early as elementary school; by the time they require inpatient treatment, the adolescents may have had years of relatively heavy use.

Most adolescents who abuse or who become dependent on mind-altering drugs experience major changes in their moods, personalities, and behaviors. Medical complications may also occur; these tend to arise either from the direct effects of alcohol and other drugs or indirectly as a result of trauma incurred during intoxication. Thus, the ability to perform a thorough medical examination and to address significant medical conditions is a basic requirement of an inpatient level IV adolescent treatment unit. The medical staff must be experienced in treating adolescents and addressing their unique needs.

Substance abuse by itself can produce symptoms that are indistinguishable from psychiatric disorders. In addition, psychiatric conditions independent of substance abuse are prevalent in the adolescent population. One of the critical tasks of the treatment program is to accurately distinguish between primary and secondary psychiatric disorders. One way of making this distinction is based on the chronology of the development of symptoms and behaviors. Primary psychiatric disorders often precede substance abuse or persist long after abstinence has been achieved. Secondary psychiatric disorders usually begin after the start of substance abuse and tend to abate with abstinence. Distinguishing between primary and secondary psychiatric conditions is not the only critical diagnostic determination. The program must also be able to correctly identify the symptoms that mimic psychiatric disorders but are caused by addictions and to identify psychiatric disorders that mimic the behaviors indicative of addictions.

The adolescent's functioning may be impeded by a range of learning disabilities or a lack of educational attainment due to substance abuse. Learning disabilities, reading difficulties, and functioning below expected grade level are common in this population. Therefore, not only must individualized treatment take such problems into account in the addiction or abuse treatment plan but the program also must be able to provide remedial and special educational services.

Substance-abusing adolescents also experience problems in their spiritual development. This is often correlated with the degree of psychological trauma seen clinically in both the adolescent and his or her family members. Addressing spiritual deficits can enhance the overall treatment outcome. In this context, the term *spiritual* is not to be confused with religion or faith-based programs embedded within a given religion. The term *spirituality* in the treatment context is closer to Eastern philosophies that involve the search for inner peace and tranquility. It also tends to be more closely associated with a sense of connection to a group or philosophy beyond the isolated self. The concept of spirituality is more fully developed in Chapter 14.

The level IV adolescent substance abuse inpatient unit provides specialized treatment using the combined skills of psychiatrists, other physicians, nurses, psychologists, other mental health workers, social workers, substance abuse counselors, individual and family therapists, group therapists, recreational therapists, educational diagnosticians, and teachers. It is useful to have a mix of recovering and nonrecovering treatment staff. The unit itself needs to be set up and maintained using firm behavioral controls to ensure that the patients have a drug-free environment in which to recover. Treatment modalities include individual and group counseling, family therapy, psychopharmacological treatment, family education about addictions, specialized activity programs, and recreational therapy. Educational evaluations, special education services, and an accredited school program are critical. Participation in 12-step programs such as Alcoholics Anonymous and Narcotics Anonymous is also essential to the success of the program.

It is important to set up the program correctly from the very beginning. Treatment failures can and will result if the program is begun without anticipating the myriad ways in which adolescent patients can manipulate staff and sabotage their own treatment. A lack of structure and programming makes it much easier for drugs, alcohol, and other contraband to flow undetected into the unit. For this reason, most individuals involved in treating severe adolescent substance abuse and dual-diagnosis patients prefer to have a locked unit. Patients must not be permitted to leave the unit undetected; all windows and screens must be secured in such a way that patients cannot disassemble them and exit the hospital in search of drugs or alcohol. The staff must be on constant watch for any signs of tampering with the windows and screens. Bedroom and bathroom fixtures and furniture should be regularly inspected to decrease the risk of escape and to prevent patients from hiding drugs or sharp objects with which they can harm themselves or staff members. If any irregularities are found, they must be attended to immediately to prevent potentially dangerous problems.

Any unusual event or behavior pattern must be regarded as a possible sign that the adolescents are sabotaging their treatment. This sabotage may be accomplished through nonparticipation, rule violations, or disruptive actions. It can also occur when adolescents plot secretly to destroy property in the treatment unit. The nursing and staff protocols should be such that a daily check is made for any broken furniture or fixtures and for holes in screens. Such protocols ensure that safety is constantly maintained on the unit.

Any unusual odors must be investigated as possible signs of marijuana, solvent, or other drug abuse. Fragrances or perfumes may be used to cover up the use of drugs. If the index of suspicion is high enough, urine drug screens should be performed and physical searches of the patients and their rooms should be conducted. On rare occasions it may be necessary to call in local law enforcement personnel with dogs trained to sniff out illegal substances. Although such measures may seem draconian to the inexperienced observer, failure to have adequate response contingencies in place poses a serious threat to the integrity of the unit and the safety of both staff and patients.

Because substance-abusing adolescents are accustomed to living in a chaotic and uncontrolled manner, it is important to provide structure for them. One of the most effective ways to do this is by establishing written unit rules and regulations that are simple, clear, and concise. A behavior modification program should be based on a daily point system, level program, or both to monitor the patients' progress in treatment and provide them with immediate feedback about their behavior. The program should be designed so that the patients progressively earn more privileges as they move through the treatment program. It is important to have a program that employs positive reinforcement and to avoid using negative reinforcement and punitive measures. On some occasions adolescents will behave violently or dangerously, and it is important to have a "time-out" system in place.

Having the adolescent substance abuse unit separate from a comparable adult unit is recommended for several reasons. Many adolescents who are heavily abusing substances have not fallen into the full pattern of severe addictive behavior. If they are mixed with adult patients, they often learn new and undesirable skills that were previously not in their repertoire. The developmental and educational needs of the adolescents require specialized services that are not part of the typical adult unit. The therapeutic needs, socialization issues, and family relationships of the adolescents are also quite different from those of most adult patients.

Adolescent substance-abusing patients tend to live with their parents and are dependent on them for support and emotional reassurance to a much greater extent than adult patients. Much greater emphasis must be placed on restoring family relationships as well as habilitating the patient to higher levels of functioning than previously achieved. This is quite different from the goal of rehabilitating previously higher-functioning adults.

Adolescent patients are much more likely to respond to peer pressure than are adult patients. The importance of peers cannot be overstated. Peer pressure is a major influence on adolescents. It is critically important to maintain positive peer pressure on the unit directed toward recovery (Morrison and Smith 1987; Smith and Margolis 1991). For all of these reasons, it is important to have a separate and specialized adolescent substance treatment unit with a dual diagnosis approach to enhance the probability of treatment success.

Environmental Change

Along with the locked unit and behavior modification, it is often important to change the patients' environment and behavior to separate them from the drug culture. This can include a change in personal habits, including his or her overall appearance, clothes, and hairstyle. Several programs insist on a change in music away from "drug-oriented music." Some programs ban video music channels such as MTV from being shown to patients while in the hospital. Although these measures may be extreme, it is important to screen out music and literature associated with drugs, suicide, and self-destructive behaviors. Some patients may be involved in unusual cults, including Satanism, and these activities should be discouraged. In short, any behavior or belief that may be associated with drug abuse or the drug culture is usually vigorously discouraged in successful treatment programs.

Habilitation

Many patients suffer a developmental lag or arrest starting around the same time as their drug abuse. They may be chronologically much older than their immature or impulsive behavior would indicate. Adult programs focus on rehabilitation, the goal of which is to help patients return to their previous functioning levels. Most severely affected adolescents have never functioned well, and the focus of adolescent programs is on habilitation. This is accomplished by teaching the adolescents new living skills and new ways of coping with situations; they are encouraged to identify and think about their emotions before they act on them, to think about the consequences of their actions, and to choose the most appropriate action before taking any action at all. These skills are particularly useful for decisions about how to deal with their parents, boyfriends and girlfriends, and situations in school settings.

One of the most important tasks of the habilitation effort is asking patients to develop new attitudes and methods for handling stress. Patients are asked to change from an immediate short-term gratification orientation to a longer-term perspective in which they consider distant goals and objectives. They are also encouraged to find new ways of enjoying themselves without using drugs. This effort can include exposing patients to a wide variety of recreational activities as well as helping them find new creative outlets that will help substitute for the instant gratification and quick high of drugs.

Staffing an Adolescent Substance Abuse Program

As noted previously, a quality level IV inpatient program requires a diverse group of professionals to address the full range of problems and issues presented by this challenging adolescent patient population. The question of diversity extends to cultural competency and the optimal mix of recovering and nonrecovering staff.

The question of using recovering versus nonrecovering staff has been intensely debated. Arguments are persuasive on both sides. We suggest that the best way to staff this type of unit is to use staff who approach patients from different vantage points. Recovering staff members may be better able to pick up certain subtleties of the substance abuse disorder, whereas nonrecovering staff members are better able to diagnose behavioral and psychiatric problems. Regular staff meetings to help the unit work smoothly and efficiently and without rancor are encouraged. We believe that combined perspectives provide a more comprehensive treatment approach.

Leadership

The primary leadership in a level IV dual-diagnosis program usually rests with the medical director, the program director, and the nurse manager. There may also be a counselor who is designated as the chief substance abuse coordinator.

Medical Director

The minimal standard for the medical director position in our opinion is that this physician be a psychiatrist, preferably one trained in child or adolescent psychiatry as well as trained and certified in addiction medicine or addiction psychiatry. Failing that, an adult psychiatrist who is fully versed in the evaluation and treatment of substance abuse disorders may be acceptable, especially if that person works closely with experienced psychologists, social workers, nurses, or other clinicians trained in adolescent substance abuse treatment.

It is important that the medical director be available to advise and supervise other attending physicians and be familiar with as many patients on the unit as possible. The medical director should also be available to treatment teams, for inservice education, and for consultation on the day-to-day operations of the unit.

Program Director

A program director is usually necessary, especially if the medical director can give only a limited amount of time to the unit. The program director should be a full-time employee and should be an experienced mental health professional who has experience in both adolescent substance abuse and psychiatric disorders. The program director may be a psychologist, social worker, or senior counselor. A masters degree and certification in substance abuse counseling (Certified Addictions Professional [CAP], Certified Addictions Counselor [CAC], Certified Substance Abuse Professional [CSAP]) is desirable. It should be emphasized, however, that experience in treating substance-abusing adolescents is far more important than any other factor in the selection of a program director.

The program director and medical director must work in tandem and rely on each other's expertise and judgment. They should discuss program and patient issues on a regular basis. Disagreements should be worked out in a manner that discourages staff splitting and dissension. If either the program director or the medical director is a recovering individual, he or she can help set a positive tone for substance abuse recovery. It is also important for both the medical director and the program director to understand and agree that psychiatric medications can be useful in carefully evaluated cases.

Nurse Manager

The nursing staff members play a critical role on the adolescent substance abuse unit and are the only staff members that have 24-hour contact with the patients. Nurses provide initial assessments and help with medical monitoring of the patients, medications, evaluations, and treatment. In general, the nursing staff ensures that quality medical treatment is provided. These staff members enforce the behavioral program. They must have a tough, no-nonsense approach to the patients while simultaneously having a therapeutic and understanding manner.

The nurse manager must work closely with the program director and medical director in both treatment planning and the day-to-day operation of the unit. Nursing staff can provide a means of ensuring continuity and communication among the diverse treatment team.

Other Staff

The social work staff plays a key role in helping to obtain the most detailed understanding of the patient's family history and dynamics. These staff members participate regularly in the staffing and treatment team meetings and help to set reasonable individual and family goals as well as aftercare planning.

Adolescent drug abuse counselors are vital to the program's success but it can be very difficult to find qualified individuals who possess in-depth experience treating substance-abusing adolescents. These counselors are often recovering individuals who can relate their own struggles to become abstinent to the adolescents. They can also give valuable suggestions for the adolescent's recovery. It is important to help these counselors understand and support the use of psychiatric treatments and medication when such treatment is appropriate.

Recreational therapists also play an important role on the unit. One of their primary functions is to show the patients how to have a good time without getting high. They also help the adolescents with relaxation techniques, stress management, control of aggressive tendencies, and to better cope with drug urges when they occur. Physical exercise once or twice per day during the hospitalization helps prevent emotional outbursts and allows the adolescents to focus more on their treatment. Recreational therapy exercises that emphasize trust and learning about oneself are often an invaluable adjunct to treatment.

Educational specialists have a major role because a significant block of time during treatment is spent in the school environment. Most substance-abusing adolescents have had difficulties in school. Many have failed or have dropped out of school all together. They often have undiagnosed learning disabilities or have a number of special education requirements. A special education teacher rounds out the treatment team and can help to identify and remediate these academic failures. The education staff can provide a sense of hope as well as improved self-esteem for such adolescents, who in the past had little expectation of success or mastery.

Outside Physicians and Therapists

It is advisable to keep the staff on the adolescent substance abuse treatment unit as cohesive and consistent as possible, allowing adolescents to work with key staff members on a daily basis. When outside physicians and therapists are used, the medical staff is an open model. It is mandatory to educate these staff members thoroughly about the unit's expectations and guidelines, including attendance at treatment teams. Often it is not possible for outside therapists or other physicians to participate actively in the team approach. When this is the case, it may be useful for that outside therapist to turn over control of the patient's care while the adolescent is on the unit. This can become a ticklish problem if the outside mental health professional feels threatened. Usually these issues can be worked out with a frank and open discussion of the issues involved.

Unitary Rounds

Once the leadership is in place, it is mandatory that clear and effective communication take place as frequently as possible. We have found that one effective method is by having unitary rounds daily for the treatment staff and patients combined. Staff members from all disciplines attend these rounds. All routine work for the day is evaluated and divided up at that time in accordance with the various roles of the regular treatment staff as outlined above. The adolescents are also given specific therapeutic work assignments. Results from the previous day's assignments are reported and a daily assessment of the patients' progress is made. If a patient is not making sufficient progress, he or she can be confronted about resistance to treatment and the need to improve. If the unitary rounds process is effective, the treatment plan for each patient is clear and unambiguous. It also allows staff daily opportunity to identify, address, and correct any distortions, attempts at manipulation, staff splitting, or other problems on the unit. It is also easier to spot problems of failure in therapeutic assignments and for the united staff to react appropriately. Some consequences may include a drop in level or restriction in privileges. An alternative approach to unitary rounds may involve staffings and rounds with the members of the treatment team twice or three times a week on each patient.

Behavioral Management

As outlined above, most of the burden of behavioral management falls on the nursing staff, counselors, and mental health workers. It is important to have a unit rule handbook that clearly and simply spells out the expected behaviors.

No matter how well the program is working, conflicts will occasionally arise between patients and staff. This is to be expected. Patients will test the willpower and the resolve of the staff in an attempt to identify any inconsistencies or weaknesses. Such testing of limits should be dealt with therapeutically by the staff at the time of the incident and then again in individual therapy with the specific adolescent. If the level of disruptive behavior is severe, it may result in placing the patient in time-out or, in the case of a particularly disruptive patient, on "relapse status." When on relapse status, adolescents are isolated from other patients and activities so that they can concentrate on their resistance to treatment and can begin to earn their way back to full treatment status. This particular limit setting is critical, especially among substance-abusing adolescents who have been out of control or violent. Associated family work will help the parents provide disciplinary consistency as well as help them impose limits compatible with the inpatient program. It also restores the parental model of rules and guidelines to which they will return when discharged.

Naturally, when consequences are imposed by the staff it is important that these consequences are logical and related specifically to the adolescent's behavior and actions. Arbitrary actions are counterproductive and are to be avoided whenever possible. Reflexive, illogical, or punitive staff actions often erode the trust that has been built up between the patient and the treatment program.

After abnormal, disruptive, or self-defeating behavior occurs, it is important to follow-up with an analysis of the causes of the behavior and the negative impact that it may have had on both the patient and the therapeutic community. It is important to address the patient's behavior in the individual treatment plan as well as in the community at large. On occasion, a separate community meeting must be called to discuss the abnormal behavior. The adolescents and staff members use this meeting as an opportunity for growth.

Behavior Modification

A behavior modification program that uses a point system is designed to increase appropriate behaviors and to decrease inappropriate behaviors during and after treatment. It allows the substance-abusing adolescent to meet the specific expectations of the treatment team. A properly administered point system ensures that a therapeutic milieu will be maintained despite changes in personnel or the whims of an individual staff member. It incorporates a consistent set of simple and explicitly stated behavioral expectations and consequences that positively reinforce therapeutic behaviors and extinguish inappropriate behavior. The point system is explained to the parents and patient by a staff member and/or a senior peer in the community at the time of the adolescent's admission to the unit. A daily point total is recorded by the nursing staff and is used to decide the level of treatment for each patient. The past and current record of points earned for appropriate behavior and consequences levied for inappropriate behaviors is a good way to measure the progress of each patient. Each patient must earn a designated number of points to be eligible for privileges and to be able to advance to the next level. One of us (R.J.A.S.) is involved in a program in which patients must obtain at least 85 points per day out of 100 possible points to be eligible to receive privileges. The privileges themselves often depend on the phase or level of treatment achieved by the adolescent. The levels of treatment may be designated as

Level I: Admission
Level II: Compliance
Level III: Acceptance
Level IV: Recovery maintenance and discharge planning

Alternatively, a level system may be designed as part of the behavior modification program. In this system, the adolescents must reach a specific step in the 12-step program, such as step 4 (i.e., "We made a searching and fearless inventory of ourselves"), to receive privileges.

Level I is the orientation and admission status wherein adolescents show responsibility for taking part in all community activities, identify themselves as substance abusers, and begin to work on their first step in the 12-step program. Privileges associated with this level include parental visiting and making supervised telephone calls to parents.

Level II is a treatment phase in which the substance-abusing adolescent presents his or her first step in the appropriate group therapy session, receives feedback from other group members, and demonstrates a willingness to explore his or her perceptions and feelings about step 1. Privileges at this level include having a radio or headset in their rooms, two supervised telephone calls, and a later bedtime.

In level III, patients accept their substance abuse disorders and learn to identify their own major defense mechanisms when used, to confront others appropriately, and to identify how their disease has inhibited them in their maturation and overall development. In this phase, there should be clear evidence of the patients' ability to be honest with themselves and others, to articulate their feelings, and to formulate their own treatment goals. Adolescents in this phase of treatment should demonstrate areas of clear progress in all of their therapeutic work. Privileges at this level involve several phone calls to parents and other family members, including contact with a sponsor or another person in a 12-step program. Visitation is more liberal and bedtime is 30 minutes later. Adolescents may go to classes and activities unescorted.

In the final phase, level IV, the adolescent helps develop a written aftercare plan and shares this in a group with the other patients in treatment. This aftercare plan emphasizes recovery goals in both psychiatric and substance abuse areas, the ability to identify signs and symptoms of relapse, and appropriate steps to take. The level IV patient has a knowledge and understanding of the first three steps in the 12-step program and at this point should have demonstrated willingness to speak up in a 12-step meeting. Added privileges in this phase include leaving the unit without staff escort, having appropriate therapeutic passes with the approval of the treatment team, and a later (30 minutes) bedtime. Phone calls during this phase of treatment are more liberal and may include calls to selected peers approved by the treatment team. It should be emphasized that the daily point system and earning the 85 points per day for the required behaviors is essential for progress. If the points are not obtained for 2 days in a row then the patient is placed back on the previous level.

It is important to have a list of unacceptable behaviors available either in a handbook or handout on the unit. Unacceptable behaviors include assaultive behavior, destruction of property, drug intoxication, possession of contraband, being in the room of another patient when it is not authorized, stealing, verbal abuse, offensive language, sexual contact, being in an unauthorized area, and being absent without approved leave. There is no smoking on the unit; thus, having cigarettes is also unacceptable. Noncompliance with treatment is not tolerated. For instance, refusal to attend a scheduled activity or complete school assignments and any disruptive behaviors result in consequences decided by the treatment team. These consequences may range from therapeutic time-out to seclusion, social restriction, or probationary status in which all privileges are lost and bedtime is 1 hour earlier. If noncompliance continues for 2 days, a level drop occurs as previously described.

The written program description should be given to the adolescent and his or her parents at admission. It should include a careful explanation of how the program is scheduled, the treatment objectives, and the behavior modification system.

Unit Freeze

On occasion, many patients on the unit may band together to oppose all treatment efforts and to attempt to ruin the therapeutic environment for every patient. The entire unit at that time may be placed on "relapse status" or a unit freeze. The purpose of this is to reestablish the effectiveness of the treatment milieu. It forces the adolescents to examine their own resistance to treatment and to confront those peers who are trying to undermine the treatment process for themselves and others. Parents must be called and informed of the unit freeze. All patients are restricted to the unit and an early bedtime is imposed. No meals are eaten off the unit and there are no off-unit activities. All privileges are suspended and no therapeutic passes are given. Visitors and telephone calls are not allowed. The television and radio are off-limits. The patients are given therapeutic assignments to work on during this time. Frequent therapy sessions lasting 2–8 hours/day focus on the patients' resistance to treatment and on how to resume work on their therapeutic issues. For those patients who do not respond to this measure a complete reevaluation is indicated, and other treatment options must be explored. Discharge may be necessary for those adolescents who instigate or perpetuate the negative therapeutic environment on the unit.

Psychotherapies

A wide variety of therapies is provided in a level IV program. These therapies should embrace both the psychiatric and substance abuse treatment areas. The unit relies heavily on group therapies, which may be divided into psychologically oriented groups and specialized substance abuse and chemical dependence groups. We recommend two to three group sessions per day, one a more traditionally oriented group therapy and the other a substance abuse treatment group. These group sessions should be conducted 7 days/week. The length of each group session should be 1–1½ hours. The traditional psychotherapy groups should have multiple goals that include reducing symptoms, reducing interpersonal and social dysfunction, improving communication skills, improving treatment attitude and behavior, enhancing trust, reducing "acting out behaviors," reducing self-defeating behavioral patterns, connecting behaviors and feelings, developing insight into impaired areas of adolescent identity and self-concept, and processing past and present trauma.

The substance abuse groups are usually divided into educational groups, 12-step groups (including Alcoholic Anonymous, Narcotics Anonymous, Cocaine Anonymous, and Co-dependent Anonymous), and substance abuse process groups. The objectives are to understand the patients' substance abuse and/or dependence and how it relates to their psychosocial problems. The groups are designed to help decrease denial and improve the possibility for a full recovery. Codependency groups and children of alcoholics groups are very important, and meetings should occur at least once per week.

Individual therapy helps patients understand the emotional, behavioral, and substance abuse problems that led to treatment. Individual therapy can be conducted by a qualified psychiatrist, clinical psychologist, clinical social worker, or other licensed clinician three or four times per week. The number of individual psychotherapy sessions is determined by the adolescent's needs in each particular case. Individual therapy is often focused on symptom reduction, such as reducing depression and anxiety, understanding maladaptive patterns of behavior, and improving overall psychosocial adjustment. Areas of resistance are explored and family conflicts are reviewed in detail. It is important for the therapist to try to tailor the individual treatment to the objectives of the adolescent substance abuse program. The individual therapist can also explore areas of coexisting psychopathology with the substance use disorder that could interfere with recovery or precipitate relapse.

Family psychotherapy is a vital part of the overall treatment program. It is desirable for all adult and adolescent family members to be involved in once- or twice-weekly therapy. This therapy should evaluate whether the family is dysfunctional and whether it is a significant factor contributing to the pathology in the substance-abusing adolescent. One of the goals of family treatment is to restore and maintain healthy family functioning. In most programs, family education groups provide information to parents and other family members about the drugs that their adolescents are abusing. The reasons why each drug is dangerous and addicting are reviewed as are the signs of relapse. Parents are educated about how they can help promote their child's recovery. Information is given on how to handle home contracts with their adolescents in preparation for discharge. Multifamily groups, in which all patients' families are invited to participate, focus on shared mutual concerns, problems, and therapeutic issues. The entire family therapy component of treatment usually requires a 5–6-hour/week time commitment by the family members. Parental resistance can be reduced by explaining to the family members that this time can make the difference between sustained abstinence and relapse.

Coordinating the therapies listed above is often difficult. At least two or three team meetings per week in which all treatment professionals are present is helpful. A number of details must be worked out, especially if specific authorization for each therapy is required by an insurance company. For example, limitations are frequently placed on the amount of individual and group therapies that are reimbursed. It is important to determine which therapies are authorized for payment and who will perform them. If the clinical needs of the patient exceed the services authorized, then it may be useful to contact the insurance company for additional authorization of services. In any case, the clinical needs of the patient must be met independent of the reimbursement.

Staff Training and Development

Staff training and development is another important part of ensuring the quality of the level IV program. It is important to maintain a good mix of recovering and nonrecovering staff. On occasion, this mix of staff can lead to intrastaff conflicts. Regular meetings of the treatment team along with staff development meetings are important to reduce friction.

Recovering staff are often attracted to this type of treatment program, but there are some risks. For instance, boundary issues can develop in which recovering staff members become excessively involved in the treatment issues of individual adolescent patients. There is a danger that they may overgeneralize from their own recovery experiences to the point of clouding their therapeutic objectivity. Because of this, it is important to carefully monitor staff members in the early stages of recovery and to have an educational mechanism for addressing these issues as rapidly as possible when they arise.

Nonrecovering staff members have their own potential problems. They may not operate on as intense an emotional level as recovering staff, and it may be difficult for them to empathize with substance-abusing adolescents at the "gut" level. Nonrecovering staff may unintentionally hinder the adolescent's treatment because they tend to believe what the adolescent says rather than focus on the adolescent's actions.

In all cases it is useful to have regular staff development meetings to process problems identified in these areas. When both recovering and nonrecovering staff learn to listen to each other's information and knowledge, each discipline enhances the treatment on the unit.

Regular educational programs focusing on difficult case presentations, accompanied by selected articles from the literature and selected books, assist greatly in staff development. Continuing education programs and workshops should be provided to facilitate such development.

School

School is an integral part of the hospital day for adolescent patients. All educational efforts are integrated into the overall treatment plan. The teacher coordinates the educational aspects of the individual adolescent's program. This routinely begins with an educational evaluation that includes determining the patient's intellectual strengths and weakness and measuring achievement levels, learning aptitudes, perceptual development, and possible learning disabilities. The director of education communicates with the school system to identify educational problem areas and special educational needs. The educational staff usually assists with a smooth transition back to community-based school. It is particularly important to diagnose and remediate learning disabilities that can contribute to negative self-concept and behaviors.

Other Treatment Areas

Activity and recreational therapies use a wide range of activities to create positive changes in the physical, social, cognitive, and emotional functioning of adolescents. Depending on the needs of the patients, activities therapy can help improve functional abilities, teach new leisure skills, facilitate social interactions, and help remediate perceptual motor dysfunction. Usually, activities therapy takes place within—but is not limited to—a group setting. Individual sessions can be conducted to enhance areas of self-esteem, self-awareness, trust, leisure time enjoyment, and physical self-image. Many programs incorporate art and music therapy into the therapeutic evaluation and recovery process. Work in these artistic areas can uncover repressed material that can help with understanding the adolescent's defenses and ego strengths. Both art and music therapy can help measure a patient's progression in treatment.

12-Step Recovery

We believe that 12-step recovery groups can be a critical component of recovery. Depending on the length of treatment, it is hoped that adolescents will work on the first four steps while they are on the inpatient unit and day partial hospital program. Regular attendance at 12-step recovery meetings at the hospital or in the community is expected. It is well documented that when adolescents continue their 12-step meetings after leaving the hospital the likelihood of maintaining abstinence is greater (Bergmann et al. 1995; Harrison and Hoffmann 1987). Adolescents usually attend community 12-step meetings accompanied by a staff member. Toward the end of their hospital stay, they are asked go to a meeting while they are out on a pass and to find a temporary sponsor. They are expected to attend 12-step meetings regularly on an outpatient basis. Parents and significant others in the home are strongly encouraged to attend 12-step meetings as well. A useful tool for helping adolescents understand the 12-step process is the *Step Workbook for Adolescent Chemical Dependence Recovery: A Guide to the First Five Steps,* which is a guide intended to help teenagers to work the first five steps of their own 12-step substance abuse treatment program (Jaffe 1990).

Discharge Planning

Discharge planning, regardless of the length of stay, is critical to ensure abstinence and continuing recovery of the adolescent. One of the most important tools is the "home contract," which documents in writing the behaviors expected of the adolescent and the consequences for both the patient and his or her family of not complying. The home contract should include

- Total abstinence from all mind-altering drugs
- Attendance at scheduled aftercare meetings
- Participation in 12-step recovery meetings, including locating and using a sponsor
- Weekly random supervised urine drug screens
- Participation in individual, group, and family therapy as recommended by the treatment team
- Compliance with rules and specific guidelines at home such as agreements about friends, curfew hours, chores, homework, and other mutually agreed upon expectations
- Clearly defined consequences if there is a breach of contract, including restrictions such as not leaving home, no television or radio or stereo, earlier bedtime, time-out, loss of use of the car, or even readmission to the hospital when indicated

Any breach of the home contract made at the time of discharge should be reviewed by the family, the adolescent, and the primary therapist. Decisions should be made on a case by case basis. Frequently, more intensive treatment is needed.

Selected Areas of Concern

Several areas of added concern exist for substance-abusing adolescent inpatients, including coexisting psychiatric illness; aggression and violence; suicide risk; and the impact of managed care on lengths of stay.

Coexisting Psychiatric Illness

Substance-abusing adolescent inpatients have a high rate of coexisting psychiatric illness (Bukstein et al. 1989, 1992; Deas-Nesmith et al. 1998; Deykin et al. 1992; Hovens et al. 1994; Stowell and Estroff 1992). The essential practical point is that when substance-abusing adolescents enter inpatient treatment, their substance use and psychiatric disorders should be evaluated simultaneously and the treatment implications thereof should be recognized.

Aggression and Violence

Special consideration is given to individuals who are aggressive and potentially violent. An aggressive or violent adolescent on the unit demands immediate and effective intervention. From a practical standpoint, it is imperative to have staff members who are trained to handle out-of-control and violent adolescents. Seclusion, restraints, and appropriate medication such as hydroxyzine, lorazepam, or haloperidol may be used on an immediate basis. Therapeutic processing after an aggressive or violent outburst is critical in addition to setting up appropriate behavioral management techniques. Neurological and neuropsychological testing is useful in determining the etiology of certain types of aggressive behavior.

The association between the abuse of alcohol and other drugs and aggressive and violent behavior is multifactorial (Horowitz et al. 1992). This problem emphasizes the need for multimodal strategies of intervention and prevention. A complex interaction occurs between a particular drug's pharmacological effects and its dosages, the psychological and biological characteristics of substance-using individuals, and the situational context in which the violent event occurs. Substance abuse among fathers, especially abuse of substances other than alcohol, is important in predicting severe aggression and conduct disorder among their adolescent children (Moss and Tarter 1993).

Suicide

It is important to recognize the higher frequency of completed suicide among substance-abusing adolescents. The typical adolescent at risk for suicide in the United States is a white male who is likely to be intoxicated and to commit suicide using a firearm without ever seeking treatment (Gabel and Shindledecker 1993). Psychopathologies such as depression, conduct disorder, and personality disorder accompanied by precipitating events are frequently present, especially in the presence of substance abuse or dependence. Emerging recognition of dual-diagnosis patients may prevent potential suicides by identifying and treating the coexisting psychiatric disorder contributing to this higher risk of suicide.

The prevalence of depressive disorders among substance-abusing adolescents is three times that reported for nonreferred groups of similar age (Kaminer 1992). There is also a much higher incidence of adolescents who have been abused emotionally, physically, and sexually during their childhoods. All of these factors must be carefully evaluated in the process of working with depressed, suicidal, and substance-abusing adolescents.

Managed Care

A final area of concern is the impact of managed care on the length of stay in this type of treatment program. Across the country, the lengths of inpatient psychiatric stay for adolescents have decreased from several weeks down to 1 week or less. The impact and implications of this are formidable. Refusal to pay for extended inpatient care has forced a reconceptualization of the delivery of services for this type of adolescent population (Dobkin et al. 1998). Three types of substance-abusing adolescents are currently being admitted: those who are evaluated, rapidly stabilized, and discharged within 3–5 days; those who are in brief inpatient treatment for 5–14 days; and those who require extended inpatient treatment. When discharged from inpatient treatment, all substance-abusing adolescents are placed in a day hospital/partial hospital program where treatment continues.

The shift to markedly shorter lengths of stay has meant that programs must now have the capacity for rapid stabilization. This often requires critical changes in the programming, a few of of which include the following:

1. The patient and family must be told at the outset about the intensity and short stay guidelines. Expectations are conveyed about a probable brief length of stay. Families are given the treatment team's recommendations about the treatment issues and the probable length of stay within 48–72 hours after the patient is admitted.
2. The utilization review department representative on the treatment team must be much more active with the myriad complex managed care company regulations and must give rapid, efficient feedback to these companies.
3. Medication for associated psychiatric and behavioral disorders must be considered earlier.
4. A coordinator for the treatment team meetings must be designated. The utilization reviewer is best suited to make sure all of the verbal and written reports are available at staff meetings, whereas the clinical unit manager is best suited to make sure that each treatment provider and staff person participates in the treatment team meeting.
5. A checklist should include all of the required data for the team discussion. This is reviewed by the team twice per week. The list includes reports, either verbal or written, from the physician/psychiatrist, individual therapist, family therapist, substance abuse counselor, social worker, educational diagnostician, nursing staff member, and/or counselor; any consultations; laboratory findings; and psychological test results.

Transfers from inpatient to partial hospitalization programs as well as to intensive outpatient programs have risen dramatically. It is important to make certain the families and the adolescents themselves have a detailed knowledge of the amount of time involved in evaluation and of the goal of rapid stabilization. This is especially true during the initial phase of treatment. A greatly increased amount of time is spent dealing with managed care groups and companies. It is therefore important to be in touch with the gatekeepers at the managed care groups and to coordinate on clinical issues as well as share information about the programming.

Conclusions

Even with the best of efforts in working with level IV substance-abusing adolescents, recidivism appears to have increased. Many adolescents return within the first months after discharge from the inpatient or partial hospital level of care. The challenges of providing quality care for these patients are clearly greater today than ever before. Even if the inpatient evaluation has been carefully performed and a clear treatment plan formulated, abstinence is not guaranteed. The adolescent and his or her family must be committed to achieving and maintaining abstinence. This is not an easy task. It is made easier, however, when the adolescent's problems have been clearly spelled out and recovery tasks and goals have been clearly explained to them and their families.

Currently, a substantial effort is being made to improve all aspects of evaluation and treatment for this population in less intensive settings. There are increasing numbers of new instruments and technologies, including more standardized diagnostic testing, as well as promising medications for both psychiatric and substance abuse problems in adolescents. The system cannot work unless efficiently designed day and evening partial hospital programs provide ongoing treatment continuity for the substance-abusing adolescent leaving the inpatient setting.

References

American Society of Addiction Medicine: Patient Placement Criteria for the Treatment of Substance-Related Disorders, 2nd Edition. Chevy Chase, MD, American Society of Addiction Medicine, 1996

Bergmann PA, Smith MB, Hoffmann NG: Adolescent treatment: implications for assessment, practice guidelines, and outcome management. Pediatr Clin North Am 42:453–472, 1995

Bukstein OG, Brent D, Kaminer Y: Comorbidity of substance abuse and other psychiatric disorders in adolescents. Am J Psychiatry 146:1131–1141, 1989

Bukstein OG, Glancy LJ, Kaminer Y: Patterns of affective comorbidity in a clinical population of dually diagnosed adolescent substance abusers. J Am Acad Child Adolesc Psychiatry 31:1041–1045, 1992

Deas-Nesmith D, Campbell S, Brady KT: Substance use disorders in an adolescent inpatient psychiatric population. J Natl Med Assoc 90:233–238, 1998

Deykin EY, Buka SL, Leena BS: Depressive illness among chemically dependent adolescents. Am J Psychiatry 149:1341–1347, 1992

Dobkin PL, Chabot L, Maliantovitch K, et al: Predictors of outcome in drug treatment of adolescent inpatients. Psychol Rep 83:175–186, 1998

Gabel S, Shindledecker R: Parental substance abuse and its relationship to severe aggression and antisocial behavior in youth. Am J Addict 2:48–58, 1993

Harrison PA, Hoffmann NG: CATOR 1987 Report: Adolescent Residential Treatment Intake and Follow-Up Findings. St Paul, MN, Ramsey Clinic, 1987

Hoffmann NG, Halikas JA, Mee-Lee D: The Cleveland Admission Discharge and Transfer Criteria. Cleveland, OH, Greater Cleveland Hospital Association, 1987

Hoffmann NG, Halikas JA, Mee-Lee D, et al: Patient Placement Criteria for the Treatment of Psychoactive Substance Use Disorders. Washington, DC, American Society of Addiction Medicine, 1991

Horowitz HA, Overton WF, Rosenstein D, et al: Comorbid adolescent substance abuse: a maladaptive pattern of self-regulation. Adolesc Psychiatry 18:465–483, 1992

Hovens JG, Cantwell DP, Kiriakos R: Psychiatric comorbidity in hospitalized adolescent substance abusers. J Am Acad Child Adolesc Psychiatry 33:476–483, 1994

Jaffe SL: Step Workbook for Adolescent Chemical Dependence Recovery: A Guide to the First Five Steps. Washington, DC, American Academy of Child and Adolescent Psychiatry/American Psychiatric Press, 1990

Kaminer Y: Psychoactive substance abuse and dependence as a risk factor in adolescent attempted and completed suicide: a review. Am J Addict 1:21–29, 1992

Morrison MA, Smith OT: Psychiatric issues of adolescent chemical dependence. Pediatr Clin North Am 34:461–480, 1987

Moss HB, Tarter RE: Substance abuse, aggression, and violence. Am J Addict 2:149–160, 1993

Smith HE, Margolis RD: Adolescent inpatient and outpatient chemical dependence treatment: an overview. Psychiatr Ann 21:105–108, 1991

Stowell RJA, Estroff TW: Psychiatric disorders in substance-abusing adolescent inpatients: a pilot study. J Am Acad Child Adolesc Psychiatry 31:1036–1040, 1992

11 Use of Medications With Substance-Abusing Adolescents

Steven L. Jaffe, M.D.
Todd Wilk Estroff, M.D.

Psychiatric medications have been used for children and adolescents since the 1940s when Bradley, in New Hampshire, and Bender, in New York City, began using amphetamine and dextroamphetamine (Benzedrine) for children and adolescents with behavior disorders. Research studies have demonstrated that psychotropic medications can be useful in the treatment of many psychiatric disorders of childhood and adolescence. A marked increase in the acceptance of this treatment has occurred over the past few years among clinicians and parents. Controlled research studies have demonstrated the efficacy of stimulant medication for attention-deficit/hyperactivity disorder (ADHD) (Greenhill and Setterberg 1993). There is now widespread acceptance of the use of antidepressants for depressive disorders, antipsychotics for psychotic disorders, and mood stabilizers such as lithium, sodium valproate (Depakote), and carbamazepine (Tegretol) for bipolar disorders. Carbamazepine, lithium, sodium valproate, and beta blockers are also used to treat aggressive outbursts among children and adolescents. There are four major clinical situations in which psychopharmacological treatment of substance-abusing teenagers can be beneficial: 1) treatment of an overdose and intoxication; 2) treatment for detoxification and withdrawal; 3) treatment to prevent relapse; and 4) treatment of comorbid psychiatric disorders.

Least-Risk Rules

General risk management rules must be applied when prescribing any medication. This entails balancing the medication's benefit while avoiding practices that will place patients at undue risk. This benefit/risk analysis also considers the natural course of the adolescent's illness and the risk of not using any medication. A decision is then made that uses a least-risk/maximum-benefit approach.

Overdose

In emergency situations when an adolescent has overdosed, the ingested substance is unknown, and the adolescent is lapsing into coma, least-risk rules dictate first giving an opiate antagonist such as intravenous naloxone (Narcan). This should occur only after basic life support measures are in place. If opiates are in any way partially or wholly responsible for the patient's altered mental status, he or she will respond rapidly. If opiates are not involved, no harm will be done and opiate overdose will be ruled out. There is no risk to using naloxone and the benefit can be lifesaving. If there is no response to naloxone and continued life support is necessary, then flumazenil (Romazicon), a benzodiazepine receptor antagonist, may be given. Although an overdose of benzodiazepines is not fatal, many overdoses involve a combination of drugs and reversal of the benzodiazepine's effects will help support vital functions. Other medical complications should be treated symptomatically—i.e., seizures with benzodiazepines or barbiturates and arrhythmias with lidocaine or propranolol (Inderal).

Detoxification

It is infrequently necessary to detoxify adolescents from alcohol or drugs. Teenagers, unlike adults, tend to use alcohol and drugs episodically and are usually in fairly good physical health. Heavy abuse of opiates and sedative hypnotics is less common among adolescents. Although rare, physical addiction and life-threatening withdrawal can occur. For these reasons the treating physician needs to be familiar with the diagnosis and treatment of these withdrawals and to always use least-risk principles.

Alcohol and Sedative Hypnotics

It is much more common to encounter an adolescent who is dependent on alcohol than on sedative hypnotics. Use of medication for stabilization and detoxification is similar for both classes of drugs, except for certain atypical sedative hypnotics described below. Benzodiazepines are usually used for this purpose because they involve the least risk. If a patient is accidentally overdosed with a benzodiazepine, he or she will simply fall asleep. There have been no reported fatalities from benzodiazepine overdose alone, and diazepam dosage has exceeded 7,000 mg. On the other hand, if the patient is untreated or undertreated for alcohol and/or sedative hypnotic withdrawal delirium tremens, seizures, and respiratory arrest can occur, possibly resulting in a fatality. The least-risk rule in this situation is to err on the side of overmedication. Long-acting benzodiazepines such as clorazepate (Tranxene), oxazepam (Serax), diazepam (Valium), lorazepam (Ativan), and chlordiazepoxide (Librium) are the benzodiazepines of choice. They are given as needed every 1–2 hours until signs of withdrawal disappear or the patient becomes sedated. The total daily dosage is added together and given in divided doses three or four times per day on the following day. Once stabilized, the dose is tapered 10%–20% per day. It is critical when treating alcohol abuse to also administer thiamine 100 mg/day.

Ethchlorvynol (Placidyl) and glutethimide (Doriden) are the two most commonly abused sedative hypnotics that are not fully cross-tolerant with benzodiazepines, barbiturates, and alcohol. There is substantial risk of withdrawal if benzodiazapines are used for detoxification from these substances. It is best to use ethchlorvynol and glutethimide themselves or phenobarbital for stabilization and detoxification. It is important to keep in mind that overmedication with these alternative medications is much more dangerous than benzodiazepine overdose. Overdose, abuse, and dependency of stimulants, lysergic acid diethylamide (LSD), marijuana, and inhalants generally do not require detoxification with medication. They should be treated symptomatically.

Opiates

Heroin or other opiate dependence is rare among adolescents (Millman et al. 1978). It is most likely to occur among inner-city youth of large metropolitan areas. Contrary to popular myth, opiate withdrawal is not dangerous. No patient has ever died from simple opiate withdrawal. It is certainly uncomfortable and unpleasant. Various medications can be used to ease the fear and discomfort of uncontrolled opiate withdrawal.

Methadone is a long-acting orally effective opiate that can be used to treat the symptoms of withdrawal. It is given in 5–10-mg doses every 2 hours for the signs of opiate withdrawal. The total daily dose for the previous 24 hours is then added together and given once a day. Additional as-needed doses can be given to supplement the standing dose until the patient is no longer in withdrawal. Once stable, the dose is then gradually reduced 10% per day over the next 10 days to 2 weeks. The last few milligram decreases are often the hardest to accomplish because of increased withdrawal signs and symptoms.

The least-risk rules of methadone stabilization are clear. It is best to medicate only the signs of opiate withdrawal. Symptoms in the form of the patient's complaints must never be medicated unless they are accompanied by the corresponding physical signs of withdrawal. Therefore, using the least-risk rule, it is best to undermedicate opiate withdrawal with methadone. Using this approach, the patient can become somewhat uncomfortable until the next dose, but unless the patient shows the signs of withdrawal he or she should not receive another dose of methadone. If the rule is ignored, the patient could be accidentally overdosed, develop a respiratory arrest, and die.

An alternative approach is that once the methadone maintenance dose is established, it can be stopped entirely and clonidine started. Clonidine is an alpha-adrenergic agonist that works at the locus caerulus and blocks sympathetic nervous system–mediated symptoms of opiate withdrawal. It is given for the signs of withdrawal in 0.2-mg doses every 2 hours as needed. The maintenance dose is established as described above and is gradually reduced over the next 2 weeks. Skin patches can be substituted for oral clonidine. It is important to remember that this is not a panacea. Problems, if they arise, occur early in the treatment, and detoxification proceeds relatively smoothly afterward.

Some clinicians have given patients naltrexone, a long-acting orally effective pure opiate antagonist. This immediately throws the patient into full-blown opiate withdrawal. Clonidine is then added to ameliorate the withdrawal symptoms. With this method, detoxification can be accomplished in 4–5 days. Other physicians use this or similar techniques with patients under general anesthesia. They claim full detoxification in 1 day.

Physicians who fail to acknowledge that drug addicts are likely to be addicted to more than one drug may start patients on clonidine only. By doing so, they violate the least-risk rule by believing the patients' self-reports of the drugs they have used. In this fashion, physicians can miss a second life-threatening withdrawal that is not adequately covered by the clonidine.

Some "old-fashioned" drug treatment programs do not treat opiate withdrawal but simply insist that patients withdraw "cold turkey." This approach is unwise. It will feed directly into the addict's worst fear of being forced into uncontrolled withdrawal and the resulting pain and discomfort. It can also miss a second, more dangerous withdrawal.

Drug Combinations or Unknown Withdrawals

Least-risk rules are most valuable when the patient is withdrawing from a combination of drugs or when the substances abused are unknown. In this situation, the rule is to undermedicate with opiates and overmedicate with benzodiazepines. In this way all the risks of dangerous or fatal reactions are avoided and the chances of helping the patient remain comfortable and safely detoxify are maximized.

Relapse Prevention

Several medications can be used to prevent relapse among patients who are motivated but cannot resist their intense drug cravings as the day wears on. Early in the day, these patients are capable of doing whatever it takes to remain abstinent. By afternoon or evening, however, their resistance fades and they again relapse. This cycle repeats the next morning. Understanding this process can be advantageous.

Three categories of pharmacologic agents can be used to resolve the relapse cycle: antagonists, agonists, and noxious agents. The decision to use these agents should be made using the least-risk approach most appropriate for that particular individual. Each of these medications is administered in the morning when the patients are most motivated to help themselves. With these agents, the patients can remain abstinent even after their own resistance has departed because the medications block any feeling of pleasure or euphoria from further substance abuse. Other medications, such as disulfiram for the treatment of alcoholism, block euphoria by producing distinctly negative consequences if there is further alcohol abuse.

Antagonist Prevention Therapy

The classic antagonist therapy is the use of opiate antagonists that block all of the opiate receptors in the body and make the addicted individual chemically unable to have opiate-induced euphoria for 24–48 hours afterward. More recently, naltrexone has been used to prevent relapse among severely alcoholic patients. It appears to work in a similar manner with opiate dependence.

Specific benzodiazepine receptor blocking agents such as flumazenil have been used in overdose situations, and when longer-acting medications are developed they could similarly be used to block sedative hypnotic– and alcohol-induced euphoria.

Agonist Prevention Therapy

Classic agonist therapy for opiate dependence uses methadone maintenance to block all opiate receptors. The methadone is usually given as a once-daily dose in the morning. If the dose is sufficiently high, all receptors are blocked for 12–24 hours at a time and are therefore unavailable for generating euphoria. Total receptor blockade requires higher daily doses of methadone than is normally prescribed in methadone clinics. Individuals receiving these lower doses can and do experience additional euphoria when more opiates are ingested. This does not happen at higher methadone doses. Even when the methadone dose is sufficiently high the situation is not perfect because the dependent individual can successfully abuse any other nonopioid substance such as cocaine, sedative hypnotics, and alcohol. Several new kappa receptor opiate agonists produce pain relief without generating euphoria.

Noxious Agent Therapy

As a last resort and only in special circumscribed instances, the treating physician may be forced to employ noxious agent therapy. Disulfiram (Antabuse) is the prototypical model for these agents. In most instances it is innocuous when taken on a regular basis, but if the addicting agent—in this case alcohol—is used, severe physical illness results. Use of disulfiram in adolescents remains controversial and rare (Meyers et al. 1994). Its use should be restricted to those alcoholic adolescents who have failed in multiple treatment settings. Similarly, it can be used to treat those who do not have the intellectual capacity to develop crisis and prevention strategies to resist their own urges and the taunts of others. Because there are safety and compliance problems with disulfiram, it should be given to teenagers only under direct adult supervision and as a part of an entire treatment plan. As with all of the above medications, it is possible to successfully use and abuse other drugs while taking these prescriptions.

Treatment of Comorbid Psychiatric Disorders

There is a controversy over whether psychotropic medications are appropriate for treating individuals recovering from a substance abuse disorder. On one side of the debate are those who believe the use of any mood-altering substance is contraindicated and that "clean and sober" means not even taking aspirin. On the other side are those clinicians who take a more open viewpoint. With the recognition of a high incidence of dual and triple diagnoses among substance-abusing adolescents, the benefits of using medication to treat comorbid psychiatric disorders is increasingly being recognized. This, of course, must be done only after careful evaluation and as part of a multimodal treatment program. Factors to be considered when contemplating the use of psychotropic medications include a family history of psychiatric disorders, whether the psychiatric disorder preceded the substance abuse (Geller et al. 1998), the nature and severity of the psychiatric symptoms during periods of abstinence, and the motivation of both the adolescent and his or her family to take the medication in a reliable manner. The psychiatrist must also consider issues of safety related to further addiction, overdose, and drug interaction if relapse occurs.

Few controlled pharmacologic studies exist of substance-abusing adolescents with psychiatric disorders (Bruner and Fishman 1998; Geller et al. 1998; Weinberg et al.1998). In spite of this, there is a wealth of clinical experience in treating teenagers. Depressive disorders may be found in 20%–50% of the population of teenagers hospitalized with a primary diagnosis of substance dependency. DeMilio (1989) showed that two-thirds of substance-dependent adolescents hospitalized with major depressive disorder continue to have major depressions even after 2–3 weeks of abstinence from drugs. This suggests that the use of antidepressants for comorbid depressive disorders may be helpful.

Medications that can be considered include the selective serotonin reuptake inhibitors (SSRIs) fluoxetine (Prozac), fluvoxamine (Luvox), sertraline (Zoloft), paroxetine (Paxil), and citalopram (Celexa), which have little cardiac effect. Tricyclic antidepressants (TCAs) may be used, but possible cardiac arrhythmias and other unpleasant side effects need to be considered. Monoamine oxidase inhibitors (MAOIs) are usually avoided because of the possibility of a fatal hypertensive crisis if the adolescent relapses into cocaine or amphetamine abuse or eats tyramine-containing foods. Trazodone (Desyrel) may be used at bedtime, especially if severe initial insomnia is present. Stowell and Estroff (1992) demonstrated an incidence of almost 10% of comorbid bipolar disorder; for these patients, lithium (Geller et al. 1998), carbamazepine, or valproic acid, alone or in combination, should be considered.

Comorbid anxiety disorders such as panic disorders and posttraumatic stress disorders may be helped by various medications, including antihistamines, buspirone, TCAs, trazodone, anticonvulsants, and the SSRIs. Benzodiazepines, especially alprazolam (Xanax), are to be avoided because of their short duration of action and resultant high addictive potential. Comorbid bulimia nervosa may be helped by TCAs or the SSRIs.

Substance-abusing adolescents with ADHD present a particularly difficult and perplexing problem. Stimulants are quite effective for improving their attention span but are problematic because of their high abuse potential; there are two case reports of methylphenidate dependence in teenagers with ADHD (Jaffe 1991). Stimulants are not totally contraindicated, however; they may be used gingerly if the patient meets the following fundamental criteria:

- Patient has no history of stimulant abuse
- Specific criteria of ADHD in adolescence are present
- Reliable family members agree to monitor the medication
- Patient has a history of stimulant response in childhood

In addition, the teenager must be abstinent and in stable recovery. We differ on how long a wait is necessary before a stimulant can be used; S.J. considers methylphenidate after 2–3 weeks of inpatient or partial hospitalization, whereas T.W.E. prefers sodium pemoline (Cylert) and would not consider using it until after many months of unquestioned recovery. We agree, however, that neither amphetamines nor methylphenidate should be used if the adolescent experiences any "highs" or euphoric effects. Other medications that may be effective for adolescent ADHD symptoms include TCAs, clonidine, bupropion, and the SSRIs (American Academy of Child and Adolescent Psychiatry 1998; Bukstein 1997). Carbamazepine, valproic acid, and lithium may be useful for aggressive outbursts such as those that occur in intermittent explosive disorder.

Teenagers treated in inpatient or residential programs may be started on psychiatric medications at or shortly after admission. We believe that this is unwise except when the patient has a clear-cut psychotic disorder or severe depression that preceded the substance abuse. In these rare cases the adolescent may have been self-medicating a primary psychiatric disorder.

Determining how long to wait to medicate other psychiatric disorders is controversial. It is clear that the comorbid psychiatric disorder cannot be successfully treated while the teenager continues to use alcohol and/or drugs. Opinions on how long to wait before starting nonstimulant medications range from a few days to a full year of observation. If the patient can be observed in day treatment or outpatient therapy, a longer period of time is available to evaluate and resolve these difficult diagnostic dilemmas. The greatest problem with outpatient treatment is that the treating physician is never certain that abstinence is being maintained.

In summary, comorbid psychiatric disorders are a major cause of treatment failures and relapse in teenagers. Psychopharmacological treatments are an important part of a multimodal treatment program and can be an essential tool in relapse prevention.

Case Examples

Case 1

Patient H was a 15-year-old white female in the ninth grade who was admitted to the hospital after a suicide attempt. She had been fighting verbally with her family members and had had increasing depression with suicidal ideation for 2 months prior to admission. She experienced decreased energy, decreased sleep, total insomnia, anhedonia, decreased appetite, and decreased concentration. She also admitted to using marijuana daily for the 4 months prior to admission. She was a heavy binge alcohol abuser, and when nothing else was available she would abuse inhalants—especially correction fluid.

The patient also admitted to various psychotic symptoms in which she saw, heard, talked to, and could touch her father, who had died 8 months prior to her admission. She also admitted to olfactory hallucinations at another time. She shared many of her psychotic features with her mother, including the belief that they could read each other's mind and that they could see the dead father at will.

Mental status examination showed that the patient was a pleasant, verbal, cooperative, white female. Affect was flat, mood was euthymic, thought content revealed a mild thought disorder with no suicidal or homicidal ideation, but she did not look forward to living. She reported olfactory, auditory, tactile, and visual hallucinations as previously mentioned. The initial diagnostic impression under DSM-IV (American Psychiatric Association 1994) was

- Axis Ia, Major Depression with Psychotic Features
- Axis Ib, Cannabis Abuse
- Axis Ic, Alcohol Abuse
- Axis Id, Inhalant Abuse
- Axis Ie, Possible Schizoaffective Disorder

- Axis If, Shared Delusional Disorder (*folie à deux*)
- Axis II, No Diagnosis
- Axis III, Rule Out Partial Complex Seizure

The patient demonstrated dramatic mood swings with continuation of the psychotic features. Electroencephalography was performed that revealed partial complex seizures. She was placed on carbamazepine and showed a dramatic response to this medication; her mood improved so that she was no longer depressed or suicidal. However, her substance abuse problem had not been addressed, and while out on a pass with her mother, she obtained correction fluid and brought it with her into the hospital, where she abused it with other patients.

For several days after she abused this inhalant the patient's mood took a dramatic turn for the worse. It returned to the previous improved state only after she was stabilized on the carbamazepine. At this point her psychotic symptoms resolved. She remained well and participated in treatment while receiving carbamazepine. Her condition was controlled well enough for her to remain abstinent and participate in 12-step substance abuse groups. Final diagnosis was

- Axis Ia, Substance (cannabis, inhalant, alcohol) Induced Mood Disorder
- Axis Ib, Cannabis Abuse
- Axis Ic, Alcohol Abuse
- Axis Id, Inhalant Abuse
- Axis II, No Diagnosis
- Axis III, Partial Complex Seizures

Comment

This unlucky patient had substance abuse, psychiatric, and neurologic disorders simultaneously, all of which contributed to her symptoms. She was obviously a very complicated and complex patient who did very well as long as she was not exposed to illicit drugs. However, the moment she was able to obtain any abusable substance, she proceeded to use it and underwent a rapid and dramatic decline in her psychiatric and functional status. It was clear that she needed treatment for her psychiatric, substance, and neurologic disorders from the very beginning. However, the psychiatric symptoms far outweighed the substance abuse problems, so they were addressed and treated first. Once the psychiatric symptoms were brought under control, the patient's substance abuse problems emerged and reasserted themselves, at which point they were treated. Unless all of her problems were addressed and treated, relapse could be rapid and severe.

Case 2

Patient I was a 16-year-old white female who had been transferred from an adolescent substance abuse treatment facility after attempting suicide by hanging. She was found in the bathroom with a towel wrapped around her neck and her face turning purple. Two days prior to this attempt she had attempted to cut her wrists, and she had made three attempts previously to run away from the treatment facility.

The patient stated that she wanted to end her life because she did not feel she could live her life without alcohol. She claimed to have started drinking heavily at age 12 and to have made her first suicide attempt at age 14. After that attempt, she was hospitalized on an adolescent psychiatric unit, but because she did not improve, she was sent to a long-term residential treatment facility in Texas where she spent 1 year. She was returned home 4 months prior to her next suicide attempt. She had immediately started drinking heavily and abusing marijuana and correction fluid. While at home she deteriorated further, eventually reaching a point at which she became intoxicated and started to cut her wrists. She was admitted again to the local psychiatric hospital where she was diagnosed as having a dual-diagnosis disorder and transferred to a substance abuse treatment facility.

Immediately after her admission to the treatment facility she began to demonstrate "weird" behavior with tangential thoughts. She had started picking at her clothes and skin and felt her body was stretched and paralyzed. At times, she had claimed to have unusual sensations or to be unable to move. During this time she would have racing thoughts and then would suddenly wake up with a start and be fine. She described sensations coming out of her body and demonstrated rapid shifts of subjects. She had also stated three times that she was going to kill herself.

The patient had been sexually abused by a neighbor at approximately age 14. She readily admitted to extensive alcohol abuse (one to two six-packs per day), inhaling correction fluid and gasoline, and smoking four to five joints of marijuana a day. Her mental status examination revealed anger with a constricted affect and depressed mood but no other psychotic features. The diagnosis was

- Axis Ia, Rule Out Substance-Induced Mood Disorder
- Axis Ib, Rule Out Mood Disorder Due to Partial Complex Seizures (Mixed)
- Axis Ic, Conduct Disorder
- Axis Id, Rule Out Bipolar Disorder
- Axis Ie, Alcohol Abuse
- Axis If, Inhalant Abuse (correction fluid and gasoline)
- Axis Ig, Cannabis Abuse
- Axis II, Mixed Personality Disorder Traits
- Axis III, Rule Out Partial Complex Seizures

During the course of her current hospitalization the patient had a behavioral outburst in which she became enraged and had to be restrained. It was noted that she had extremely irregular respiration during this period of time. She appeared to lose consciousness and had no recollection of the event afterwards. In addition, during the time she was restrained she demonstrated fasciculations of her chin and other parts of her face. An electroencephalograph was immediately performed and revealed a temporal lobe focus. She was treated with carbamazepine and showed dramatic improvement in her mood, and she experienced no further behavioral outbursts.

After the patient was stabilized psychiatrically and medically, it became clear that she still needed treatment for her substance abuse disorders. She was transferred in stable condition to the adolescent substance abuse unit for further treatment. Final diagnosis was

- Axis Ia, Substance-Induced Mood Disorder (Mixed)
- Axis Ib, Mood Disorder Due to Partial Complex Seizures (Mixed)
- Axis Ic, Posttraumatic Stress Disorder (sexual abuse by neighbor)
- Axis Id, Alcohol Abuse
- Axis Ie, Inhalant Abuse (correction fluid and gasoline)
- Axis If, Cannabis Abuse
- Axis II, Mixed Personality Disorder Traits
- Axis III, Partial Complex Seizures

Comment

This patient is a striking example of a triple-diagnosis patient—that is, she had medical, substance abuse, and psychiatric disorders simultaneously. This unfortunate young woman was hastily and incorrectly diagnosed at four different facilities. The first facility focused simply on her behavioral disorder and assumed it was due to psychiatric problems. Her lack of improvement was blamed on her resistance to psychiatric treatment, when in fact it was due to the failure to diagnose her extensive substance abuse disorder. As a result, even after 1 year of residential psychiatric treatment she immediately relapsed into severe substance abuse when she returned home.

When rehospitalized, the patient's substance abuse disorder was correctly diagnosed but her psychiatric disorders and the possible medical/neurological causes of her disordered behavior were not appreciated. She was transferred to a facility that focused on the substance abuse disorder while minimizing the possibility of other disorders. This almost resulted in her death.

When the patient was finally completely reevaluated, it became clear that she had psychiatric, substance abuse, and medical/neurological problems, all of which were contributing to her failure to improve. Because of the impossibility of treating all of these disorders simultaneously, it was decided to treat them in a hierarchical fashion—treating the most severe disorders first. This was accomplished first by treating both the possible affective disorder and her partial complex seizure disorder with one medication—carbamazepine. This resulted in dramatic improvement, but as she improved it also became clear that her drug cravings were getting worse. Thus, once she was stabilized, she was transferred to a facility that would pay attention to all three of her diagnoses simultaneously.

This example is somewhat extreme, but it is not uncommon for dually and triply diagnosed patients to relapse because they have been inaccurately or incompletely diagnosed and treated. This again demonstrates the value of a thorough, comprehensive medical, biological, and psychiatric and substance abuse approach to the diagnosis of all adolescents with behavioral disorders.

Case 3

Patient J was a 16-year-old white male who had failed ninth grade twice. He was transferred from an outpatient residential treatment center where he had been treated for 8 months. He was referred because the attending psychiatrist thought he had developed new, severe psychiatric problems that prevented him from making any progress in his recovery.

At age 11 the patient had been caught by the police for shoplifting and for using drugs. He had displayed no further symptoms until age 14, when he started abusing marijuana, alcohol, hashish, phencyclidine hydrochloride (PCP), and LSD. His parents had started finding empty cellophane drug bags throughout the house. During this time the patient became angry, oppositional, and defiant and was arrested several times, once for breaking into a car and again for breaking into a department store. After the latter incident he had been referred to a mental health center for treatment, but this resulted in failure.

The patient was arrested a third time, for disorderly conduct, making obscene gestures, and simulating sexual acts, and afterward his parents refused to allow him back into the house. The welfare authorities were called, but the patient refused to cooperate when offered foster care. At that time he was reported to be a facile liar and very oppositional. His desperate parents took him to the outpatient residential program where he was treated for 8 months but made no progress. While in the program he had trouble relating to the other children and adolescents. During his last month in the program, his behavior became increasingly disturbed, and his therapists insisted that his parents remove him. His parents indicated that the patient had not been in this state when admitted into the program 8 months previously; the angry, hostile, conduct-disordered son they had sent for substance abuse treatment had, by the time he was discharged, become a bizarre, posturing person with a gross thought disorder. They described being shocked when they first saw him after his discharge. He was a totally different individual and would make strange gestures and assume unusual postures. At various times he would hold his hands outside the window of the car, position his hands and arms across his chest while walking, or hold his neck with both hands. When asked to carry his baggage, he held his hands in front of his clavicle and carried the suitcase in that unusual position while walking. This created a very bizarre and unusual picture.

Mental status examination revealed a thin white male who was obviously psychiatrically disturbed. He had bizarre posturing at times and at other times answered questions in an unusual or idiosyncratic fashion. His affect was flat, and his mood was depressed. He displayed a thought disorder with circumstantiality and tangentiality and some loosening of associations. Echolalia and clang associations were present, and asked direct questions he would reply in a manner that was often difficult or impossible to understand. When he filled out his daily diary on the unit, his responses were also idiosyncratic and bizarre. The patient denied any hallucinations, depersonalization, derealization, or illusions. He was oriented to person, place, and time. The patient admitted to smoking marijuana from the age of 12 progressing up to more than one joint per day and also admitted to drinking twice per week.

The initial diagnostic impression obviously was quite complicated and extensive. It included

- Axis Ia, Rule Out Major Depression
- Axis Ib, Rule Out Bipolar Disorder
- Axis Ic, Rule Out Schizophrenia
- Axis Id, Rule Out Mood Disorder Due to Medical Illness, Neurologic Disorder, and Inborn Error of Metabolism
- Axis Ie, Rule Out Substance Induced Mood Disorder
- Axis If, Cannabis Abuse
- Axis Ig, Alcohol Abuse
- Axis II, Schizoid and Schizotypical Personality Disorder Traits
- Axis III, Rule Out Medical Illness, Neurologic Disorder, and Inborn Error of Metabolism

A Schedule for Affective Disorders and Schizophrenia for School-Age Children (K-SADS) was performed. The diagnoses on that semistructured interview were

- Axis Ia, Possible Schizophreniform Disorder
- Axis Ib, Possible Schizophrenia, Catatonic or Disorganized Type
- Axis Ic, Possible Substance Induced Psychotic Disorder
- Axis Id, Conduct Disorder, Solitary/Aggressive/Severe
- Axis Ie, Cannabis Abuse
- Axis If, Alcohol Abuse
- Axis II, Schizoid and Schizotypical Personality Disorder Traits

IQ testing revealed a verbal IQ of 86, performance of 68, and full-scale IQ of 76. None of the tests for unusual organic illnesses proved to be positive, including 24-hour and sleep-deprived electroencepalographs. Because of the severity of his psychosis, the patient was started on fluphenazine (Prolixin), but this had to be changed to intramuscular injection because of his opposition to treatment. The patient's psychosis responded well, but he remained depressed, and he was placed on a low-dose antidepressant. His dose was slowly increased every other day to avoid causing him a more severe mania or psychosis. As his antidepressant dose reached therapeutic levels, he began to make gradual and steady progress.

Throughout treatment the patient continued to identify himself as a drug addict. He was not willing to pay attention to his severe psychiatric problems. Because of the severity of his psychiatric illness and the fragility of his ego, it was impossible to treat his substance abuse disorder as an inpatient, but it was addressed through his attendance at 12-step programs and by continuing his medications. Final diagnosis was

- Axis Ia, Schizoaffective Disorder
- Axis Ib, Possible Schizophrenia, Catatonic or Disorganized Type
- Axis Ic, Possible Substance Induced Psychotic Disorder
- Axis Id, Conduct Disorder, Solitary/Aggressive/Severe
- Axis Ie, Cannabis Abuse in Remission
- Axis If, Alcohol Abuse in Remission
- Axis II, Schizoid and Schizotypal Personality Disorder Traits
- Axis III, No Diagnosis

Comment

This was a true dual-diagnosis patient in whom the original symptoms of severe drug abuse and oppositional behavior were overwhelmed by the onset of a new and severe psychotic disorder. It is unclear whether the psychotic disorder would have emerged all by itself or whether it was something induced by drugs of abuse in a vulnerable individual. An alternative explanation is that this psychotic disorder was caused by a treatment program that was overly punitive and harsh and not sensitive to the psychiatric issues of this patient. At no point during his entire 8-month treatment was he allowed to go to school or visit alone with his parents. He was permitted to see his parents only monthly and only at a distance in group meetings because he had failed to achieve the proper status in the program to allow parental visits.

A major sign that something was overlooked by the original treatment program occurred when the patient passed the usual length of stay without making progress. Utilization and length of stay reviews of this the patient should have picked his case up as an outlier months earlier. This mechanism was not in place at that time but was subsequently instituted because of incidents such as these. He was identified when a new psychiatrist became involved with the program who had the patient transferred for a complete reassessment, which helped clarify his diagnosis and helped in the decision about which symptoms required immediate treatment.

Because the patient's psychotic and affective symptoms clearly overwhelmed his initial drug abuse problem, those symptoms had to be treated first. Medications were chosen carefully, avoiding any that could be addictive. As the psychotic symptoms cleared, a great deal of depressive psychopathology remained. The patient was carefully treated with initial low doses of antidepressant medication and he responded well.

This patient could have easily wound up on the back wards of a state hospital or in prison if either the psychiatrist had not picked up the severe psychiatric nature of his illness or the parents had been unwilling to pursue the best treatment available for their child.

References

American Academy of Child and Adolescent Psychiatry: Summary of the practice parameters for the assessment and treatment of children and adolescents with substance use disorders. J Am Acad Child Adolesc Psychiatry 37:122–126, 1998

American Psychiatric Association: Diagnostic and Statistical Manual of Mental Disorders, 4th Edition. Washington, DC, American Psychiatric Association, 1994

Bruner AE, Fishman M: Adolescents and illicit drug use. JAMA 280:597–598, 1998

Bukstein OG: Practice parameters for the assessment and treatment of children and adolescents with substance use disorders. American Academy of Child and Adolescent Psychiatry. J Am Acad Child Adolesc Psychiatry 36(10, suppl):140S–156S, 1997

DeMilio L: Psychiatric syndromes in adolescent substance abusers. Am J Psychiatry 146:1212–1214, 1989

Geller B, Cooper TB, Sun K, et al: Double-blind and placebo-controlled study of lithium for adolescent bipolar disorders with secondary substance dependency. J Am Acad Child Adolesc Psychiatry 37:171–178, 1998

Greenhill LL, Setterberg S: Pharmacotherapy of disorders of adolescents. Psychiatr Clin North Am 16:793–814, 1993

Jaffe SL: Case report: intranasal abuse of prescribed methylphenidate by an alcohol and drug abusing adolescent with ADHD. J Am Acad Child Adolesc Psychiatry 30:773–775, 1991

Meyers WC, Donahue JE, Goldstein MR: Disulfiram for alcohol use disorders in adolescence. J Am Acad Child Adolesc Psychiatry 33:484–489, 1994

Millman RB, Kuhri ET, Nyswander ME: Therapeutic detoxification of adolescent heroin addicts. Ann N Y Acad Sci 311:153–164, 1978

Stowell AJ, Estroff TW: Adolescent dual diagnosis: a pilot study of inpatient substance abusing adolescents. J Am Acad Child Adolesc Psychiatry 31:1036–1040, 1992

Weinberg NZ, Rahdert E, Colliver JD, et al: Adolescent substance abuse: a review of the past 10 years. J Am Acad Child Adolesc Psychiatry 37:252–261, 1998

12 Adolescent Psychiatry and 12-Step Treatment

J. Calvin Chatlos, M.D.
Todd Wilk Estroff, M.D.

This chapter may be considered basic by those who are already familiar with Alcoholics Anonymous (AA), Cocaine Anonymous (CA), Narcotics Anonymous (NA), and other 12-step approaches to the treatment of addictions. Unfortunately, 12-step programs are poorly understood by many physicians, psychiatrists, psychologists, social workers, and other mental health professionals. This is particularly true if these professionals have not experienced addiction themselves or among their family or friends. Twelve-step programs are often believed to be illogical, unscientific, and overly "spiritual." Successful 12-step treatment is an experiential process that is often difficult to describe in words to the outside nonparticipating observer. The 12-step approach is often unfamiliar to many psychiatrically oriented mental health practitioners because no comparable treatment technique exists in the fields of psychiatry and psychology. As a result, therapists are often skeptical about whether it actually works. Twelve-step treatment is frequently viewed as "voodoo," "mumbo jumbo," "psychobabble," or "self-help jargon." This attitude has led to the rather widespread belief that the 12-step approach to treatment of addictions is not compatible with standard psychiatric treatments. This chapter explains the therapeutic techniques, values, and the particular language of the 12-step experience in order to make it simple and understandable.

Twelve-step treatment is simple and effective. At their most fundamental level, the 12 steps as a whole provide a progressive plan for treatment. The steps will not help individuals who cannot or will not admit that they have a problem or who will not commit themselves to change. They require a certain level of intelligence, discipline, and basic trust in order to be effective. Individuals lacking the required trust, commitment, and persistence account for high dropout rates over time. Despite these weaknesses, the 12 steps themselves can be used both to guide treatment and as a way to evaluate an individual's progress toward recovery.

Scientific data have indicated that regular attendance at 12-step meetings greatly reduces relapse rates among substance-abusing adults and adolescents (Harrison and Hoffmann 1989; Hoffmann and Estroff 1998a, 1998b; Hohman and LeCroy 1996). In addition, mounting scientific evidence shows that a combination of professional services and 12-step support is more effective in achieving abstinence than either method alone (Hoffmann et al. 1998; Zywiak et al. 1999). The combination of psychiatric and 12-step strategies provides more effective treatment for dually diagnosed individuals. The 12-step support is useful both during the acute treatment phase and for the long-term prevention of relapse (Hoffmann and Estroff 1998a, 1998b). It can help identify specific personal and emotional barriers to successful treatment. Once identified, these barriers are dealt with as flaws in thinking or behaviors that must be mastered before the addiction can become controlled and stable. Recovering adolescents often view the 12 steps as a way of thinking and behaving that is useful regardless of their religious orientation. Because of this, it is advantageous for practitioners who work with substance-abusing adolescents to become familiar with the literature of the 12 steps and 12 traditions (Alcoholics Anonymous 1981). Little information exists that helps explain the value of 12-step treatment to mental health professionals (Bean-Bayog 1991; Ehrlich 1987; Evans and Sullivan 1990; Nace 1992; Schulz 1991). *The Recovery Book* is a practical guide for patients and families that can also help practitioners understand the 12-step process (Mooney et al. 1992).

Treatment

After the DSM-IV (American Psychiatric Association 1994) diagnoses are made and an assessment for level of care has been determined using patient placement criteria, various considerations are important (American Society of Addiction Medicine 1996; Hoffmann et al. 1987, 1991).

12-Step Techniques to Engage the Adolescent

Most substance-abusing adolescents do not want treatment. Outside forces are often necessary to initiate care. Initial abstinence often requires environmental control, which may include admission to a residential treatment program to separate the adolescent from the people, places, and activities that reinforce his or her substance abuse. Judicious use of leverage arising from the adolescent's school, a court, a job, or a family intervention can make the difference between treatment and continued addiction.

Intervention

An intervention is frequently necessary. The purpose of the intervention is to get the adolescent into treatment. Interventions often involve confronting the teenager about his or her substance abuse. With that purpose in mind, the adolescent's family, friends, therapist, and clergy gather together and tell the adolescent how worried they are and urge him or her to enter treatment. During the intervention, the parents are asked to tell the child how his or her drug or alcohol use has affected them. The family intervention should be facilitated by a skilled therapist as participants present their concerns to their adolescent. A successful intervention will strengthen the family's commitment to treatment and dispel the adolescents' fantasies that their parents will rescue them from treatment. In addition, the family intervention can often break through an adolescent's grandiosity and denial and at the same time establish the family's firm commitment to treatment. During the intervention the adolescents often express guilt, shame, and disappointment that they covered by their substance abuse. In more disturbed families, the "family" intervention may include extended family members and other interested parties while simultaneously excluding immediate family members who contribute to or encourage the adolescent's substance abuse (Fishman 1993). Once the intervention has been effective, treatment can begin. Continuing interaction with the family and the adolescent can ultimately transform the family from one that initiated and maintained addiction to one that supports and maintains abstinence.

Written Contract

Adolescents entering treatment are asked to make a commitment to abstinence. In treatment this commitment is often formalized with the use of a mutually agreed upon written behavioral contract. This contract specifies attendance at self-help meetings (AA/NA) and treatment; agreement for ongoing urine monitoring; the people with whom the teenager will and will not associate; the homes and specific locations that will be avoided; and the adolescent's responsibilities at home and school. The parents' commitment to treatment is also spelled out in the contract. The agreement provides new behavioral expectations for both the parents and their child. It creates a supportive family recovery environment and provides the structure the family needs to commit to their child's abstinence.

Preparation for Step 1: Drug Chart and Life Story

The 12-step process for adolescents begins with the individual writing and presenting a comprehensive personal drug chart. This assignment reviews all alcohol and drug use from first use to current use. The chart also reviews the progression and harmful consequences in physical, emotional, social, sexual, and spiritual areas of the adolescent's life. This comprehensive drug history often leads to clarification of both the substance abuse and psychiatric diagnoses as the adolescent becomes more honest and open while working with his/her therapists. It is useful to have the drug chart presented to other adolescents in a group session for supportive critical comment and acceptance. Jaffe's (1990) *Step Workbook for Adolescent Chemical Dependence Recovery: A Guide to the First Five Steps* is available specifically for work on the adolescent's drug chart and each of the first five steps of AA. This workbook continues to promote the recovery process by having adolescents write and present their "Life Story." They are expected to include details of events that led to the initiation of their drug use, the events during their progression of use, and their current life situation. All areas of their lives are examined including problems, strengths, and goals.

The commitment to abstinence and the use of the 12 steps are often difficult for adolescents in the early stages of drug dependence. It is helpful to point out that this commitment begins as a single day's declaration that is renewed "one day at a time." The first five steps also provide a sequential guide to the recovery process. Because it is unrealistic to expect teenagers to be capable of making and keeping lifelong commitments early in recovery, the adolescent is only expected to make a commitment to complete of each of the first five steps in succession.

Completion of each step occurs when a cognitive, emotional, and behavioral shift is noted. During this time, adolescents attend AA and NA meetings such as Young People's AA or age-appropriate NA meetings. They are expected to obtain the phone numbers of other members to begin building their own support network. The recommended frequency of attendance ranges from two to four meetings per week depending on the stage of recovery, intensity of other treatment, and the adolescent's commitment to treatment. Some programs encourage "90 in 90," which refers to a commitment to attend 90 12-step meetings in 90 days. Group members are encouraged to obtain a sponsor after 1–2 months of attendance at meetings. Only about half of the adolescents who complete treatment in inpatient settings continue to attend meetings after discharge (Harrison and Hoffmann 1989), but those substance-abusing adolescents who do attend 12-step meetings are more likely to have had prior treatment, friends who did not use drugs, less parental involvement while in treatment, or more feelings of hopelessness (Hohman and LeCroy 1996).

As teenagers make progress in their treatment, it is not unusual for them to have emotional and behavioral reactions. They tend to repeat previous patterns of behavior. These old patterns may inhibit the recovery process. Exploration of these reactions can uncover old emotions and memories that are related to the later stages of their substance use disorder. Some of the most difficult therapeutic work involves identifying these events in detail, reexperiencing the thoughts, feelings, and behaviors associated with the event, and determining in the present how they can produce a different outcome.

These thoughts and feelings are often associated with powerful urges to use drugs or alcohol or to repeat other self-destructive activities such as unprotected sex, bingeing and purging, violence, suicide, or self-mutilation. Understanding and changing these automatic, sometimes unconscious, counterproductive behaviors is a key element toward successful recovery. Compulsions to use mood-altering drugs are often out of awareness and can be addressed only after they have been identified and worked through during a period of abstinence.

It is important for treatment professionals to recognize that the use of the 12 steps in an intensive adolescent treatment program may be different than their use in AA/NA support groups. These differences are related to an increased intensity of treatment necessitated by the shortened lengths of time allowed for therapy. Detailed 12-step work with adolescents has been described at length (Chatlos 1989, 1991a, 1991b, 1996; Evans and Sullivan 1990). Once the adolescents have started treatment they must be introduced to the 12 steps in a manner in which they can easily understand.

It is important to remember that the 12-step program was originally designed for the unquestionable alcoholic patient. This was then applied to those who are dependent on other mood-altering substances. The founders of AA were considered "hopeless" alcoholics and approached the task of recovery as helping the desperate or hopeless case. The steps may be useful for abusers as well as dependent individuals, but this initial perspective should be kept in mind.

The 12 Steps

Step 1

> We admitted we were powerless over alcohol (our addiction) and that our lives had become unmanageable.

The first step is probably the most misunderstood concept in AA and other 12-step programs. It does not mean that the individual is powerless to change, but rather that he or she acknowledges having a problem. In severe cases, the problem is the inability to moderate the use of alcohol or other drugs. The adolescent must accept that he or she is different from "normal people" who are able to use small amounts of alcohol or drugs and stop. In short, the individual is giving up on the futile goal of continued use without consequences (i.e., powerlessness). However, when treating adolescents it is important to deal with the concepts stated in step 1 in the reverse order. Therefore, the initial work should focus on acknowledging how their lives have become unmanageable and not on convincing them of their powerlessness over drugs and alcohol.

Activities associated with step 1 center around education about the nature of addictions. Reading assignments help members accept that they are addicted and therefore "different" with respect to their use of alcohol and other drugs. The recognition that addiction is a lifelong disease can help support a commitment to abstinence.

The concept of powerlessness is often difficult for adolescents. Their fear of being powerless is often confused with issues of authority and discipline. When they feel powerless they can demonstrate cognitive distortions and paranoia. Some adolescents complain of being brainwashed. As firm limits are set, therapists and law enforcement personnel are often perceived as punitive adults with whom they have had previous unpleasant experiences. Replacing this suspicious point of view with trust, honesty, and acceptance is critical to the realization that their lives are out of control. As they make progress they begin to realize that their inability to regulate their emotions and behavior is directly related to their substance abuse disorder. With this recognition the difficult transformation of their lives can begin.

Psychiatric Issues in Step 1

Because psychiatric disorders often complicate the addiction process and contribute to the unmanageability of the adolescents' lives, an integrated approach to the first step is helpful. Persistent, severe distortions or paranoia may indicate an underlying psychotic disorder. Under the intense experience of drug abuse treatment, adolescents with schizophrenia or schizophreniform disorders can begin to display psychotic thinking. These patients must be placed in a more supportive therapeutic environment. They may have limited ability to benefit from the 12-step recovery process until antipsychotic medications are used. Adjustments to the 12-step approach may be necessary (Evans and Sullivan 1990).

Initial Use of Medications

Teenagers rarely need detoxification with medications. However, abstinence is necessary to accurately diagnose the presence or absence of a comorbid psychiatric disorder. Severe psychiatric symptoms such as mania, auditory hallucinations, severe depression, or suicidal ideation often require the immediate use of psychotropic medications regardless of a definitive diagnosis. However, as noted in prior chapters, a later trial without medication may be indicated after psychiatric reassessment.

Case Examples

Bipolar Disorder During Step 1

Patient K was a 16-year-old female with extensive cocaine and alcohol abuse. She was admitted for treatment. She was mildly depressed and guarded but cooperative and engaged in treatment. During the subsequent 10 days, her affect became more depressed and tearful, with psychomotor retardation, paranoid ideation developing into delusions, ideas of reference, and a morbid preoccupation with her own death and the past deaths of her relatives. These symptoms of major depression with psychotic features led to a trial of nortriptyline. As the doses were increased, her mood responded and her psychomotor retardation abated. However, her mood rapidly progressed to euphoria, inappropriate laughing and giggling, and flight of ideas. She was diagnosed as having bipolar disorder, although she had no history of hypomanic or manic episodes and did not satisfy the time criteria for the disorder. She responded well to lithium and completed treatment while maintained on lithium.

The diagnosis was

- Axis Ia, Cocaine Abuse
- Axis Ib, Alcohol Abuse
- Axis Ic, Bipolar Disorder
- Axis II, No Diagnosis
- Axis III, Asthma

The medication prescribed was lithium carbonate, 300 mg three times daily.

Comment

If during the first 1–2 weeks of abstinence the patient reveals persistent and severe psychiatric symptoms, then medications may be indicated. It should be emphasized that drugs should be used only in the early stages of treatment when the symptoms are severe and the treating physician's hand is forced. In this case, the persistence and intensity of the patient's symptoms dictated that medication management was necessary early in the course of her illness. Because few studies demonstrate specific efficacy of medication in drug- and alcohol-addicted teenagers, medication interventions must be guided by clinical response and research experience with adults and non-substance-dependent adolescents.

Adolescents with borderline personality disorder maintain more organized thought processes with confrontation (Davanloo 1980; Davis 1989). However, they can develop overwhelming urges to use drugs, have sex, binge or purge, commit suicide, self-mutilate, be violent, or run away. With the structure of treatment, an "abandonment depression" can develop (Masterson 1972). Loneliness and depression can begin as adolescents contemplate their life without drugs, without drug-using "friends," and without the self-destructive behaviors previously used to cope with their feelings of loneliness and alienation. The degree of alienation that they experience is often related to the severity of their drug use and their social withdrawal.

Adolescents with severe conduct disorders or antisocial personality disorder are more easily identified early in treatment. They have a limited ability to experience guilt and shame. For some patients, the development of intense mistrust without depression can be indicative of secrets about unexposed criminal behavior or issues of past child abuse. These must be addressed before treatment can continue, so it is often necessary to reassure the patients that confidentiality will be maintained. The presence of persistent depressive symptoms with psychomotor retardation or psychotic symptoms must be evaluated for an underlying major depressive disorder. Carefully selected substance-abusing teenagers have responded well to antidepressant medications.

Conduct Disorder During Step 1

Patient L, a 16-year-old male with a diagnosis of conduct disorder, was admitted to an inpatient program for marijuana and mixed substance dependence. He had a history of parental separation beginning at age 2 with his mother's remarriage and his stepfather's subsequent leaving when the patient was 7 years old. His medical history included several years of left-sided headaches associated with flashing lights and nausea that had been diagnosed as migraine headaches when he was 13. An electroencephalogram and a computed tomography scan were normal.

In treatment the patient initially was guarded and presented a "macho" image. Early on, work revealed his issues with authority. He developed mood lability with angry episodes that terminated with migraine headaches. He acknowledged severe drug urges and the desire to run away. During one of these attacks he stated that when the therapist was talking to him it was like the therapist was beating something into his head. He recalled how his stepfather had hit him in the head and repeatedly criticized him by calling him a wimp. He recalled wishes to hit his stepfather but his inability to act because of his own fears of annihilation. His headaches worsened as more anger was directed toward the therapist. A breakthrough occurred when he identified the disappointment of not having a father who was emotionally available. After gaining this insight he cried for the first time in treatment. He tearfully related how he wanted his father and stepfather to be proud and to admire him as being a strong son. As he revealed his wishes he smiled and the migraine headache abated. The migraine headaches did not return throughout treatment.

The patient was subsequently able to recognize how his arguments, runaway behaviors, headaches, anger, disappointment, and poor relationships with his family were related to his drug and alcohol use and how these behaviors were a part of the "unmanageability" of his life. He also recognized that his "macho" image masked his feelings of "powerlessness." The diagnosis was

- Axis Ia, Cannabis Dependence
- Axis Ib, Mixed Substance Dependence
- Axis Ic, Conduct Disorder, Undifferentiated Type
- Axis II, Narcissistic Personality Traits
- Axis III, Migraine Headaches

No medications were prescribed.

Comment

Other psychiatric barriers to treatment may indicate developmental arrests or deficits. This may explain some of the severe regressive and childlike behaviors that can occur during treatment of these adolescents.

Completion of step 1 is often the goal during a short-term inpatient treatment. Step 1 leaves people open to the possibility of receiving help with their powerlessness and unmanageability. Adolescents with attention-deficit/hyperactivity disorder, learning disabilities, and prior social and school failure frequently experience overwhelming feelings of defeat. They frequently equate treatment with school and staff members with critical parents or teachers. Reading and written assignments are especially difficult and frustrating. When addressed properly with remedial support and development of alternative coping strategies, treatment can become one of their first successes and a very rewarding experience. Unfortunately, many substance-abusing adolescents with mental retardation are unable to understand—let alone benefit—from any 12-step treatment.

Step 2

> We came to believe that a power greater than ourselves could restore us to sanity.

Step 2 refers to a belief in a loving, caring force greater than addiction. The essence of this step is the individual's acknowledgment that outside assistance is required because willpower alone is insufficient. The hallmark of addiction or substance dependence is the pattern of relapse to use in addition to the lack of control once use is initiated. Many addicted persons look to the alcohol or drug as a higher power, and many will comment that giving up the substance is like losing a cherished friend. This "loss" can be ameliorated by finding another source of strength and support. Most dependent individuals require some outside assistance or reliance on a power greater than themselves to achieve lasting and durable recovery.

Belief in a higher or external power can help the addicted person recover from destructive patterns of behavior. "Being restored to sanity implies being able to do what one needs to do and not what one wants to do" (Jaffe 1990, p. 32). Step 2 is the first step to introduce a spiritual—not religious—focus (see Chapter 14). It includes work with values and ethics. It requires examining the adolescent's disturbing past, including damaging religious episodes that may be emotionally and spiritually destructive and produce negative cognitive distortions of how a higher power can help them. Some skeptical adolescents find that use of the acronym GOD—for Good Orderly Direction—facilitates the spiritual experience of a higher power without invoking a deity or religion. This allows them to consider a higher power in relation to principles and rules rather than as a distinct or guiding being. This spiritual process involves examining personal relationships with powers greater than the self. Examples of these powers include family members and other individuals who have had a significant (good or bad) impact on the adolescent's life. Step 2 assignments include sharing the comprehensive drug chart with parents, which helps break through family denial and opens the family to rebuilding damaged relationships.

The adolescents' faith in alcohol and drug use to solve their problems is explored while they examine their damaged relationships. They feel betrayed and often reexperience their losses and broken relationships. Parental divorce and separation shatter their idealized models of family and parental caring. Some of their most painful feelings are related to the loss of trust and self-worth they experienced as a result of physical or sexual abuse. They often feel victimized in all aspects of their lives by unsuccessful treatment and by past therapists. Working on these unresolved trust-related issues is a necessary and important part of step 2 treatment.

It is important to note the adolescent's strengths and to focus on safety (Evans and Sullivan 1990). Education helps explain that "sanity is not acting on first impulses" (Narcotics Anonymous 1993), and looking at higher power issues can produce a renewed commitment to recovery. Behavioral relapses are less likely to be perceived as a disaster if they are used as an opportunity to renew commitment to abstinence and to learn better relapse prevention strategies (Gorski and Miller 1986; Jaffe 1992; Marlatt 1985). These strategies may include identifying high-risk situations that precipitated the relapse-related behaviors and assessing the antecedents to these behaviors in the form of relapse warning signs (Bell 1990).

Part of relapse prevention must deal with the "insanity" of urges that can occur at any time and often precede and precipitate relapse. Drug urges can include a desire to get high or escape feelings or a desire for self-punishment in order to feel pain. Work with adolescents requires helping them understand that urges and cravings are often "feelings in disguise." Identification and expression of the feelings they previously managed with drug abuse can lead to a breakthrough into a new level of awareness of the process of recovery (Chatlos 1991b; Lane and Schwartz 1987). Therapeutic work then involves learning a new coping strategy that will result in different actions. Many recurrent behaviors and urges are triggered by the recovery process itself. Linking earlier behavioral disasters to the adolescent's alcohol and drug use can transform addiction treatment from being a burden to liberation.

The spiritual focus in treatment assists adolescents involved in negative spiritual activities such as Satanic worship. Other cultlike activities can lead to intense rage, hatred, and sadistic revenge. This part of their "insanity" is often associated with painful issues of power and humiliation as well as covering feelings of inadequacy and mortifying shame. Intense emotional issues that arise in dealing with some teenagers at this stage require a strong emphasis on reality testing with understanding of the psychological processes of projection and identification. A psychiatric perspective of these issues can help clarify diagnostic and therapeutic issues during step 2. This is useful in guiding the psychotherapeutic process while at the same time carefully selecting those few adolescents who will benefit from psychotropic medications.

Psychiatric Issues in Step 2

A different spectrum of psychiatric disorders can emerge for the first time during step 2. The adolescent's symptoms are frequently indicative of a posttraumatic stress disorder (PTSD) or are related to being the child of an alcoholic or drug addict (parent–child disorder). It is important to recognize these symptoms as soon as they occur because they can interfere with treatment. The conditions indicated should be addressed immediately. Failure to do so may lead to premature termination of treatment, exacerbation of dangerous self-destructive behaviors, or relapse to drug use. Medication is rarely indicated initially for PTSD.

In addition to PTSD, personality disorders, anxiety disorders, paraphilias, and obsessive-compulsive disorders can be diagnosed more easily at this stage of treatment. If persistent, these disorders should be carefully treated with appropriate nonaddicting psychotropic medications.

Case Examples

Conduct and Anxiety Disorder During Step 2

Patient M was a 16-year-old female with a history of parental divorce when she was 7, followed by multiple geographic moves. She was admitted with extensive cocaine, marijuana, and alcohol abuse and was diagnosed as having conduct disorder with progressive antisocial behaviors, including poor school motivation, truancy, shoplifting, stealing, runaway episodes, and fighting using knives. She had depressive symptoms as part of her posttraumatic stress disorder and her borderline personality. She had a history of being raped at age 13 and of a suicide attempt at age 14 in which she overdosed by taking 120 aspirin tablets. She had also been involved for 2 years with Satanic worship, which included daily rituals and animal sacrifice.

The patient expressed motivation in treatment, but as she worked on her second step and examined her involvement in Satanism she developed extreme anxiety, sweating, restlessness, and palpitations. These symptoms would occasionally occur during group sessions, making it necessary to remove her from the group. Because she appeared to have a separation anxiety component, she was started on imipramine, which was increased to 100 mg/day. During the next 5 days her mood fluctuated with increasingly frightening dreams and thoughts about attacking another patient with a knife. As she became less overwhelmed on medication, the patient continued to deal in psychotherapy with her need to have power and get revenge. She experienced severe loneliness and directed her outrage toward the therapist, wanting to kill him and put a knife through his chest. She had an extreme fear of dying as well as guilt and fear that Satan would come and punish her. This was mixed with a desire to be taken by and married to Satan. Extreme feelings of love and hate were delusional and projected onto Satan. Her rage at her abusive father and her desire for power and revenge combined with her guilt and fear of dying were progressively dealt with. This led to decreased feelings of loneliness and self-hatred. She was able to continue treatment without further panic attacks even after the imipramine was discontinued.

The patient's diagnosis was

- Axis Ia, Alcohol Dependence
- Axis Ib, Cocaine Abuse
- Axis Ic, Cannabis Abuse
- Axis Id, Conduct Disorder, Solitary/Aggressive/Separation
- Axis Ie, Anxiety Disorder
- Axis II, Borderline Personality Disorder
- Axis III, Iron Deficiency Anemia

On discharge from inpatient treatment, the patient was no longer receiving any medications.

Conduct Disorder During Step 2

Patient N, a 17-year-old male with marijuana and alcohol abuse and major depressive disorder, was motivated and progressed well to completion of his step 1. Following this, his mood changed. He was not as active, was often confused, and made little progress in treatment. There was no clear explanation until he developed leg pain, for which no physical signs of a problem were present. He then revealed that he had had an injury in which he broke a leg during a soccer game. The injury destroyed his dreams of becoming a professional athlete. He had never performed as well in athletics after this injury as he had previously. This disappointment for his father and himself had not been resolved and had resurfaced to block his treatment. The disappointment and self-pity associated with this event prevented his ability to commit to step 2 and were part of his "insane" behaviors. Once this issue was identified and examined, he was able to successfully continue treatment. His diagnosis was

- Axis Ia, Cannabis Abuse
- Axis Ib, Alcohol Abuse
- Axis Ic, Major Depressive Disorder
- Axis Id, Conduct Disorder, Undifferentiated Type
- Axis II, No Diagnosis
- Axis III, History of left knee injury

No medications were prescribed.

Step 3

> We made a decision to turn our will and our lives over to the care of God as we understood Him.

Step 3 consolidates the adolescents' treatment gains while emphasizing making mature adult choices, taking personal responsibility for their actions, surrendering opposition to external analysis and criticism of their behavior, and being willing to consider outside opinions. This step is instrumental in facilitating character transformation and overcoming past defensive patterns. It promotes changes through the adoption of new behaviors.

In this manner, step 3 deals with issues of growing up, separation, and individuation as the adolescents try new behaviors and gain autonomy. Treatment of adolescents during this step emphasizes concrete experiences with family members and focuses on resolution of major family conflicts. This may be accomplished through family therapy sessions, multifamily groups, or a more structured "Family Week" or "Family Weekend" (Chatlos 1991b). In families in which some members have untreated substance abuse or psychiatric disorders, the adolescents can be helped to recognize that their own behavior is heavily influenced by harmful family illnesses. As trust and faith in other individuals grows, the possibility opens of a deeper self-awareness and intimacy in relationships. Adolescents must be taught helpful distinctions between sex and sexuality, lust, love, and intimacy as they develop the courage and ability to pursue new relationships.

Psychiatric Issues in Step 3

When a substance-abusing adolescent has reached this stage it is unlikely that any new unsuspected psychiatric disorders will emerge, but previously revealed disorders can intensify to the point at which pharmacologic intervention is necessary. It is important to note that the chief benefit of psychiatric input at this point is limited to the diagnosis of psychiatric disorders that will not respond to medication, such as a personality disorder. The accurate diagnosis of these disorders helps by confirming that the treatment should continue focusing on psychotherapeutic and behavioral issues.

Case Example

Atypical Depression During Step 3

Patient O was an 18-year-old male with marijuana, cocaine, and alcohol abuse as well as atypical depression. His father had died of a heart attack 7 months earlier at age 42. This had occurred at the height of the patient's dependence and several months after his hospitalization due to a drug overdose. Treatment focused on his grief and guilt, in which he blamed himself for his father's death. As he progressed, he began to experience such intense guilt for surviving and for feeling good that he attempted to leave treatment. As he worked his commitment to step 3, he was afraid to face his sister toward whom he had sexual thoughts, and whom he had once approached sexually while he was drunk. He expressed great embarrassment, which again led to anger and hurt directed toward his father for not being available to help him with his sexual feelings and his social relationships with girls. He felt burdened by the responsibility of being the oldest child and growing up without a father. He had feelings of inadequacy that were associated with depressed moods. He took the third step as he gave up his overly responsible and perfectionistic attitude. He began to reach out more to others for support and guidance. He became more relaxed in his relationships with others and developed a deeper level of intimacy. He was less self-critical and his depressive symptoms resolved.

Diagnosis was

- Axis Ia, Cannabis Dependence
- Axis Ib, Cocaine Abuse
- Axis Ic, Alcohol Abuse
- Axis Id, Depressive Disorder Not Otherwise Specified
- Axis Ie, Conduct Disorder, Undifferentiated Type
- Axis II, No Diagnosis
- Axis III, No Diagnosis

No medications were prescribed.

Step 4

We made a searching and fearless moral inventory of ourselves.

Step 4 fosters personal responsibility and personal growth for continued self-motivated recovery. Courage and "rigorous honesty" are required for this process to be truly "searching and fearless." The inventory is extensive and should be written in great detail. It must include behaviors related to psychiatric and behavioral disorders as well as to drug abuse. Individual and personal assistance often enhances the structured format provided by the *Step Workbook for Adolescent Chemical Dependence Recovery* (Jaffe 1990) mentioned earlier. Step 4 aims for self-acceptance and acceptance by others. It is designed to help the individual form a trusting partnership with another human being. Openness at this point in treatment allows the teenagers to deal with issues of intimacy and sexuality as appropriate for their age.

Case Example

Depression and Bulimia During Step 4

Patient P was an 18-year-old girl with cocaine, marijuana, and alcohol dependence and psychiatric diagnoses of major depressive disorder and bulimia nervosa, which were treated with imipramine 200 mg/day. Her work with Step 4 involved multiple issues of intimacy. She was initially very outgoing and outspoken during treatment but later became fearful of closeness with her peers in group therapy. She also became frightened that her successes in treatment would not last. She identified feelings of inadequacy and jealousy in relation to getting peers' attention and also feelings of loneliness.

For her Step 4 presentation, the patient focused on a female peer who was early in recovery and was dependent on male relationships. She felt compelled to help. She demonstrated her integration of step 1 by recognizing her powerlessness over this peer and over her feelings of wanting to help this "lonely" girl. Integration of step 2 was demonstrated with recognition of her "codependent" desire to help and take care of this "helpless" girl. She was able to recognize the projection of her own insecurity and helpless feelings onto this other girl. She shared how hard it was for her to feel close to girls and how she had always confused sexual with intimate feelings.

During this process, the patient used step 2 to ask for group feedback. The group members guided her to look at differences in her relations with boys and girls. She became anxious, and the group members identified that she was probably withholding secrets. As her anxiety about sharing her secrets increased she chose to take step 3 and trust the group. She told them of her embarrassment about how she had behaved during her past relationships with males. She had engaged in acts of bondage and mild physical abuse in attempts to please her boyfriends. She admitted that "If he wasn't happy, I wasn't." When she acknowledged her male dependence and was able to express her fears that closeness with females would end in abuse, she was able to tearfully hug her female partner during the presentation.

The diagnosis for this patient was

- Axis Ia, Cocaine Dependence
- Axis Ib, Alcohol Dependence
- Axis Ic, Cannabis Abuse
- Axis Id, Major Depressive Disorder
- Axis Ie, Bulimia Nervosa
- Axis II, No Diagnosis
- Axis III, No Diagnosis

Imipramine 200 mg at bedtime was prescribed.

Step 5

> We admitted to God, to ourselves, and to another human being the exact nature of our wrongs.

Step 5 involves sharing the step 4 inventory with another person and is similar to the trust shared during psychotherapy. The emphasis is on honesty and revealing of secrets and past mistakes. These revelations are fostered by trusting the listener's integrity and commitments during this process.

One method of demonstrating progress in a treatment program is for the substance-abusing adolescents to make a step 5 group presentation. They are asked to choose a specific negative character trait that has been present within themselves throughout treatment. For instance, they may discuss their arrogance, their perfectionism, their self-pity, their need to feel that they are a victim, their fear of living, or their fear of loneliness. They then choose another patient who possesses the same character structure. In front of the peer group they detail how they used steps 1 through 3 to overcome this negative trait. If it is done successfully, a breakthrough and transformation can occur, which can be inspiring. This expression of the courage and emotions is frequently moving to all in attendance.

Step 5 can also be taken in a more private setting with a sponsor, another AA/NA member, or a clergy member. Often, a well-trained and experienced clergyperson creates a safe and trusting environment in which the adolescents can reveal their most intimate, hateful, vengeful, and evil secrets, acts, and thoughts. This then allows them to ask for and accept forgiveness.

As recovery at this stage progresses, the barriers to treatment that are encountered are often related to the developmental risk factors that originally predisposed the adolescent to alcohol and drug addiction or mental disorders. These may include vengeful reactions and resentments from past abuse or issues of separation and insults to their self-worth and dignity. As the teenagers gain experience with this process, they experience recovery as an exploration and discovery and as a life adventure that helps maintain their commitment to abstinence.

At this stage, most adolescents experience a significant improvement in their overall well-being. They have demonstrated honesty, openness, willingness, responsibility, and a decision to form a working partnership with their family, friends, and sponsors.

Psychiatric Issues in Steps 4 and 5

As treatment progresses through step 5, the psychiatric barriers to successful completion of the next step rapidly diminish. At this point the diagnosis and treatment easily differentiate substance abuse disorders from psychiatric disorders, and treatment becomes a united process. Because of this, the discussion of the last seven steps includes the psychiatric perspective.

Step 6

> We were entirely ready to have God remove all these defects of character.

As substance-abusing adolescents explore their character defects they become more aware of the harmful impact these defects have had on other lives and the role that these defects can play in fostering their own relapse. The adolescents' willingness to let go of old behaviors and rely on their higher power help them to emphasize self-discipline. Elements of steps 6–12 are often used in therapeutic work with adolescents during the earlier steps.

Step 7

> We humbly asked Him to remove our shortcomings.

Step 7 continues to provide support for the next challenge in recovery. Using introspection and hard work the adolescents can change their own characters if they sincerely want to. This may involve long and difficult periods of meditation, prayer, and sharing their feelings with their therapists, sponsors, and other AA/NA members. The most difficult part of this step, after wanting to change, is learning how to behave in satisfying, life-affirming ways when they are confronted with new and different situations.

Step 8

> We made a list of all persons we had harmed and became willing to make amends to them.

Step 8 starts the process of forgiveness. The adolescent has become ready to understand rather than to be understood. "The 8th Step offers a big change from a life dominated by guilt and remorse" (Narcotics Anonymous 1988, p. 38). The focus with this step is on developing a willingness to deal on a personal level with the people whom they, the adolescents, have made uncomfortable or whom they have actually harmed. This is an unpleasant step to take, and it is suggested that this step should be taken without consideration of step 9. Working through step 8 is often blocked by the fear of taking the actions required in step 9.

Step 9

> We made direct amends to such people wherever possible, except when to do so would injure them or others.

Step 9 continues to emphasize acceptance of personal responsibility for actions taken. Amends can range from apologizing to making restitution. Other positive behaviors may include remaining sober and responsible, holding a job, maintaining regular hours, keeping promises, spending more time with loved ones, and doing community service.

Step 10

> We continued to take personal inventory, and when we were wrong, promptly admitted it.

Disciplined behaviors are fostered with daily journal recordings, daily meditations, and a regular review of old patterns of anger, resentment, and fear. Continued action on this inventory is supported. "By continuing a personal inventory, we are set free, in the here and now, from ourselves and the past. We no longer justify our existence. This step allows us to be ourselves" (Narcotics Anonymous 1988, p. 42).

Step 11

> We sought through prayer and meditation to improve our conscious contact with God as we understood Him, praying only for knowledge of His will for us and the power to carry that out.

Prayer and meditation increase the experience of the higher power. The focus here is on "quieting the mind" and listening to the power within. The goal is to increase experience of the higher power and the ability to use it as a source of strength in life. This leads to emotional balance and restoration of confidence and courage. Seeking of peace and serenity is practiced as stated in the Serenity Prayer: "God grant me the serenity to accept the things I cannot change, the courage to change the things that I can and the wisdom to know the difference." This search for serenity leads to a new vitality in life and an intuitive trust in the process that "cannot be adequately explained in words" (Narcotics Anonymous 1988, p. 46).

Step 12

> Having had a spiritual awakening as the result of these steps, we tried to carry this message to alcoholics/addicts and to practice these principles in all our affairs.

A number of recovering individuals find that assisting others helps them reinforce and strengthen their own recovery. This step affords the opportunity for individuals to help others while helping themselves. It also provides a mechanism for disseminating the 12-step process.

It is best to describe the processes, feelings, and actions demanded by taking step 12 by quoting the descriptions of this step that are contained in the writings of AA and NA:

> The steps lead to an awakening of a spiritual nature. This awakening is evidenced by changes in our lives. These changes make us better able to live by spiritual principles and to carry our message of recovery and hope to the addict who still suffers. (Narcotics Anonymous 1988, p. 48)

> We share our experience, strength, and hope. (Narcotics Anonymous 1988, p. 49).

> We feel that our lives have become worthwhile. Spiritually refreshed, we are glad to be alive. (Narcotics Anonymous 1988, p. 50)

This completes the circle consolidating the previous Steps. "Carrying the message" assists AA integrating these principles throughout our lives. "We find joy as we start to learn how to live by the principles of recovery." (Narcotics Anonymous 1988, p. 50).

The successful outcome illustrated by these 12 steps allows adolescents to live with a sincere gratitude for being alive. This chapter is written for the purpose of facilitating the psychiatrist's role in this spiritual awakening. The faith in this process, even for adolescents, is best expressed by the quote:

"Rarely have we seen a person fail who has thoroughly followed our path" (Alcoholics Anonymous 1976, p. 58).

In summary, this chapter reviews how 12-step treatment in concert with psychiatric services can be applied to adolescents. This is particularly important for adolescents because they almost always have a combination of substance abuse and psychiatric disorders. It also illustrates how to make 12-step treatment more understandable and meaningful to substance-abusing adolescents. The adolescents' 12-step progression helps define their progress as well as provide an impetus for further treatment. The role of psychiatric disorders in the 12-step treatment process is described using an integrated dual-diagnosis treatment approach.

References

Alcoholics Anonymous: Alcoholics Anonymous, 3rd Edition. New York, Alcoholics Anonymous World Services, 1976

Alcoholics Anonymous: Twelve Steps and Twelve Traditions. New York, Alcoholics Anonymous World Services, 1981

American Psychiatric Association: Diagnostic and Statistical Manual of Mental Disorders, 4th Edition. Washington, DC, American Psychiatric Association, 1994

American Society of Addiction Medicine: Patient Placement Criteria for the Treatment of Substance-Related Disorders, 2nd Edition. Chevy Chase, MD, American Society of Addiction Medicine, 1996

Bean-Bayog M: Alcoholics Anonymous, in Clinical Manual of Chemical Dependence. Edited by Ciraulo DA, Shader RL. Washington, DC, American Psychiatric Press, 1991, pp 359–376

Bell T: Preventing Adolescent Relapse. Independence, MO, Herald House/Independence Press, 1990

Chatlos JC: Adolescent dual diagnosis: a 12-step transformational model. J Psychoactive Drugs 21:189–201, 1989

Chatlos JC: Adolescent drug and alcohol addiction: diagnosis and assessment, in Comprehensive Handbook of Drug and Alcohol Addiction. Edited by Miller N. New York, Marcel Dekker, 1991a, pp 211–233

Chatlos JC: Adolescent drug and alcohol addiction: intervention and treatment, in Comprehensive Handbook of Drug and Alcohol Addiction. Edited by Miller N. New York, Marcel Dekker, 1991b, pp 235–253

Chatlos JC: Recent trends and a developmental approach to substance abuse. Child Adolesc Psychiatr Clin N Am 1:1–28, 1996

Davanloo H: Short-Term Dynamic Psychotherapy. New York, Jason Aronson, 1980

Davis DM: Intensive short-term dynamic psychotherapy in the treatment of chemical dependency, Part I. International Journal of Short-Term Dynamic Psychotherapy 4:61–88, 1989

Ehrlich P: 12-step principles and adolescent chemical dependence treatment. J Psychoactive Drugs 19:311–317, 1987

Evans K, Sullivan LM: Dual Diagnosis: Counseling the Mentally Ill Substance Abuser. New York, Guilford, 1990

Fishman HC: Intensive Structural Therapy: Treating Families in Their Social Context. New York, Basic Books, 1993

Gorski TT, Miller M: Staying Sober: A Guide for Relapse Prevention. Independence, MO, Herald House, 1986

Harrison PA, Hoffmann NG: CATOR Report: Adolescent Treatment Completers: One Year Later. St Paul, MN, Ramsey Clinic, 1989

Hoffmann NG, Estroff TW: Documenting quality care for adults: how to document clinical treatment. Seminar presented at the 1998 Florida Summit II, Orlando, FL, September 1998a

Hoffmann NG, Estroff TW: Documenting quality care for children and adolescents: how to document clinical treatment. Seminar presented at the 1998 Florida Summit II, Orlando, FL, September 1998b

Hoffmann NG, Halikas JA, Mee-Lee D: The Cleveland Admission Discharge and Transfer Criteria. Cleveland, OH, Greater Cleveland Hospital Association, 1987

Hoffmann NG, Halikas JA, Mee-Lee D, et al: Patient Placement Criteria for the Treatment of Psychoactive Substance Use Disorders. Washington, DC, American Society of Addiction Medicine, 1991

Hoffmann NG, DeHart SS, Gogineni A: Alcohol dependence as a chronic health problem among older adults. The Southwestern Journal on Aging 14:57–64, 1998

Hohman M, LeCroy CW: Predictors of adolescent AA affiliation. Adolescence 31:339–352, 1996

Jaffe SL: Step Workbook for Adolescent Chemical Dependence Recovery: A Guide to the First Five Steps. Washington, DC, American Psychiatric Press, 1990

Jaffe SL: Pathways to relapse in chemically dependent adolescents. Adolescent Counselor 55:42–44, 1992

Lane RD, Schwartz GE: Levels of emotional awareness: a cognitive developmental theory and its application to psychopathology. Am J Psychiatry 144:133–143, 1987

Marlatt GA: Relapse prevention: theoretical rationale and overview of the model, in Relapse Prevention. Edited by Marlatt GA, Gordon JR. New York, Guilford, 1985, pp 3–70

Masterson JF: Treatment of the Borderline Adolescent: A Developmental Approach. New York, Wiley Interscience, 1972

Mooney A, Eisenberg A, Eisenberg H: The Recovery Book. New York, World Publishing, 1992

Nace EP: Alcoholics Anonymous, in Substance Abuse: A Comprehensive Textbook. Edited by Lowinson JH, Ruiz PR, Millman RB. Baltimore, MD, Williams & Wilkins, 1992, pp 486–495

Narcotics Anonymous: Narcotics Anonymous, 5th Edition. Van Nuys, CA, NA World Service Office, 1988

Narcotics Anonymous: NA—It Works. How and Why. Van Nuys, CA, NA World Service Office, 1993

Schulz JE: 12-step programs in recovery from drug and alcohol addiction, in Comprehensive Handbook of Drug and Alcohol Addiction. Edited by Miller NS. New York, Marcel Dekker, 1991, pp 1255–1271

Zywiak WH, Hoffmann NG, Floyd AS: Enhancing alcohol treatment outcomes through aftercare and self-help groups. Med Health R I 82:87–90, 1999

13 Spirituality

Martha A. Morrison, M.D.
Norman G. Hoffmann, Ph.D.
Sara S. DeHart, Ph.D.
Todd Wilk Estroff, M.D.
Paul King, M.D.

The spiritual component of recovery is an important, often overlooked, and usually misunderstood aspect of the treatment effort. This is especially true in the treatment of substance-abusing adolescents. The very personal nature of the concept of spirituality and the lack of a universally agreed upon definition fuels the confusion and misunderstanding. Of all the chapters in this book, this one has been the most difficult and controversial. No other chapter has prompted so much intense discussion, controversy, and genuine disagreements. Nowhere else are the clashes among psychiatric models, traditional substance abuse treatment approaches, and personal experiences more profound. This chapter attempts to provide nothing more than a very brief introduction to the concepts defining and relating to spirituality in the context of treatment. Those who wish to delve more deeply into the topic may wish not only to consult the literature on the topic but also to query those with personal experience in recovery.

What Is *Spirituality* in the Context of Treatment?

Attempts to apply definitions of *spirituality* derived from other sources to the context of substance abuse treatment and recovery range from misleading to humorous. Most attempts to define spirituality would invoke a dictionary definition referring to "the spirit or the soul as distinguished from the body," or as something related to religious beliefs. Others attempting to define the term may think of supernatural beings or essences. Only the most cynical would accept the definition of a liquid containing alcohol as spiritual.

It is tempting to define spirituality in terms of what it is not. It is not religion. One of the most profound realizations from the Alcoholics Anonymous (AA) model and the 12-step movement was the observation that religion itself is not enough to overcome addiction. Like willpower, religious faith alone was not enough to achieve abstinence for the chronic alcoholic patient. Nor should spirituality be confused with charismatic groups led by any "gurus" or "heroes."

In the context of adolescent substance abuse treatment and recovery, spirituality is associated with a profound personality change and the finding of an inner peace and strength. It is also highly personal and specific to the individual. During treatment, spirituality should be kept as clearly distinct from religion and religious interpretations. In the AA philosophy, the definition or identification of a higher power is left to the individual. His or her higher power can range from a traditional view of God to nature or even to the collective wisdom of the AA group. In this context, spirituality becomes a bridge to something beyond oneself. It is a way of connecting to and achieving a sense of association with a universe larger than one's personal existence. This is what is referred to as developing a consciousness of a power greater than oneself. The spiritual experiences of individuals are often extremely emotional or even mystical. Whenever this inner change occurs, there is an outward, observable change in attitude, personality, and behaviors.

Documentation of the association between this concept of spirituality and changes in personality and behaviors dates back to the beginnings of AA. In the "Big Book" of AA there are several discussions related to spirituality as a component of personality change:

> The terms "spiritual experiences" and "spiritual awakening" are used many times in this book which, upon careful reading, shows that the personality change sufficient to bring about recovery from alcoholism has manifested itself among us in many different forms. (Alcoholics Anonymous World Services 1976, p. 569)

One physician, describing the concept of the personality change that occurs among individuals who became sober through AA participation, wrote "...we observe a profound change in personality. You would hardly recognize them" (Alcoholics Anonymous World Services 1976, p. 572).

How Is Spirituality an Issue for Adolescents?

Most if not all substance-abusing adolescents enter treatment with very distorted views of spirituality. They often have overwhelmingly negative and destructive views of their lives. Spirituality is almost universally associated with the disapproval of religious authority figures. This can be exacerbated by a variety of negative experiences that have resulted in the dismissal or complete rejection of spiritual concepts.

In the most extreme form, this opposition to religion results in identification with, and glorification of, negative stereotypes. Typically this will take the form of espousing creeds of cruelty, hate, and evil. Physical manifestations include wearing black clothing, gruesome tattoos, and displaying Nazi swastikas, pentograms, upside-down crosses, and use of the number 666. These adolescents may be preoccupied with death, doom, and destruction and frequently describe feelings of profound emptiness and nothingness. This negative spirituality, for want of a better term, is often expressed as the glorification of evil through gruesome oral, written, musical, and artistic themes.

How Is Spirituality Addressed in Treatment?

Spirituality cannot be taught in a didactic fashion. It is largely an experiential, nonlogical process of association and emulation. The first exposure tends to come through the example of other recovering persons, either recovering members of the staff or members of self-help groups attended by the adolescent patient during treatment. Recovering individuals who have achieved a spiritual awakening or spiritual state appear to have a sense of calm, peace, and fullness that contrasts with the gloom and doom described above. This sense of positive serenity can stimulate curiosity for an adolescent who has never shared such an experience.

Example and knowledge alone are not sufficient to bring about the transformations necessary for recovery. As the adolescents settle into the treatment program, they are required to act in accordance with principles such as honesty and personal integrity. This promotes, and to an extent requires, behaviors that are compatible with the type of personality change noted in the AA literature. Many times the substance-abusing adolescent acts on the basis of external direction rather than out of an understanding of the spiritual or philosophical implication of the behavior. Most often, behavioral changes occur first. Understanding and internalization associated with the spiritual awakening develop gradually over time.

At this point the 12-step component of the program can be useful to begin the internalization process. For example, the first step, admitting powerlessness, is not a surrender in the military sense. Rather, it is the giving up of the pretense that there is no problem and the delusion that the addicted individual has his or her use under control. Step 2 then gives permission to seek help from someone or some power outside oneself. Having acknowledged that the problem is beyond one's ability to deal with it alone, the rational thing to do is seek assistance. The third step adds refinement in that the individual agrees to accept, or at least listen to, advice or guidance from others. In step 4, the "searching and fearless moral inventory" requires the individual to take personal stock of past behaviors as well as his or her personal strengths and weakness. This step requires the groundwork of the prior steps and begins development of a blueprint for internalizing changes. Gorski (1989) is an excellent reference for those not familiar with the steps of AA. Each of the steps requires some action on the part of the patient. The principle is that if the individual follows the required behaviors, insight and awareness will result.

In a sense, this approach to spirituality is a mentoring of the adolescents to help them find positive principles and develop the confidence to follow those principles. The "personality change" is seen as the adolescent becomes able to emulate positive role models. These changes are an indication of the spiritual awakening described in the "Big Book." As the adolescent comes to find this internalization a comfort and source of peace, the probability of lasting recovery is enhanced.

Adolescents who "work" the steps experience something greater than the sum of each individual step. They describe a growing feeling of personal vital energy, of being alive, and of having a new meaning to life. A positive attitude begins to replace the negative perspective. Along with a growing sense of confidence comes a sense of humility—that they are a part of a greater whole in which the credit for accomplishments often needs to be shared. The adolescents take credit for their own efforts and achievements, and at the same time they honestly acknowledge the assistance from others that they have received. Lasting recovery and sobriety also involve an ongoing willingness to ask for help when it is needed and to expect growth to be a continuing process. This is the essence of the spiritual awakening that recovering individuals talk about or that occurs while these individuals are in the process of achieving their profound personality change. That change, in turn, further facilitates long-term recovery.

Conclusion

Even if the reader does not understand or believe in spirituality as presented here, it can be the most important aspect of treatment and prolonged recovery for the substance-abusing adolescent. Spirituality can be a very powerful force in the initiation and maintenance of abstinence when everything else has failed. As such it must not be ignored, even if it does not appear to be logical, scientific, or explicitly articulated. Both the skeptical readers and those with personal experience in recovery are urged to keep an open and accepting mind. The objective of this admonition is that the former not reject what is unknown to them and that the latter not focus on their own path as the only one.

References

Alcoholics Anonymous: Alcoholics Anonymous, 3rd Edition. New York, Alcoholics Anonymous World Services, 1976

Gorski TT: Understanding the Twelve Steps: A Guide for Counselors, Therapists, and Recovering People. Independence, MO, Herald House/Independence Press, 1989

14 Family Treatment

Susan D. Wallace

Todd Wilk Estroff, M.D.

> The family is the basic unit of growth and experience, fulfillment or failure, illness, or health. We are all products of our experience.
>
> Nathan Ackerman

This chapter focuses on intensive family therapy and how it can increase the chances for the successful treatment of adolescent substance abuse disorders. Comprehensive family therapy uses a continuum of inpatient and outpatient gender-specific treatment for both substance-abusing adolescents and their parents. Effective family treatment plays an important part in a positive outcome. This chapter describes the characteristics of the adolescents and parents who seek treatment; emphasizes the importance of positive family participation; explores the family issues specific to substance-abusing adolescents and their parents; outlines the components of a sensible proven treatment model; and addresses the family's cognitive, behavioral, moral, ethical, spiritual, and interpersonal problems that must change.

The impact of family pathology on adolescent behavior cannot be overestimated. Adolescent drug abuse is often a result of the entire family's abnormal behavior. Parents and children from these families frequently share poor self-concept, unusual thought patterns, and negative experiences. They use similar rationalizations to justify their continued use of drugs and alcohol. They usually lack critical social skills. They grow up in family systems that are remarkable for their poor communication and lack of respect for the individual. Unfortunately, these destructive family patterns are not recognized as abnormal but often play a role in the initiation and continuation of the adolescent's substance abuse. Recognition and acknowledgment of these counterproductive behaviors as eccentric can emphasize how important parental participation can be. As difficult as it may be to change, if the parents can alter their behavior, they can play an important part in their child's recovery.

Sadly, some parents are either unmotivated or are too disturbed to be a resource. In cases in which parents are unavailable or unable to participate in family treatment, it is important to replace them with another interested individual or individuals. Mentors can fill this role. Mentors are solicited to 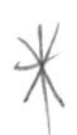 substitute for the missing family members to promote the adolescent's recovery and help him or her to become a responsible adult. Most often, concerned relatives will take on this mentoring role. Obviously, treatment is much more problematic and will regularly fail when adolescents have neither a parent nor an interested mentor guiding them.

Rationale for Gender-Specific Treatment

The development of emotions, values, and ways of dealing with the world differs for males and females. Family functioning can play a decisive role in an adolescent's self-image and behavior. Adolescents' reactions can be positive or negative depending on their life circumstances, academic competence, social acceptance, parental approval, and personal appearance. Not surprisingly, the situation becomes tenuous when substance abuse begins because it adds a distinctively negative component to the adolescents' milieu. Because of this negative factor, the adolescents' response to normal stressors can become more disturbed. They tend to have more psychiatric symptoms, tend to isolate themselves, and often react more intensely to physical, sexual, and emotional trauma.

Although there are some common reactions, males and females display their reactions to these multiple insults in far different gender-distinctive ways. For example, boys form their identity primarily in relation to the world around them. They are socialized to find their place in the world and learn how to gain power within that structure. Adolescent males often base self-esteem on physical strength and not on showing emotions. Boys have a tendency to shut down emotionally and have difficulty in expressing their feelings and emotions. This tends to result in emotional if not physical isolation. Adolescent females, on the other hand, primarily form their identity in relationship to other people. This means that they are interested in what their relationship means and how it works. Girls define themselves through the people they associate with and by how well they get along with other people. They easily express their feelings and emotions but are often unable to identify or verbalize the source of their particular emotion or behavior. They tend to be more submissive, dependent, passive, and emotional than males. They are frequently expected to conform to traditional gender roles. Worst of all, they often base their self-esteem on their own physical attributes and attention from men. When upset, they often expect adults to guess what is going on inside them, and they respond enthusiastically when an adult in their life shows an interest in exploring their feelings. Adolescent girls with substance abuse problems are often identified as being more deviant than boys who display identical behaviors. They are considered to be sicker, more problematic, and at higher risk. They also characterize themselves as having less value as people.

These gender-related feelings and behaviors are important to explore during treatment. It is important to provide separate care for male and female substance-abusing adolescents. This is best accomplished in same-gender group therapy. Separate therapy is an ideal that is not always possible.

Parent Gender Issues

It is important to note that problematic adolescents of both genders have far different ways of responding to their male and female parents. They have a greater tendency to be combative, angry, and antagonistic with their mothers but less frequently engage in these behaviors with their fathers. One adolescent explaining the difference said, "Mothers will stay with you no matter what, because mothers don't leave." Adolescents of both genders entering residential substance abuse treatment are more likely to reside with a single female parent. This is usually due to out-of-wedlock birth, divorce, or separation.

Absent fathers are the rule. They are frequently less communicative and more demanding, especially toward their sons, whereas they tend to be more permissive with their daughters except in sexual matters. They tend not to explain their reasoning to their children, responding only with "because I said so," whereas mothers attempt to answer by explaining their reasoning and sharing their emotions. Thus, parents of both genders have their own specific issues relating to their same-gender and opposite-gender children. These problems are best addressed in a supportive, accepting environment to allow for a greater understanding of distressing socialization experiences and the often unconventional communication styles. Parents need to express their thoughts and feelings in a safe setting without fear of ridicule. This is also best accomplished in a same-gender group setting.

Parent Profiles

> When I had to wrap my purse in plastic and take it into the shower to keep her from stealing, I began to get a clue that my daughter was out of control.
>
> A parent

The parents of substance-abusing adolescents who present for treatment share many characteristics with their children. Frequently they are using substances, are in recovery, or have a history of drug abuse. Often they have developed into an imperfect maturity as a result of many missed steps on the developmental path to responsible adulthood. They lack the necessary social skills to cope with difficult or problematic situations involving themselves and their children. The result is that they are unable to model responsible adult behavior for their children and are unable to parent effectively. These deficits often produce wide-ranging negative consequences for everyone in their lives. A major treatment goal, therefore, is to teach them how to become effective parents.

Mothers

Many mothers of substance-abusing adolescents report leaving their family of origin on bad terms or to avoid intolerable family conflict. They often left home during their teen years and tend to bear children before their twentieth birthday and before marriage. When treated in the safety of a single-gender therapeutic environment, they are able to characterize their early pregnancies as a desperate way to find solace and balance in their lives. Unfortunately these poor choices are rarely effective and only make the situation worse. Some mothers report feeling disconnected from their nuclear family and their children, resulting in an overwhelming sense of loneliness. They have often lived in families with long histories of social isolation, public ridicule, and inadequate parenting. Their isolation and shame ensure that significant family secrets remain secret.

These mothers frequently have as many or more problems as their children. They often present with poor physical health as a result of personal neglect or cigarettes, alcohol, or drug use. Many have lifelong histories of mental health problems and report significant histories using and abusing prescribed medication. They report being physically, sexually, and emotionally abused. Their peer relationships are similar in nature to the unrewarding patterns of their children. "Not fitting in" and seeking acceptance from a negative peer group is also part of the parental experience.

Parents of both genders report seeking out relationships for purposes other than mutual satisfaction. Mothers frequently report their involvement with men as dissatisfying experiences. Their relationships often re-create the negative experiences of their own nuclear family. They frequently describe themselves as looking for nurturing and protection but believe they will never find it.

Fathers

Fathers also report dissatisfying relationships with members of the opposite sex. They relate that they also learned their attitudes and behaviors by observing how the dysfunctional men in their families treated women. It is common for mothers to report sexual victimization; however, increasing numbers of fathers are also reporting that they too were sexually abused. These revelations optimally occur when the fathers feel safe enough to share their painful past experiences in a fathers' group.

Both parents have often missed affectionate platonic relationships with members of the same gender. This makes it difficult for them to build and teach relationship skills to their own same-gender children. Many parents have experienced school and academic failure and many dropped out before completion of high school. Both male and female parents tend to view leisure time and recreation as an unobtainable luxury. They have difficulty controlling their emotions and often feel guilty about their abusive behaviors toward their children.

By the time they bring their teenagers to residential treatment, these parents are unable to effectively deal with or parent their substance-abusing adolescent. Parents of both genders report a repetitive cycle of being too permissive and then too rigid and controlling. This cycle is the result of their own confusion about parenting and not having enough faith in themselves to make decisions and stick to them. Their desire to change the way they deal with their anger is often identified as a major treatment goal. They report feeling overwhelmed by guilt and regret and their sense of failure as parents. Most of them simultaneously verbalize love for their adolescents, fear of losing them, frustration trying to help them, and their desire to cooperate in any way they can. Most parents who participate in residential treatment have enormous difficulty understanding and accepting the following issues with regard to their adolescent:

- Accepting that some of their teenager's problems are beyond their control
- Accepting that they are part of the problem and not "blaming" their child
- Being consistent in providing models through their own behaviors—especially by not using drugs or alcohol
- Supporting and enforcing the program's rules and contracts
- Staying consistent in their resolve to guide their child during and after treatment
- Understanding adolescent relapse and not blaming the adolescent or the program
- Keeping the lines of communication open by listening to the positive as well as the negative things their adolescent has to say

However, it is not enough for these parents to accept and understand these issues. They must also deal with their own individual, parental, and family issues, including the following:

- Their own use and abuse of substances
- Their failure to take on a parenting role
- Their high tolerance for inappropriate behaviors
- Their failure to respond to unacceptable behaviors
- Their exaggerated responses to inappropriate behavior
- Their poor role modeling
- The keeping of family secrets
- Their failure to be an emotional resource for their children
- Their unrealistic view of their children's ability to thrive without guidance
- Their lack of consistency

- Their lack of vigilance
- Their avoidance of emotional issues
- Their conflicting messages (e.g.,"You can tell me anything, as long as it does not upset me.")
- Their failure to provide safety and predictability at home
- Their failure to recognize the importance of their family
- Ways in which they place their children into the middle of their own marital conflicts
- Their personal mental health issues that interfere with parenting
- Their loss of resolve that results in their surrendering to their acting-out adolescent
- Their failure to accept that parents must anticipate their adolescent's problems and plan how they will react when crises occur

Adolescent Profiles

> Make a fearless moral inventory, yeah right. You counselors and my parents would just use my honesty as a way to keep me in treatment longer.
>
> An adolescent in residential treatment

Treadway (1989) described adolescent substance abuse as "hanging on for dear life." This description is a fitting comment on what to expect when treating adolescents. By the time adolescents are in serious trouble with substance use the family, school, and community have lost effective control. When parental control is ineffective, adolescents often escalate their behavior and become even more inconsistent. Just when parents need to be more assertive with their children it becomes almost impossible to do so. Parents of troubled adolescents have the understandable fear that their child's life will end in injury, death, or suicide. This causes them to lose their resolve to be strong when confronted with their adolescents' dangerous behaviors. The result is that the adolescents find their parents rapidly cycling between firm resolve and placation. The parental experience becomes an endless cycle of anger over the teenager's unacceptable behavior coupled with fear of losing the teenager altogether.

On the other hand, when adolescents have too much freedom they feel abandoned. Escalation of their acting out behaviors is often an attempt to get parental attention or to force their parents to exercise parental control. It is normal for adolescents to struggle with their parents and other authority figures. Every family undergoes significant stress when it enters new stages of the family life cycle. Even in relatively normal families it is difficult for parents to allow their adolescents more autonomy so that they can begin the separation process.

Separation and individuation are important developmental tasks of adolescence. Substance-abusing adolescents do not have sufficient opportunity to address and resolve these adolescent rites of passage. Substance abuse blocks their emotional growth and arrests this critical step along the path to mature adulthood. Adolescents who have not developed these essential skills need to understand and hopefully correct the aberrant relationships within their family. Although adolescence is a time for learning to move toward independence, firm parental guidance is essential. Adolescents require firm adult supervision to become effective adults and parents. Ideally this will occur in a supportive family context.

Adolescent Denial

Most adolescents do not view their substance use as a problem. Consequently they lack the insight, hindsight, and foresight and thus any motivation to change their behavior. They believe that the use of substances is an issue for the older generation (25 and up) and that sobriety is for "other" people. Adolescents do not have as long a substance abuse history as adult substance abusers, and as a result they cannot reflect on their own dysfunctional behaviors or develop the insight necessary for future decision making. They are at a time in their lives in which they find substance use to be the easiest means of managing emotional pain. Adolescent substance abuse patterns and motivations are frequently different from those of adults, and thus adult treatment protocols are often not directly applicable to adolescents. Adolescents presenting with substance abuse have innumerable problems that vary from abuser to abuser. Adolescent substance abuse is not caused by a reliable cluster of personal characteristics that differentiate them from nonabusers. Substance abuse in adolescents is a function of a number of environmental and genetic factors.

Most of the adolescents in residential treatment have a history of previous treatment for multiple problems ranging from family and school problems to delinquency. Substance use and abuse are usually the last problems to be identified in an acute medical or legal setting. Adolescents hide their substance abuse. They fear not having access to their drugs and being forced into treatment imposed by their parents or the legal system. If honest, most adolescents define their use and abuse of substances as a way to feel "mellow" or "numb," which to them means finding emotional tranquility in the midst of family dysfunction and chaos. The safety provided by a treatment program encourages adolescents to express their emotional pain and share how they found solace in their substance use and abuse. Most substance-abusing adolescents surmise that the substance use kept them functioning at some level at least until they ended up in treatment. They report a pattern of early experimentation and use that turned quickly into regular abuse. At admission, they are often unable to contract for any type of sustained abstinence.

Before admission, getting high was the activity that overshadowed every other issue in their lives. Their substance abuse compromised their school, family, and social lives; their recreation; their health; and their relationships. Although many report a long history of school problems both academically and behaviorally, most believe that substance use is something positive in their lives. This makes engaging these adolescents in treatment even more difficult.

As the substance use escalates, family conflicts intensify. The adolescent's substance abuse progression also leads to other behaviors that elicit unwanted attention. These adolescents are most often the "identified patient" in the nuclear family. Most adolescents who come into treatment are living in families or have extended families whose major problems have gone unaddressed for years if not generations. They are reacting to divorce, abandonment, or physical, emotional, and/or sexual abuse. Most of the adolescents come from families in which substance abuse is an integral part of the family's identity and is the major method of coping with adverse events. These families often have extensive histories of emergency treatment and hospitalization for "accidents" and drug and alcohol overdoses. Most substance-abusing adolescents report these incidents as standard ways of getting attention from their families.

Diagnostic Issues

Most adolescents entering residential treatment have a history of both substance use and mental health issues. Accurate diagnosis of the adolescent is difficult because newly admitted adolescents typically withhold information. Getting a true assessment requires the establishment of trust with staff and peers and that often takes time. A preliminary diagnosis is frequently made in a crisis situation and at a time when the adolescent is in an acute care facility. The crisis is usually precipitated by trauma, intoxication, drug overdose, or suicidal gestures. Psychiatric considerations are often overshadowed by more urgent acute medical and safety issues. In the rush to get the adolescent out of the acute care situation as quickly as possible, the more complex symptoms are often left undiagnosed, deferred, ignored, or misdiagnosed.

Daily living in a residential treatment setting must provide the safety and security needed to build trust. Other adolescents in treatment must be clean and sober. When these conditions are met, a more accurate assessment of the adolescents' problems can be more easily elicited. They can begin to discuss their favorite drugs of abuse and how they use the drugs to self-medicate. They can compare their use and abuse to those of their parents and the other adolescents in treatment with them. Additionally, they can begin to identify their parents' and their own mental health issues even if they cannot accurately label the disorder.

Like their parents, substance-abusing adolescents often begin their substance abuse with tobacco, alcohol, and marijuana, the so-called gateway drugs. For a time, their choices are nonspecific and do not follow a pattern. As their use progresses, they tend to focus on and select a favorite drug. Most will deviate and use other substances if the price or availability is favorable. They are generally looking for stimulation or sedation and choose the substances that will produce the desired effect. For example, when anxious, they seek sedation, and when depressed, they seek stimulation and euphoria. Adolescents in group therapy settings are helped in their own self-assessment as they identify and understand their drug abuse and mental health issues. They talk about their pretreatment experiences with their family, their school, and their friends. They share stories of feeling anxious, angry, and perhaps sad and lonely. They talk of not fitting in, often isolating themselves to avoid being hurt. They share trauma, parental marital conflict, and the painful life issues that affect them. Adolescents often report finding answers in drugs as they became preteens. They also discuss how their use patterns changed over time and progressed from experimentation to regular use.

Substance abuse can produce, mask, and enhance as well as mimic psychiatric disorders among both parents and children. Withdrawal can also imitate psychiatric symptoms. It is important to have open communication with the adolescents and their parents to understand how to best treat them. Adolescents presenting at any point in time can appear to fit the symptoms of various mental health disorders. It is important not to jump in with psychotropic medications until the situation has stabilized for at least a few weeks, unless severe symptoms force an earlier decision. The most common diagnoses are mood, anxiety, and personality disorders. Most of the problems fall into a mixed affective category, which the adolescents describe as either alternating or simultaneous mixed episodes of depression and mania.

Adolescents who display criminal behaviors tend to report greater inhalant abuse (gasoline, glue, Freon, carburetor cleaner, or correction fluid), which disinhibits them and induces reckless behavior and feelings of invincibility. Most adolescents avoid lysergic acid diethylamide (LSD) and mescaline because they share a fear of hallucinogens, believing that the effects are too unpredictable. Many adolescents are reluctant to report and often minimize alcohol use because they are afraid of the stereotypes of alcoholics or because of unpleasant family experiences. The rare adolescents who are able to integrate their drug use and mental health symptoms can help their counselors to better plan their treatment.

Family Treatment Protocol

> You counselors are brainwashing our parents.
>
> A resident adolescent

The primary goal of the treatment program is to understand both parents and their adolescents in their context and tailor treatment to respond to their presenting and underlying needs. Family recovery is as important as the recovery of the adolescents. Family involvement should help shift the power dynamics from the adolescent back to the parent. Power in the family should belong to the parent. If possible, that hierarchy should be reestablished early in the treatment process.

Parental Reassurance

When parents come in to the treatment program they feel weak, battered, and powerless. As a result, they feel unable to help their child. At admission parents are often on an emotional roller coaster. They question whether the placement was the correct move and they feel guilty about having to transfer their parenting responsibility to a treatment program. It is important early on to reassure the parents and to explain the details of the program and its philosophy. They should be told that they will be both consulted and included in all phases of their child's treatment.

Sharing the treatment philosophy helps ease some of the parents' fears. In addition, some parents need to be reassured that the program counselors and other parents will understand their needs and fears. In forming alliances with the parents, the staff must also respond to the parents' own desires for nurture, structure, and predictability. Failure to recognize the parental needs during treatment can often compromise the treatment of the adolescent. Parents of substance-abusing adolescents also need time to develop strengths and skills. Addressing these parental issues is a priority because if they are not addressed, the parents' fear and frustration can severely interfere with their involvement in the adolescent's treatment.

Parental Education

Family treatment begins with parental education and orientation. This is the most important phase of treatment because it is preparation for the entire therapeutic experience. When parents first arrive they receive a "Parent Survival Manual" that outlines in humorous ways what to expect as their child settles into treatment. This orientation acts as an important motivational tool for parents, helping them to commit to and become active participants in their child's treatment. The orientation has four phases: 1) learning the program philosophy, 2) settling in, 3) predicting behaviors, and 4) understanding the program and the parental role in treatment. Orientation is based on a social support model and is taught by parents who have successfully completed treatment with their adolescents. A positive outcome is more easily achievable when parents participate in orientation and understand the concepts presented.

Orientation to the Program's Philosophy

During orientation parents are taught that life problems and uncomfortable situations cannot be planned. They learn that adolescents do not abuse substances because their parents deliberately pushed them in that direction. They learn to understand that humans do not plan on poverty, alcoholism, divorce, illness, or other major life issues that have an impact on their lives. They learn to understand that most people handle difficulty using only the behaviors that they know. They are told that parents are an important part of the solution and are crucial to a positive outcome.

The parents of other adolescents in the program teach the orientation program and talk with parents who are just beginning treatment. They talk about the issues and behaviors that cause them to feel guilty and powerless. They share issues that may have contributed to their adolescent having to be in residential treatment. The inexperienced parents are reassured that the need to place their adolescent in residential treatment does not negate their ability to parent. They are taught that their issues are fairly common among the parents of substance-abusing adolescents. A philosophy of hope and a nonjudgmental approach are emphasized. All parents are encouraged to share their problems with each other.

Settling In

After learning the overall program philosophy, parents go through a settling-in phase. They are taught that most adolescents will try to get out of treatment, and that they will encounter various amounts of emotional battering from their adolescent. This prediction helps them plan their responses in advance, at a time when they are calm and, it is hoped, rational. They are taught how to survive during this high-anxiety phase of treatment. They are reassured that the staff members will handle these situations if they (the parents) feel unable to do so or if their adolescent's behavior gets out of control.

Predicting Behaviors

The predicting phase is sometimes seen by adolescents as a conspiracy. Seasoned parents share their experiences and anecdotal stories. Parents must be helped to understand that adolescent denial is to be expected and that it is best handled with firmness and humor. They are told that most adolescents will plot to get out of treatment in a well-defined pattern.

Use of Guilt

The parents are told that initially their adolescents will attempt to use guilt. They are told to expect that everything they have ever said or done wrong in their entire lives will be thrown in their faces. An adolescent once told a parent, "If you don't take me out I'll go downstairs and tell all the parents that you're a drunk." The parent's response was, "I'll go tell them myself but you are staying here because I love you." When the guilt approach fails, the adolescent will regroup and try again by pretending to cooperate.

Pretending

The regrouping phase occurs when the adolescent becomes tired of trying to get out and appears to cooperate. They parrot 12-step sayings and appear to be extremely compliant. This is not necessarily a good sign, but it is predictable and it must often be addressed as a false commitment to treatment. When they realize it is not working, the adolescents become tired of pretending and move on to a third phase, "the last ditch effort."

The Last Outburst

At least one last major incident will occur in which the adolescent will try anything in his or her power to avoid treatment. If the parents do not succumb to this intense pressure, treatment can truly begin. By predicting these events in advance, parents are able to successfully resist their adolescent's manipulative behavior. They must be reassured that their strength is, in fact, greatly admired by their adolescent and that their firm stance advances effective treatment. The adolescent may realize this but will not admit it until a much later date.

Understanding the Family Role in Treatment

A final phase of parental education and orientation is understanding the roles they play in their child's treatment. Many parents are in treatment and recovery themselves and have a very difficult time understanding that adults and adolescents recover in different ways. They are taught that not wanting help is natural and that it is not a fault of the program or their adolescent. The differences between adolescent and adult recovery are thoroughly explained. For example, parents are taught that adolescent recovery is a long and arduous process that takes commitment and a firm sense of purpose on their part as well as their adolescent's part. Parents are helped to empathize with their teen and to remember how they thought and acted when they were the same age. Most parents realize that for their adolescent to remain clean and sober for the rest of his or her life may be unrealistic. When recovering parents are able to share their own stories about how long it took for them to become sober, they will also remember that talking about substance abuse in a positive light was normal for them when they were adolescents. They also come to realize that their adolescents must be allowed to express the positive effects of the abused substances and how they saw this as a survival tool.

Understanding the Difference Between Habilitation and Rehabilitation

The most difficult issues for family members to understand are the need for habilitation and the improbability that a 14-year-old can be rehabilitated.

Habilitation means learning new social skills and self-controls that were never present in their lives. This is in direct contrast to *rehabilitation*, the relearning of these skills that occurs during adult substance abuse treatment. Parents are helped to understand that it is up to the adolescents to learn and internalize this knowledge and to learn to make choices about their future based on what they discover during their period of habilitation. The parents are taught to encourage honesty in their adolescents, whether it is positive or negative.

For example, adolescents think that they are expected to embrace recovery regardless of how they truly feel. It is much more therapeutic for adolescents to be open and honest about what they are actually thinking. If this honesty is permitted many adolescents will openly state that they have no intention of becoming clean and sober. Expression of these honest but negative thoughts is not an indicator of treatment failure. Instead parents are taught that their adolescent must get positive feedback for honesty. They are also assured that brutal honesty from their child is hard to hear but is critical to the adolescent's recovery. When this happens, adolescents will openly talk with their parents when they feel like getting high. These moments provide parents a powerful opportunity to be supportive and earn their child's trust. When their children criticize them or their parenting skills many parents react in negative ways and blame the adolescent or the program for the criticism. They in effect "shoot the messenger" rather than learn from the truth. The important message for parents is to listen and try to understand everything their adolescent says, not just what they want to hear, and not to personalize their child's honest yet negative comments.

Parents must understand that adolescents may not sustain total abstinence during their teen years but at least they have the tools to use when they are ready. The power of their child's substance-abusing peer group is another important factor for parents to grasp. Many adolescents view "friends" as a shield and a lifeline. They view changing friends as a frightening prospect. Parents are prepared to address this issue with their adolescent by acknowledging that change is hard for everyone, especially for an age group that is already experiencing rapid physical and emotional change. The parents also learn that the desire to change one's life for the better is an adult concept. Finally, parents review the purpose of each phase of the entire program and the reasons why it is constructed that way. When the parents finish their orientation, education, and personal treatment they are better equipped to take a more active and participatory role in their adolescent's treatment.

Parental Treatment

In addition to the parents' orientation, gender-specific parent groups, individual and family therapy, and weekly 2-hour psychoeducational groups are mandatory. These groups help the parents address the problems presented by their adolescents. They learn in these groups about specific adolescent substance abuse issues and why adolescents need to be approached in different ways than adults. Psychoeducational groups analyze common dysfunctional and problematic family systems and the impact of grandparents on their current parenting methods. Communication between the parents and the therapist is emphasized as a way to learn effective parenting skills. Psychoeducational groups teach parents to understand the developmental stages of adolescence and how parenting needs to change to respond to these stages. Discussions are held on adolescent sexuality. These psychoeducational groups help parents understand about co-occurring psychiatric disorders and how these disorders can be related to their child's substance abuse. They are helped to understand why medications are prescribed for the children and the importance of open communication with the adolescent's physician. Lastly, they are educated about postdischarge program requirements and the importance of contract compliance in the aftercare program. The psychoeducational groups help enhance the parents' ability to deal with their problem adolescent and develop the skills necessary to avoid making the same mistakes with their other children.

Forming a Parenting Partnership

It is important to note the strengths of each family and to use these strengths to help the parents gain the motivation to participate. The family distress model by Cornille and Boroto (1992) is important because it describes a model that promotes family problem solving and encourages the use of social supports. It also helps families identify their strengths and encourages a sharing partnership rather than a hierarchical relationship between therapist and family. A "parenting partnership" is a concept that encourages parents to learn from the treatment staff and other parents. This is often difficult because families are often forced into treatment during a crisis, especially when their adolescent acts out in the community. In a sense, the adolescents force their family members to get them help as a direct consequence of their own negative behavior.

A positive therapeutic alliance between therapist and family is helpful.

When it occurs, counselors can model and guide rather than educate and direct. The consultative, collaborative approach to family therapy is important. When the relationship is mutual and shared, partnering outcomes are more positive. This helps lay the groundwork for families to break their dysfunctional behavioral patterns. A stepwise approach toward this partnership is important. Missed or fumbled steps while forming this relationship can result in mistrust and repetitive mistakes.

It should be obvious that effective family treatment calls for addressing issues deeper than those on the surface. Addressing these issues also ensures more positive and lasting outcomes. The objective of family treatment is for parents to become a guide for their adolescent. If successful, the positive outcome is achieved within the context of a collaborative therapeutic alliance that persists long after the families leave treatment. They continue to do well because real change has occurred.

Parents must learn to identify the issues that their adolescents must deal with by themselves and to help the adolescents learn how to set limits for themselves. Major initiatives that the parents of a substance-abusing adolescent must be prepared to undertake include

- Helping their child to remove him- or herself from a negative, substance-abusing peer group and to create an alternate positive peer group instead
- Helping their adolescent defuse a crisis
- Helping the adolescent remove him- or herself from access to or temptation to use alcohol and other drugs
- Helping the adolescent understand any emotional pain he or she is feeling
- Using the family therapist to improve family functioning and resolve the adolescent's reactions to family dysfunction
- Providing tutorial help aimed at promoting success when the adolescent is failing in school
- Providing structure, predictability, and set limits when the adolescent is out of control
- Helping the adolescent design a self-concept building program when he or she has a damaged self-concept
- Helping their child to have a basic understanding of the need for treatment when he or she does not want help
- Making choices for their teenager when he or she is making bad choices, but only until the teenager can make decisions on his or her own
- If the family is part of the problem, including the family in the solution of the problem

Summary

Substance-abusing adolescents and their parents are linked in a number of important ways. This link must be identified and explored during treatment. Often the families are as dysfunctional as the adolescent and have many of the same needs. The problems are often cross-generational.

Adolescents who are unmotivated to change their behavior react negatively to family problems. They respond positively when their family commits to working together on issues. Although adolescent and parental conflict is often very difficult to treat, these problems can be transformed when the members of each group are able to openly and honestly discuss the issues that divide them. The goal of family treatment is to empower parents and prepare them for what to expect from their adolescent. They must also understand that a positive outcome takes work and active involvement for as long as they are needed. Social supports and parent–therapist partnerships can be used as ways for parents to maintain their strength and resolve. They must learn to vigorously parent their substance-abusing adolescent, who may not want to recover. Parents need to learn that despite past difficulties they not only have the right but also the responsibility to be a strong parent. Developing these parenting and communication skills is one of the most practical approaches to successfully treating the adolescent substance abuser.

Family treatment is one of the most practical and effective approaches for adolescent substance abuse treatment. Parents learn new personal coping skills such as accepting that some of their teenager's problems are beyond their control; accepting their role in the problem and not blaming a negative peer group; being consistent in their modeling of behaviors, especially regarding substance use and abuse; supporting and enforcing the program's rules and contracts; staying consistent in their resolve to guide their child both during and after treatment; understanding adolescent relapse; and keeping the lines of communication open and listening to their adolescent's positive and negative feedback.

References

Cornille T, Boroto D: The Family Distress Model: a conceptual and clinical application of Reiss' Strong Bonds finding. Contemporary Family Therapy 14:181–196, 1992

Treadway D: Before It's Too Late: Working With Substance Abuse in the Family. New York, WW Norton, 1989

15 Relapse

Steven L. Jaffe, M.D.
Todd Wilk Estroff, M.D.

Drug abuse is now recognized as a chronic disorder for which the expectation of lifelong abstinence after just one treatment episode is unrealistic for adults. This is especially true among adolescents, for whom maturity, judgment, peer influences, and dysfunctional family members can contribute to the relapse risk. There is also a growing recognition that drug addiction is a brain disease and that addicted individuals can experience uncontrollable drug cravings long after abstinence has been achieved. These cravings can often lead to relapse (Leshner 1997a, 1997b). Relapse among adolescents must be viewed as both a common and normal event in what may be an eventual stable recovery. For these reasons, when relapse does occur, it is important not to become angry, upset, or discouraged. Rather, the response should be to determine what caused the relapse and what can be done to help prevent further relapses.

Follow-Up Studies and Relapse

Longitudinal research and treatment evaluations provide the perspective to distinguish between the idealized goals of addiction treatment and realistic expectations for adolescent treatment. The goal of treatment is that the adolescent will achieve lifetime recovery from the point of initiating treatment onward. While a laudable goal, it is unlikely to occur, and in most instances disappointment will occur if continuous lifetime recovery is the only acceptable outcome.

The outcome literature provides a more realistic picture of what is likely to be achieved rather than just the ideal. The risk for at least a brief relapse is high, and relapse will occur in most cases. A significant but much smaller minority achieve protracted periods of continuous abstinence. The important point of the outcome literature is that about half the adolescents who receive treatment have long-term favorable outcomes. The odds can be improved by the commitment of both the parents and the adolescent to stay in treatment.

Difference Between Abstinence and Recovery

It is important to distinguish between abstinence and recovery. Abstinence means only that the adolescent is not using drugs or alcohol. Forced abstinence can be achieved if adolescents are confined to their homes, a juvenile detention center, or a residential treatment setting. Abstinence does not mean that the adolescent is in recovery. If the teenager simply resumes using drugs after forced abstinence, relapse has not occurred; the adolescent is simply continuing his or her previous pattern of abuse or dependence. Although the line between abstinence and recovery is somewhat ambiguous, forced abstinence is clearly not recovery.

To achieve a state of recovery, adolescents must not only abstain from substance use but also make a commitment to sobriety—striving not to use alcohol or drugs for the rest of their lives (Jaffe 1996). Recovery requires the active participation of the substance-abusing adolescents in making honest efforts to recognize and deal with their long-term illness. If recovery does not ensue, then the adolescent cannot relapse. Only if the teenager achieves a state of recovery is relapse possible.

Minor and Major Relapses

A *minor relapse* is a brief relapse into use of alcohol/drugs after some level of recovery has been achieved. As defined by most studies and researchers, this type of relapse is a brief period of use lasting no more than 30 days. Brief relapses are very common among substance-abusing teenagers and often occur as the teenager tries one more time to see if he or she can use drugs or alcohol in moderation. A minor relapse is often referred to as a "slip" or "lapse." Parents, therapists, and others must accept that slips and lapses will occur from time to time. They need to give the teenager increased support and guidance in order to quickly return him or her to an abstinent recovery state. It is critical for the parents, the therapists, and the adolescent to learn from the experience, analyze what caused the relapse, and determine how future relapses can be prevented. If the return to use of alcohol and drugs is more severe than a simple slip or lapse or persists over a period of more than 1 month, then a *major relapse* has occurred.

Several major follow-up studies have been done of substance-abusing adolescents treated in hospital or residential treatment programs. Dobkin et al. (1998) reported that of 280 Canadian inpatient adolescent substance abusers, 128 (46%) did not complete the 2-month inpatient phase of treatment. Of the remaining 152 adolescents who did complete treatment, 69 were followed up 1 month postdischarge and were divided into two groups—one that did well and one that relapsed. The group that did not improve had more social anxiety, depressive symptoms, and troubling thoughts at intake. Concomitant problems may have precipitated relapse or been a result. Co-occurring conditions are addressed later in this chapter.

Another major follow-up study of adolescents treated for chemical dependency was done in San Diego (Brown 1993). Adolescents who completed residential treatment and were diagnosed with chemical dependency without a concomitant psychiatric diagnosis were given semistructured interviews at 3 months, 6 months, and 1 year after discharge. One hundred adolescents participated in the study. Because the subjects were paid for their interviews there was almost 100% follow-up participation.

The findings demonstrated that although relapses were common, almost one in three of the adolescents remained alcohol and drug free for the first year after treatment. When relapse occurred, it tended to happen shortly after treatment. This is evidenced by the fact that 33% of the subjects relapsed within the first month, and at the 1-year follow-up, 48% had become major relapsers (returned to heavy use). Of the sample, 23% were in the minor relapse category (transient lapses with a total of less than 30 days of alcohol/drug use during the follow-up year) and 29% were abstinent all year. Thus, 52% (abstinent plus minor relapsers) were considered to be doing well at 1-year follow-up.

Of the patients who were doing well, 38% were attending self-help groups regularly, whereas 14% had positive outcomes without support group attendance. Within this 14% there were two groups. One consisted of younger adolescents whose families were nonabusers and had high family participation. The other group was made up of older adolescents who became independent of their unsupportive substance-abusing families, often through extensive school and work involvement. Thus, those adolescents with positive outcomes who were not using formal support systems had other types of support networks. Other findings in this follow-up study were 1) that social pressure was the predominant factor of relapse; 2) that heightened vigilance for the risk of relapse was associated with better outcome; 3) that behavioral coping strategies (rather than cognitive) seemed more effective; and 4) that those who abstained experienced enhanced self-esteem and improvement in family and school functioning during the follow-up year.

Similar findings were reported in a large treatment evaluation study with outcome data on 493 adolescents from 11 facilities in 7 states (Harrison and Hoffmann 1987). Only two-thirds (69%) of the original adolescent population of 915 patients completed the hospital/residential treatment program. The follow-up sample contacted at 6 and 12 months postdischarge included 58% of the treatment completers and only 44% of the noncompleters. The group that could not be reached for follow-up was also analyzed and was found to have been more impaired on admission to the program and to have had more traumatic past histories. During the year after treatment, 44% of the followed patients reported total abstinence, and an additional 22% reported at least 3 months of abstinence during each of the two 6-month follow-up intervals. The remaining 35% had relapsed to prolonged or multiple periods of use.

Treatment completion was significantly associated with recovery as 48% of treatment completers versus only 29% of noncompleters reported total abstinence. Abstinence was also associated with regular 12-step support group attendance by the adolescents and support group attendance by their parents. Adolescents who went to two or more meetings per week were six times more likely to report total abstinence than nonattenders. If their mothers attended a 12-step support group regularly, the adolescents' abstinence rate rose to 54% compared with 40% if their mothers did not attend. If their fathers attended a 12-step support group, the adolescents' abstinence rate went to 63% compared with 42% if their fathers did not attend.

A larger study of treatment completers that followed up with 924 adolescents for 1 year posttreatment found similar results (Harrison and Hoffmann 1989). Almost half of the treatment completers attended self-help groups at least weekly, and of these individuals 61% reported abstinence compared with less than 20% for those who either did not attend or stopped going to support group meetings. Clearly, the treatment evaluation studies support the conclusion that even residential treatment can provide only a beginning for recovery and that sustained effort by the adolescents and their families is required for continued abstinence.

The importance of continuing care, self-help group attendance, and parental involvement was also found in a multivariate study of 2,317 adolescents followed for 1 year (Hsieh et al. 1998). The extent of aftercare attendance and self-help group involvement by both adolescents and parents during the initial 6 months after treatment were the most significant predictors of abstinence at 1 year posttreatment. Interestingly, the pretreatment characteristics of the adolescents were not significantly related to abstinence 1 year after treatment. This would suggest that regardless of how involved the adolescent may be with drugs before receiving treatment, the greater the extent to which he or she can be engaged in treatment and ongoing aftercare, the greater the likelihood of abstinence.

From these studies it is clear that treatment and continuing care compliance are essential for promoting recovery for substance-abusing adolescents (American Academy of Child and Adolescent Psychiatry 1998; Bukstein 1997; Weinberg et al. 1998). Noncompliance and failure to use self-help support networks dramatically increase the likelihood of relapse.

Evaluation of the Relapse

Once relapse is suspected or has occurred, it is critical to retain an overall perspective of the situation, to ensure that the adolescent is safe from harm, and to stabilize the situation. After safety and stability are established, it is critical to perform a failure analysis to determine why the adolescent relapsed and how it can be prevented in the future. Emotion has no place in this reevaluation. It must be done in as cold and calculating a manner as possible. The objective is always to find the mechanisms by which the adolescent relapsed and what can be done to disrupt the process. It is not to fix blame. Instead, everyone involved the adolescent's care must change their focus from faulting the adolescent's behavior to identifying what they themselves have failed to recognize and/or treat and how they can help the adolescent avoid relapse in the future.

Relapse Is Not a Disaster

It is important to remember that relapses, especially brief relapses, are common. Brief relapses are so common that they should be viewed as a painful yet normal part of the illness of substance dependency. It is important to remember that a substance use disorder is an illness that is difficult to treat precisely because it is a chronic and relapsing disease. Studies of adults with chronic medical illnesses such as asthma, diabetes, and hypertension have rates of noncompliance and relapse similar to those of the addictions. As a result it is neither unusual nor unexpected to find relapses occurring during a course of treatment or periodically during the maintenance phase of treatment. Relapse can become a beneficial learning experience if it is caught early and used as a tool to analyze and fine-tune the adolescent's treatment, relapse prevention, and recovery strategies. Parents and mental health professionals often need to process their own feelings of anger and failure when their adolescent relapses before they can approach the teenager in a calm yet firm and supportive manner.

Marlatt and George (1984) studied the immediate precipitants of relapse among motivated adult addicts. Among the adults, the most common precipitants were interpersonal negative emotional states (35%), social pressure (20%), and interpersonal conflict (16%). Teenagers who acknowledge they are addicts and struggle to remain abstinent tend to relapse through similar pathways, but the frequency of the immediate precipitant is different and the path to relapse involves several adolescent developmental issues.

Immediate Treatment Decisions After Relapse

After a relapse has occurred and the severity and length of the relapse are fully evaluated, changes in care and recovery strategies must be made. These changes can take several forms depending on the adolescent's condition and the situation. Depending on the severity of the relapse a more intensive level of treatment is often indicated. If the relapse is minor and the teenager is still motivated toward recovery, then a further trial of more intensive outpatient treatment is often indicated. Increased attendance at 12-step meetings and individual, group, and family therapy can help adolescents reestablish their recovery. Working another first step often increases motivation for sobriety (Jaffe 2001). More frequent urine screens are often indicated. These can serve to promote return to recovery not only by providing heightened vigilance for use but also by helping the adolescent resist peer pressure to again use drugs. Enrollment in day and evening programs provides increased structure and more intensive treatment. Some teenagers, especially those with weak motivation or who experience prolonged or severe major relapses, may require hospitalization or other residential placement. Substance-abusing adolescents who become suicidal or homicidal also require immediate hospitalization or placement in a structured environment.

12-Step Compliance

Analyzing the cause of the relapse and preventing it in the future are critical to maintaining recovery once abstinence is reestablished. Working a 12-step program, finding a recovering peer group, and trusting a sponsor also help reestablish abstinence. Unfortunately, many adolescents feel uncomfortable in adult 12-step meetings and would rather attend a meeting that focuses on their age group. These Alateen meetings are very difficult to locate and attend in both rural and urban settings. In the rural areas, it is often difficult to find enough adolescents to hold a meeting on a regular basis. In the urban scenario enough adolescents attend, but once the groups are formed they often fall apart after a short period of time. The oldest members tend to grow up and move beyond adolescent issues. As they do, they tend to move over to regular adult-oriented meetings. It is extremely difficult for substance-abusing adolescents to organize and keep an Alateen meeting going without outside help. The only ongoing meetings we are aware of are those that are organized and supervised by adults.

Pathways to Relapse

Failure to take medications or attend psychotherapy sessions, oppositional behavior, and poor decision making can all contribute to relapse. Multiple pathways to relapse have been identified. Four general types are among the more prevalent: 1) a conscious decision to resume use; 2) multiple problem interactions; 3) omnipotent attitudes; and 4) setting oneself up for relapse through seemingly irrelevant decisions. As noted earlier, only after recovery has been instituted can an adolescent relapse back into substance abuse. This perspective should be kept in mind during the following discussion.

A common route of relapse involves teenagers who consciously decide to again use drugs. These adolescents have worked some parts of a program and are abstinent. They frequently are in the early stages of recovery, but during aftercare, they decide that they are not really addicted and that they can control the use of small amounts of alcohol or drugs. Others are not convinced that their substance abuse disorder requires total abstinence. Still other adolescents relapse after contemplating their lives without drugs or alcohol. The expectation that life without mood alteration is too hard to endure prompts them to return to drugs and alcohol. Each of these groups of teenagers make conscious decisions to again use drugs and alcohol. Unfortunately this usually leads to relapse. Teenagers who make a conscious decision to resume substance abuse tend not to complete the first five steps during treatment. They are more emotionally detached from other adolescents, their sponsors, and their families. Such warning signs and lack of treatment progress should be considered in assessing relapse risks.

Another pathway to relapse is the broad category of dual-diagnosis patients. This group consists of substance-abusing teenagers who simultaneously have psychiatric disorders such as bipolar, psychotic, or affective disorders, attention-deficit/hyperactivity disorder (ADHD), or posttraumatic stress disorder (PTSD) and concomitant substance abuse disorders. The presence of an undiagnosed or undertreated concomitant psychiatric disorder is the second most frequent cause of adolescent substance abuse relapse (Jaffe 1992). Numerous studies (Bukstein et al. 1992; Hovens et al. 1994; Stowell and Estroff 1992) have demonstrated a high incidence of affective disorders (bipolar disorder, major depression and dysthymia), ADHD, learning disabilities, anxiety disorders (especially PTSD), and physical/sexual abuse. A thorough psychiatric reevaluation should be performed whenever a teenager has relapsed. Concurrent psychiatric disorders should be treated with appropriate nonaddicting medications when indicated (see Chapter 12).

A third mechanism of relapse is the most frequent path among adolescents. In this situation the recovering teenagers realize that they are addicted, yet believe that they can associate with their drug-using friends and still not abuse drugs or alcohol. The grandiose and omnipotent thinking of adolescence contributes to their view that they will not relapse. This cognitive distortion persists even after they have been warned multiple times, both during treatment and in aftercare, that stable recovery is not possible in the face of continued association with substance-using and substance-abusing peers. They continue to persist in the beliefs that they have sufficient willpower to resist the lure of addictive substances and that they will be the first person to successfully handle these difficult situations. This thought process is best described as a *cognitive omnipotent decision*. In other words, the decision to continue to socialize with their alcohol- and drug-using friends often moves them to the point at which they cannot resist the social pressures, temptations, and urges to use drugs or drink. If they do decide to try just a little bit of drugs or alcohol, relapse often occurs even though they are highly motivated to remain abstinent. More than half the teenagers studied relapsed via this pathway (Jaffe 1992).

The previously cited studies (Brown 1993; Jaffe 1992) have shown that continuing contact with an alcohol- and drug-abusing peer group is the most common pathway to relapse. Most well-motivated teenagers who are intently working on their recovery program will eventually relapse if they continue to associate with their substance-abusing acquaintances. Thus, evaluation of the teenagers' peer group is essential. Exposure to these drug-using peers increases urges and temptations as well as direct and indirect peer pressure. This is often more than a recovering teenager can handle. Once relapse occurs, the teenager must again attempt to cut off all contact with these peers. A new non-drug-abusing peer group must be established. These individuals are often found within the 12-step programs. A 12-step sponsor can help the relapsed teenager make contact with other teenagers who are successfully working their own recovery programs. Many high schools have aftercare groups in which recovering teenagers can meet and socialize with other recovering teenagers. They can help each other avoid drug-using peers and situations.

A fourth route of relapse occurs when teenagers unconsciously or naively create situations in which exposure to alcohol or drugs will occur and relapse will often ensue. One or a series of unsound decisions set up high-risk situations in which social pressure combines with temptation and easy access to drugs and alcohol. Marlatt and George (1984) called this process the making of *seemingly irrelevant decisions*. This process occurs much more commonly among adults and is rather infrequent in adolescents (Jaffe 1992). It is important to note that it is possible for an adolescent to relapse, to determine precisely the causes of the relapse, and to institute a new relapse prevention program and still relapse again. In these cases serious consideration needs to be given to the possibility that the adolescent is untreatable. If this is a serious consideration, a complete review of the entire clinical case is mandatory before the teenager is dropped from therapy. This process is described in more detail along with specific case histories in Chapter 17.

Summary

The frequency of relapse, especially brief relapse, makes the event normative among substance-abusing adolescents. If the situation is properly managed, a relapse need not be a disaster. Analysis of why the relapse occurred is critical. The most important task when relapse occurs is identifying which pathway or combination of pathways have led to the relapse. Analysis of the causes of the relapse helps set the course for revised and more effective treatment and adjustments to recovery strategies for the adolescent. The issues of which peer group the adolescents continue to associate with, whether they have been faithfully working a 12-step program, and whether those and other conditions have been participating in their concurrent psychiatric treatment are the keys to evaluating, treating, and preventing future relapse.

References

American Academy of Child and Adolescent Psychiatry: Summary of the practice parameters for the assessment and treatment of children and adolescents with substance use disorders. J Am Acad Child Adolesc Psychiatry 37:122–126, 1998

Brown S: Recovery patterns of adolescent substance abuse, in Addictive Behavior Across the Life Span: Prevention, Treatment and Policy Issues. Edited by Baer J, Marlatt G, McMahon R. Beverly Hills, CA, Sage, 1993, pp 161–183

Bukstein OG: Practice parameters for the assessment and treatment of children and adolescents with substance use disorders. J Am Acad Child Adolesc Psychiatry 36 (10, suppl):140S–156S, 1997

Bukstein OG, Glancy LJ, Kaminer Y: Patterns of affective comorbidity in a clinical population of dually diagnosed adolescent substance abusers. J Am Acad Child Adolesc Psychiatry 31:1041–1045, 1992

Dobkin PL, Chabot L, Maliantovitch K, et al: Predictors of outcome in drug treatment of adolescent inpatients. Psychol Rep 83:175–186, 1998

Harrison PA, Hoffmann NG: CATOR 1987 Report: Adolescent Residential Treatment Intake and Follow-Up Findings. St. Paul, MN, Ramsey Clinic, 1987

Harrison PA, Hoffmann NG: CATOR Report: Adolescent Treatment Completers: One Year Later. St. Paul, MN, Ramsey Clinic, 1989

Hovens JG, Cantwell DP, Kiriakos R: Psychiatric comorbidity in hospitalized adolescent substance abusers. J Am Acad Child Adolesc Psychiatry 33:476–483, 1994

Hsieh S, Hoffmann NG, Hollister CD: The relationship between pre-, during-, post-treatment factors, and adolescent substance abuse behaviors. Addict Behav 23:477–488, 1998

Jaffe SL: Pathways to relapse in chemically dependent adolescents. Adolescent Counselor 55:42–44, 1992

Jaffe SL: Preventing relapse: guidelines for the psychiatrist. Child Adolesc Psychiatr Clin N Am 5:213–220, 1996

Jaffe SL: Adolescent Substance Abuse Intervention Workbook: Taking A First Step. Washington, DC, American Psychiatric Press, 2001

Leshner AI: Addiction is a brain disease, and it matters. Science 278:45–47, 1997a

Leshner AI: Drug abuse and addiction treatment research. Arch Gen Psychiatry 54:691–694, 1997b

Marlatt GA, George WH: Relapse prevention: introduction and overview of the model. British Journal of Addiction 79:261–173, 1984

Stowell RJA, Estroff TW: Adolescent dual diagnosis: a pilot study of inpatient substance-abusing adolescents. J Am Acad Child Adolesc Psychiatry 31:1036–1040, 1992

Weinberg NZ, Rahdert E, Colliver JD, et al: Adolescent substance abuse: a review of the past 10 years. J Am Acad Child Adolesc Psychiatry 37:252–261, 1998

16 Adolescent Development and Substance Abuse

Stuart A. Copans, M.D.
Jean Kinney, M.S.W.
Todd Wilk Estroff, M.D.

When the interaction between adolescent development and adolescent substance abuse is contemplated, several basic questions arise and must be addressed. First, is there a relationship between the normal steps of adolescent development and the initiation of adolescent substance abuse? Second, what is the effect of adolescent substance abuse on the course of normal adolescent development? Third, what is the developmental course of adolescent substance abuse itself? Does abuse develop in a predictable way? If it does, what are the stages in its development and what are the markers of each stage? The following discussion focuses on these issues as they pertain to normal adolescent development.

Children from very disturbed and traumatic backgrounds are much more susceptible to substance abuse. Even in the absence of other serious disruptions, substance use and abuse pose consequences for adolescent development. Teenagers' development is already so abnormal that any discussion of the effects of drug and alcohol abuse on their maturation becomes inseparable from the effects of their other stressors.

Normal Adolescent Development and Substance Abuse

Drug abuse among children is virtually unknown. Before puberty, most children experience drug-induced euphoria as unpleasant and something to be avoided. One of the main reasons this occurs is brain maturation. As the adolescent's brain develops it creates the increased ability to experience the pleasure of drug-induced euphoria. At the same time this brain maturation allows adolescents the intellectual ability to devise a plan to repeatedly obtain and use drugs and alcohol. As they begin to enter puberty, adolescents begin to take chances and experiment with previously prohibited activities. The risk of initiation of drug and alcohol abuse dramatically rises with age. These developing capabilities often interact with other risk factors, including the adolescents' inborn genetic predisposition to become addicted and environmental stressors that increase the chance that they will try drugs or alcohol. There is also the popular attitude that many personal problems can be solved by taking a pill or medication (Jaquier et al. 1998). The unfortunate result is that drug and alcohol experimentation is the rule among today's adolescents. It is normative (i.e., not abnormal) for high school students in the United States to have drunk alcohol and smoked marijuana at some time during the past year. Among younger children and adolescents, price, availability, and social acceptance often dictate which specific substances are used and abused. As teens age they start to focus in on a particular substance or combination of substances that they prefer to use. Drug and alcohol experimentation in combination with rising adolescent sexual drives is often used to facilitate sexual activity. The drug or alcohol is used either as a way of decreasing a potential partner's inhibitions or as a way of enhancing sexual pleasure (Fergusson and Lynskey 1996). There is evidence that abusing alcohol leads to unplanned first intercourse among adolescents and that it is inversely related to whether the first intercourse was planned. In effect, those adolescents who planned their first intercourse ahead of time were less likely to drink or abuse drugs (McLean and Flanigan 1993). The risks do not end there, however, because adolescents who use alcohol or drugs are more likely to be sexually assaulted by someone they know (Muram et al. 1995).

Peer pressure and even intimidation can be intense and can play a central role in the initiation and continuation of adolescent substance abuse. However, these are not the only correlates of substance abuse. Webb et al. (1991) examined the relationship between risk factors and the initiation of alcohol use over a 15-month period among a cohort of seventh graders who were abstinent at the time of initial testing. Rejection of parental authority and deviant behavior were both related to initiation of alcohol use.

Substance-abusing adolescents describe a number of developmental topics that they believe lead to the initiation and continuation of their drug and alcohol abuse. Substances are frequently abused on a dare or to relieve painful feelings. Drugs are often used as a way to experiment with different identities, to distance themselves from their parents' control, or to assert their ability to think and act independently. Rationalizations abound.

Copans (1985) suggested that the increasing incidence of adolescent substance abuse is also directly related to a lack of adult guidance and support while the adolescent is going through the basic tasks of development. It is interesting that typical teenage drug and alcohol abuse and teenage sexual activities support this idea. This is especially true when it is noted that these behaviors are most likely to occur in the adolescents' own bedrooms between the end of school and dinner time (Sussman et al. 1998).

Drug Use and Abuse Do Not Mean Certain Addiction

Just because an adolescent has tried drugs does not mean that addiction will automatically ensue. In many cases a period of heavy adolescent drug abuse is replaced by little to no use in adulthood. Despite this encouraging information, the risk of adult addiction after adolescent exposure to drugs and alcohol is elevated. This increased risk can result in three possible adult scenarios. The first is of consistently moderate alcohol use throughout adolescence and early adulthood. The second is heavier drug or alcohol abuse during adolescence and dramatically decreasing use in adulthood. The third scenario has the worst result: heavy alcohol and drug abuse in adolescence continues into adulthood and produces an addiction (Bates and Labouvie 1997).

Early onset of continuous substance abuse has a worse prognosis than substance abuse disorders that begin in adulthood (Clark et al. 1998). In a prospective study of 480 alcohol-abusing adolescents followed over a 9–10 year period, it was found that chronic alcohol use in adolescence was related to higher alcohol use, alcohol-related problems, aggressive behavior, theft, and suicide ideation in young adulthood (Duncan et al. 1997)

Effects of Adolescent Substance Abuse on Development

The effects of adolescent substance abuse on normal adolescent development have been discussed for years. The cardinal rule is that a developmental arrest or delay occurs around the chronological age when the adolescent's substance abuse begins. During treatment, adult drug addicts are taught that "If you started drinking at 14, then you are still 14 years old emotionally."

Unfortunately, few studies clearly demonstrate a cause and effect relationship between adolescent substance abuse and retardation of emotional and moral development. However, adult data do exist. Valliant (1983), in a longitudinal study of adults, was able to demonstrate that adults used more immature psychological defenses when actively abusing substances and more mature and higher-developmental-level defenses when sober. Relapse was accompanied by the reappearance of the immature patterns of behavior and the disappearance of the more mature defenses.

Beginning in the mid-1970s, Bentler (1992) studied early and mid-adolescence drug use patterns, personality patterns, and behavioral correlates in a large sample of normal youths. Teenage drug use was found to disrupt many critical developmental tasks of adolescence and young adulthood. Tendencies to use many different drugs as an adolescent led in young adulthood to increased drug-related crimes, decreased college involvement, increased job instability, decreased income, increased psychotic episodes, and increased theft.

Adolescent substance abuse is not necessarily a uniform phenomenon. Mezzich et al. (1993), in a study involving 43 adolescents, identified two separate and distinct groups. Cluster 1, the smaller group, was characterized by more negative affect. Most subjects belonged in Cluster 2, which was characterized by behavioral dyscontrol and hypophoria—i.e., a history of suicide attempts. Cluster 2 subjects demonstrated more severe alcohol and drug use problems, more behavioral disturbances, more general psychopathology, lower prevalence of depressive symptoms, and less severe anxiety disorders. These results suggest two variants of adolescent alcohol abuse and dependence that may affect the adolescent's development.

Developmental Stages of Adolescent Substance Abuse

Several studies on the development of adolescent substance abuse have suggested a sequence of progressive drug involvement across multiple ethnic groups. The exact sequence of which drug is taken in what order is not fixed. In the early stages of use, drug choice may depend on price and availability more than anything else. The progression appears to be both unidirectional and cumulative.

Andrews et al. (1991) constructed a Guttman scale from 2 years of self-reported data from substance-abusing adolescents. The study supported the notion that adolescent substance abuse developed in regular stages, moving from alcohol use to cigarette use, to marijuana use, and finally to harder drugs. Blaze-Temple and Lo (1992) conducted a survey of 1,093 13–17-year-olds that showed that the Guttman model held for both genders and for all ages, although it was more predictive for older individuals. More general drug use and an expanding drug repertoire occurred increasingly with age. Eventually, multiple drug use was widespread. Interestingly, the authors found that marijuana abuse was not a necessary step for the progression to other illicit drug use. The "stepping stone" hypothesis was supported for the licit substances of tobacco and alcohol but not for marijuana in a Spanish population of adolescents (Adrados 1995). Of the subjects in this study, 29% of current abusers of any illicit drugs reported never using marijuana. The relative risk rate for use of marijuana or other illicit drugs was especially high if the abuser was a current tobacco smoker. Alcohol and tobacco were both implicated as important gateway drugs, but tobacco use was found to be more predictive of progression to further drug abuse than alcohol.

Cocaine abuse and dependence is an excellent model for drug abuse occurring in stages. It also strongly suggests that addictions progress more rapidly in adolescents than in adults. Schwartz et al. (1991) studied 464 largely white, middle-class, suburban, drug-abusing teenagers. Of the 130 (28%) who smoked crack, 87 (67%) were designated as "experimenters." They had used crack 1–9 times during their lives. Twenty (15%) were in an intermediate group who smoked crack 10–50 times in their lives, and 23 (18%) were heavy users who smoked crack more than 50 times in their lives. Of heavy users, 60% rapidly progressed from initiation of crack use to at least weekly use in less than 3 months, which is much more rapid than with most adults. Almost 50% of the 87 experimenters and nearly all the 23 heavy users reported preoccupation with thoughts of crack, rapid loss of ability to modulate their use of the drug, and rapid development of pharmacological tolerance. Of the 87 experimenters, 7% had injected cocaine intravenously, compared with nearly 25% of the 43 who smoked crack more frequently. Use of crack by middle-class adolescents is associated with rapid addiction and serious behavioral and medical complications. Clearly, the stages and rapidity with which the addiction develops can be heavily influenced by the pharmacological characteristics of the drugs being abused.

In clinical practice, staging is often used to evaluate the level of abuse or addiction in adolescents. Staging evaluates various factors including the frequency of use, the amount of use, the effect on peer functioning, and any associated antisocial behaviors. There are few data about these stages, although it is generally accepted that adolescents move through the stages of addiction far more rapidly than adults (Clark et al. 1998). These stages as outlined are as follows (MacDonald 1984):

Stage one: Experimentation/learning the mood swing
Stage two: Regular use/seeking the mood swing
Stage three: Daily preoccupation/preoccupation with the mood swing
Stage four: Dependency/using to feel normal

Dual and Triple Diagnosis

An additional factor complicating analysis of the effects of adolescent substance abuse on development is the heavy overlap of substance abuse with other psychiatric disorders. The causes and effects of each disorder on the other are basically bidirectional; they can be envisioned as a two-way street in which childhood and adolescent psychiatric disorders predispose adolescents to substance abuse (Geller et al. 1998) while at the same time substance abuse predisposes adolescents to psychiatric disorders.

Studies of adolescents entering inpatient treatment because of a primary substance use disorder demonstrate a high incidence of psychiatric disorder (Hovens et al. 1994). Stowell and Estroff (1992) found that 82% of these patients met DSM-III-R (American Psychiatric Association 1987) criteria for an Axis I psychiatric disorder. Of this population 74% had two or more psychiatric disorders. Mood disorders were found in 61%, conduct disorders in 54%, and anxiety disorders in 43%. Substance-induced organic mental disorders were found in 16%. These data strongly argue that adolescent substance abuse can have profound effects on the development of adolescent psychiatric disorders and thus on the adolescent's development. These psychiatric effects exacerbate the developmental arrest and delay associated with substance abuse.

Clinical Implications

This chapter has attempted to answer several basic questions posed in the introduction. Based on the available evidence, the conclusions are as follows:

1. A relationship exists between the normal steps of adolescent development and the initiation of adolescent substance abuse.
2. Adolescent substance abuse affects the course of normal adolescent development.
3. There is a developmental course of adolescent substance abuse that progresses in a predictable way.
4. When adolescent substance abuse disorders develop, there are stages in the development and markers of each stage.

For these reasons, comprehensive developmental assessment is an essential part of the assessment and treatment of adolescents with substance abuse problems.

References

Adrados JL: The influence of family, school, and peers on adolescent drug misuse. International Journal of the Addictions 30:1407–1423, 1995

American Psychiatric Association: Diagnostic and Statistical Manual of Mental Disorders, Third Edition Revised. Washington, DC, American Psychiatric Association, 1987

Andrews JA, Hops H, Ary D, et al: The construction, validation and use of a Guttman scale of adolescent substance abuse: an investigation of family relationships. Journal of Drug Issues 21:557–572, 1991

Bates ME, Labouvie EW: Adolescent risk factors and the prediction of persistent alcohol and drug use into adulthood. Alcohol Clin Exp Res 21:944–950, 1997

Bentler PM: Etiologies and consequences of adolescent drug use: implications for prevention. J Addict Dis 11:47-61, 1992

Blaze-Temple D, Lo SK: Stages of drug use: a community survey of Perth teenagers. British Journal of Addiction 87:215–225, 1992

Clark DB, Kirisci L, Tarter RE: Adolescent versus adult onset and the development of substance use disorders in males. Drug Alcohol Depend 49:115–121, 1998

Copans SA: Tasks of adolescent development and their relationship to alcohol use and abuse in college. Symposium presented at the Dartmouth–Cork College Alcohol Conference, Stowe VT, May 1985

Duncan SC, Alpert A, Duncan TE, et al: Adolescent alcohol use development and young adult outcomes. Drug Alcohol Depend 49:39–48, 1997

Fergusson DM, Lynskey MT: Alcohol misuse and adolescent sexual behaviors and risk taking. Pediatrics 98:91–96, 1996

Geller B, Cooper TB, Sun K, et al: Double-blind and placebo-controlled study of lithium for adolescent bipolar disorders with secondary substance dependency. J Am Acad Child Adolesc Psychiatry 37:171–178, 1998

Hovens JG, Cantwell DP, Kiriakos R: Psychiatric comorbidity in hospitalized adolescent substance abusers. J Am Acad Child Adolesc Psychiatry 33:476–483, 1994

Jaquier F, Buclin T, Diezi J: Automedication chez l'adolescent. Schweiz Med Wochenschr 28:203–237, 1998

MacDonald DI: Drugs, drinking and adolescence. Am J Dis Child 138:117–125, 1984

McLean AL, Flanigan BJ: Transition-marking behaviors of adolescent males at first intercourse. Adolescence 28:579–595, 1993

Mezzich A, Tarter R, Kirisci L, et al: Subtypes of early age onset alcoholism. Alcohol 17:767–770, 1993

Muram D, Hostetler BR, Jones CE, et al: Adolescent victims of sexual assault. J Adolesc Health 17:372–375, 1995

Schwartz RH, Luxenberg MG, Hoffmann NG: "Crack" use by American middle-class adolescent poly drug abusers. J Pediatr 118:150–155, 1991

Stowell RJA, Estroff TW: Psychiatric disorders in substance-abusing adolescent inpatients: a pilot study. J Am Acad Child Adolesc Psychiatry 31:1036–1040, 1992

Sussman S, Stacy AW, Ames SL, et al: Self-reported high-risk locations of adolescent drug use. Addict Behav 23:405–411, 1998

Vaillant G: The Natural History of Alcoholism. Cambridge, MA, Harvard University Press, 1983

Webb JA, Baer PE, McLaughlin RJ, et al: Risk factors and their relation to initiation of alcohol use among early adolescents. J Am Acad Child Adolesc Psychiatry 30:563–568, 1991

17 Untreatable Substance-Abusing Adolescents

Todd Wilk Estroff, M.D.

In medicine, no one talks about untreatable patients. This topic is avoided because most physicians believe that there is always something they can do to help. The nearest physicians get to discussing untreatability is with regard to the right of competent adult patients to refuse treatment. However, this situation is different in the field of substance abuse disorders.

Untreatable substance-abusing adults and adolescents do exist. These patients are classified as untreatable when all treatment options, maneuvers, and techniques have been exhausted or thwarted. In effect, there is no winning move that will lead to their recovery. When this point is reached, difficult decisions must be made, and they must not be made in haste or anger or mistakes will follow. Forcing an adolescent out of therapy can at times be therapeutic, as long as it is done calmly, without emotion, and with a clear message that the adolescent may return when he or she is ready for treatment.

Major reasons for classifying adolescents as untreatable include severe sociopathy/personality disorder, severe oppositional defiant behavior, and not wanting to stop abusing as well as parental factors such as lack of commitment and/or sabotage. Teenagers who enter substance abuse treatment through the criminal justice system may be simply seeking an easy way out of jail. They often view treatment as a way to bide their time or to slide through the system. If this happens in a program, then something is wrong. An effective program will identify and confront these patients. When substance-abusing adolescents find that drug treatment is not easy, they often rebel at the requirements. They may demonstrate their untreatability by simple noncooperation and nonparticipation with their evaluation and treatment. They can also engage in active sabotage of the treatment program manifested by inappropriate sexual behavior, violence, actively seeking drugs, bringing drugs and alcohol into the treatment setting, or open defiance of the treatment rules. Other adolescents may want treatment but are untreatable because their parents refuse to acknowledge their problems and/or remove them from treatment. Parents can also sabotage their child's treatment by refusing to participate (see Chapter 15).

Therapeutic Discharge

Although it may be painful to do so, it is often best to discharge the untreatable substance-abusing adolescent. The decision to discharge should never be taken lightly. It should be made only after the adolescent has been classified as untreatable. Any consideration of discharging an adolescent or of labeling him or her as untreatable should prompt a complete relapse reevaluation to determine what has been missed (see Chapter 16). It is tempting to get rid of failures as quickly as possible and not to think of what other treatable problems the adolescent may have, what might have been overlooked in the evaluation, or what else might be done to help the patient.

Danger of a Missed Diagnosis

There is a significant danger of a missed diagnosis if the evaluating staff member is angry or frustrated. Undetected withdrawal, severe drug cravings, and bipolar disorders often cause disturbed behavior in which the adolescent appears untreatable. For these reasons, it is important to have a general rule to never discharge a patient in anger. In most cases, patients are untreatable only when staff members are feeling angry, defeated, and depressed. It is the duty of the treatment professional to always step back and ask, "What treatable thing have I missed?"

When the Decision Is Made to Discharge

When the adolescent has been classified as untreatable, he or she must be discharged as quickly as possible. However, good judgment and least-risk principles must be used. One of the most difficult issues at this point is *how* to discharge these patients from the program. This situation is much less complex in adult substance abuse programs because these programs can simply discharge disruptive, unmotivated, or uncooperative patients; if such patients do not agree to become fully compliant and surrender control, they are rapidly shown the door. There is a higher standard of care for adolescents. Because adolescents are not adults and cannot think or care for themselves in an adult manner, their precipitous discharge from treatment is neither advisable nor wise. Nothing is more frightening or infuriating to a parent than receiving a sudden phone call saying "Come and get your child. We cannot provide any further treatment and you need to remove them now!" This kind of phone call does untold damage to the reputation of the program; it indicates inadequate communication with the parents and a failure to warn parents of a problem or of the possibility that discharge or transfer may be necessary. Discharges of this sort are often done in a fury and in such a pejorative manner that a maximum of ill will is produced. Both the patient and the parents feel abandoned in this situation, and parents may even refuse to come to and pick up their adolescent.

It is also important to discharge patients without prejudice. Reassure them that they are welcome back *when and if* they decide they want treatment for their substance abuse disorder. Because not all patients can be or are treatable, discharge under these conditions can be therapeutic for both the patient and other patients who remain in treatment and are motivated. It is important to note that in a desire to help substance-abusing adolescents, staff members may overlook the fact that some individuals are not and will never be amenable to treatment. Such individuals belong in the criminal justice system and have no place in substance abuse or psychiatric treatment systems unless their motivation radically changes.

How to Discharge the Untreatable Adolescent

Untreatable adolescents must be told firmly and quietly that because they are not interested in further treatment, arrangements are being made for discharge, that they will be discharged as soon as possible, that no further acting out is necessary, and to remain calm until discharge planning has been finalized. What to do with these patients prior to their discharge depends on the individual. If the patient is nondisruptive, he or she can be kept on unit but isolated from the other patients to prevent disruption of other patients' treatment. Disruptive patients should be immediately removed from any contact with the other adolescents in treatment and may need to be transferred to the most secure part of the program. In general, drug-addicted and criminal patients can maintain excellent behavior when they know they will be discharged; patients with psychiatric disorders cannot behave. It is important to remember that when discharging the untreatable substance-abusing adolescent, haste causes disasters. It is wise to slow the process down and to think carefully and calmly about what is being done and why.

The parents, legal authorities, and school officials should all be given the same information. If they will listen, it is important to meet with the parents to explain why the patient is untreatable and to present this as a mutual problem. At this conference it is important to lay out as specifically as possible all the potential negative consequences of the child's continued substance abuse. This conference is designed not to frighten but rather to forewarn the parents about unwarranted optimism and to not ignore their severely disturbed child's needs. Including them in the disposition decision process helps them understand and helps diffuse a lot of their anger and frustration at their own child, the staff, and the program. Some remarkable attitude changes can occur after discharge when loving parents use this information and what is left of the parent–child relationship to persuade their adolescent to accept treatment.

These patients may have legal charges pending, so it may be mandatory to contact court officers. A patient's case may be so extreme that the court authorities will not allow discharge and will insist that the adolescent be held for transport back to jail or to a detention center.

This discussion is not meant to imply that it is unreasonable to discharge untreatable patients. Discharge is often the only rational choice. After discharge it is important to discuss the situation with the other adolescents in the program. It is disruptive for patients to see someone sitting around not working a program and not making progress. They must be told the patient's exact status and why the treatment is so different for this particular patient.

It is unethical to maintain a patient in treatment once it is decided that the patient is making no progress, that treatment has been ineffective, and that the patient should be discharged. The only exception to this would be during the time that disposition planning is finalized, which should be done as rapidly as possible.

Discharging the untreatable patient has other benefits because it frees up resources for patients who are more likely to benefit from treatment. This is a significant advantage because many programs have waiting lists and often waste resources in vain attempts to help untreatable patients. It is not wise to expend resources when other, more motivated patients can benefit from the additional treatment.

Case Examples

Following are case examples of hospitalized patients. These case examples illustrate the least-risk/maximum-benefit rules for dealing with untreatable patients. Each case also describes the multiple second chances given to substance-abusing adolescents and the many attempts made to engage these adolescents in treatment before their final discharge from therapy.

Case 1

Patient Q was a 16-year-old white male who had been court ordered for evaluation and treatment. The patient had an extensive history of abusing alcohol, crack cocaine, mushrooms, heroin, ecstasy, and lysergic acid diethylamide (LSD). On mental status examination, the patient was cooperative and showed no evidence of any thought disorder, psychosis, or depression. He entered treatment and was initially cooperative, but his behavior gradually deteriorated to the point at which he was disrupting other patients' treatment and was unwilling to participate in his own therapy.

His probation officer was contacted, and the patient was told that if he did not complete the program he would be returned to jail. He decided to go to jail and was discharged from the program. After 3 weeks in jail, he contacted the program director and asked if he could return to treatment. He was reevaluated at the jail by the program director. It was believed that the patient had undergone a change of attitude and had improved motivation. He appeared sincere, and it was believed that his behavior was not an attempt to manipulate the program and get out of jail. A specific written contract was signed that outlined the conditions under which he would be allowed to return to treatment. It was also clearly stated in writing that if he failed to meet any of these conditions he would be returned to jail.

The patient was accepted back in to the program and made a satisfactory adjustment. His initial behavior was compliant; however, he again became defiant and uncooperative over time. He was openly oppositional and refused to follow through with any of the contract conditions. A urine drug screen was positive for cocaine. His negative behavior escalated until staff members decided that he was not gaining anything from treatment and would further disrupt the treatment of the other patients.

The court officer and the patient's mother were notified and the situation was explained to them. The patient continued to refuse to cooperate even under intense pressure from both his mother and the parole officer. He was discharged and returned to jail. His final DSM-IV (American Psychiatric Association 1994) diagnostic impression was

- Axis Ia, Alcohol Abuse
- Axis Ib, Cocaine Abuse
- Axis Ic, Hallucinogen Abuse (mushrooms, LSD)
- Axis Id, Opiate Abuse (heroin)
- Axis Ie, Amphetamine Abuse (ecstasy)
- Axis If, Conduct Disorder, Group Type
- Axis Ig, Possible Major Depressive Disorder
- Axis II, Antisocial Personality Disorder
- Axis III, No Diagnosis

Comment

This type of case is one of the most difficult and upsetting to deal with because the patient is essentially untreatable. It is important to note that the patient failed twice during his treatment despite powerful court-created leverage. Both times it was made clear to the patient, his parents, and the hospital staff that if the patient did not complete treatment he would be returned immediately to jail, but the patient's pathology was so severe that he preferred going to jail over working on his problems.

As mentioned earlier, it is important that once a patient is deemed untreatable, he or she should suffer the consequences as rapidly as possible. In this case, the patient had a very specific agreement in writing and he broke it. A rapid, careful, and dispassionate decision was made that the patient would never comply with his agreement and that he was, at that point, untreatable. His parents and the court were informed of his refusal to cooperate. Under these circumstances the best solution was to discharge the patient back into the criminal justice system, and his transfer to the county jail ensued immediately.

Readmission of this patient into treatment can be questioned, especially in retrospect. At the time he negotiated his second treatment, he did indeed seem motivated and cooperative. Despite his second failure in treatment the door was left open to further treatment when the patient was sufficiently motivated. This was clearly explained to the patient, his parents, and the parole officer. The unanswered question is whether such individuals are simply young criminals who are refractory to any treatment at any time or if they can be treated given sufficient commitment to treatment.

Case 2

Patient R was a 17-year-old white male who was court ordered into treatment of drug abuse. The patient's father had found him passed out on the kitchen floor on the weekend prior to entering treatment. He reportedly had been beaten so badly that he could not recall the events of the previous evening. In addition, he had a positive urine drug screen for marijuana. He had been truant from school, had demonstrated violent behavior, and had dropped out of the ninth grade. The patient had initially been admitted to a hospital in which he spent most of his first 3 months of treatment in seclusion and restraints. He relapsed immediately after discharge by smoking marijuana and drinking.

Six years previously the patient had displayed various antisocial behaviors including destruction of a neighbor's lawn, stealing, vandalism of a motor vehicle, fighting, expulsion from school, arrest for possession of illegal drugs with intent to sell, and abuse of alcohol, marijuana, and LSD. He had been diagnosed at age 7 as having attention-deficit/hyperactivity disorder and had been given Ritalin (methylphenidate). He had been noted to be an extremely withdrawn child who had difficulty interacting with his peers.

During his reevaluation he denied any current alcohol abuse but admitted to daily drinking 1 month previously. He was smoking two to three joints of marijuana per day up to the day of assessment. He denied depression, mania, or panic disorder symptoms. The family history was positive for severe substance abuse and psychiatric disorders, with nine of ten parental siblings reported to be alcoholics. There was extensive alcoholism and mental illness on his mother's side.

Mental status examination showed the patient was slightly depressed with no psychotic features. Laboratory testing was normal except for a positive urine drug screen for cannabinoids. The initial diagnostic impression was Axis IA, cannabis abuse; Axis IB, alcohol abuse; Axis IC, conduct disorder; Axis ID, rule out bipolar disorder; Axis IE, rule out major depression; Axis II, rule out antisocial personality traits; and Axis III, no diagnosis.

The patient's stay in the hospital was stormy from the start. He demonstrated no signs of withdrawal and did not require detoxification. He remained guarded, oppositional, angry, and depressed. He refused to participate in any treatment. He stated "I want to go home" and submitted a 72-hour notice of right to release. When that expired, his parents refused to pick him up. The staff did not think discharging this minor patient to an uncertain fate was reasonable. It was decided not to release him until a safe disposition could be arranged that ensured that a responsible adult was taking responsibility for him. Because of this, the child abuse authorities were notified of the situation and the patient was discharged to them.

At the time of discharge it was believed that this was a dual-diagnosis patient with major components of an affective disorder, probably bipolar, and several substance abuse disorders. However, because of his extreme opposition and resistance to any treatment efforts and because he did not meet the criteria for commitment, it was not possible to keep him in treatment. It was explained to him that the staff thought that he was ill and needed further treatment and that they would take him back under certain negotiated conditions. His diagnosis at that time was

- Axis Ia, Probable Bipolar Disorder
- Axis Ib, Possible Major Depressive Disorder
- Axis Ic, Possible Substance (marijuana, LSD, alcohol) Induced Mood Disorder
- Axis Id, Cannabis Abuse
- Axis Ie, Alcohol Abuse
- Axis If, LSD Abuse
- Axis Ig, Conduct Disorder
- Axis II, Antisocial Personality traits
- Axis III, No Diagnosis

After his discharge from the hospital, the patient was taken by the child abuse authorities and handed over to his father, who brought the patient back to the hospital 24 hours later. The patient begged to be readmitted and agreed to be treated for his psychiatric and substance abuse disorders. He was admitted directly to a dual diagnosis unit, where it became clear that his extreme irritability and oppositional behavior was accompanied by hyperactivity and pressured speech. The diagnosis of a bipolar disorder was made and he was placed on lithium carbonate.

The patient's behavior improved markedly for several weeks while on lithium. He then became very oppositional again and refused to take it anymore. At this point his negative behavior escalated and he refused to cooperate in any way. He threatened other patients and staff members and had to be isolated from the other patients. The staff members decided that he was untreatable on the dual diagnosis unit, and his father was called in to discuss the matter. The father became enraged at the staff and demanded that additional treatment measures be taken before his son was discharged.

The medical director of the hospital was consulted, and it was agreed to take the patient back to the evaluation unit for reevaluation of possible mania or another psychiatric disorder that had been missed. The patient agreed to be transferred back to the evaluation unit and also agreed to take lithium while he was there. He took it for several days but with time again refused to take it. He remained oppositional and defiant, refusing to cooperate in any way with any and all attempts to help him.

At this time it was clear to everyone that the patient was untreatable. His father was again contacted, and he again refused to pick the patient up. Arrangements were made for the patient to return to live with his mother.

Comment

This case demonstrates the need for a higher standard of care for adolescent patients. Because they are not adults, they cannot be discharged as rapidly as possible. Arrangements must be made for a safe, reasonable transfer into the care of a responsible adult. In this patient's case his nearest relative refused to cooperate. Because he did not meet the criteria for commitment, the patient was released to the child abuse authorities. It is unclear how or why the patient was returned back to his father. However, a major mistake was made when the patient presented to the hospital again asking to reenter treatment: a written contract should have been negotiated and signed before he was allowed to return.

When the patient again became disruptive in the hospital, the case was completely reviewed. Because he did not cooperate with the terms of his transfer back to the evaluation unit, and because he could not be committed against his will, he was again released. His discharge was delayed for several days until proper arrangements could be made to discharge him to the care of a responsible adult. It is important to note that he was not allowed to disrupt the program on the dual diagnosis unit and was instead transferred back to the evaluation unit, which was better able to cope with his severe emotional or behavioral outbursts.

Some therapists advocate a waiting period or "cooling-off time" during which the patient cannot be readmitted to the hospital. There have been numerous instances in which patients have been readmitted rapidly and have done well. This case is an exception to that rule.

Case 3

Patient S was a 17-year-old black male who was admitted for his third drug abuse hospitalization because he was again using drugs, drinking, and running away from home. He admitted to extensive use of alcohol, cocaine, amphetamines, and heroin. His urine drug screen 1 month prior to admission had been positive for marijuana, but his therapist had not believed this was a significant development and thus had not admitted the patient. The patient had significant depressive symptoms with some paranoid ideation and feelings that his pregnant girlfriend was sexually involved with another individual. He had previously been diagnosed as having a major depressive disorder.

The patient's mental status examination was significant for restricted range of affect and depressed mood as well as evasiveness and extreme guardedness. Laboratory testing was negative except for a urine drug screen, which was again positive for cannabinoids. He was admitted, stabilized, and transferred to the outpatient dual diagnosis treatment unit, where he continued to demonstrate depression. He was treated with an antidepressant and had good response. However, after 2 weeks he refused the medication because he was experiencing side effects. He could not be persuaded to try another antidepressant with a lower side effect profile.

The patient appeared to make progress in his psychotherapy and his substance abuse treatment, but his once negative urine drug screen again became positive for marijuana. He was confronted and relapse reevaluation was initiated. He appeared to cooperate but did not return to treatment after a weekend trip with his family. His parents were contacted. They did not support any further treatment and he was discharged.

The final diagnosis was

- Axis Ia, Major Depression
- Axis Ib, Possible Substance Induced Mood Disorder (Depressed)
- Axis Ic, Amphetamine Abuse
- Axis Id, Heroin Abuse
- Axis Ie, Cannabis Abuse
- Axis If, Cocaine Abuse
- Axis II, Antisocial Personality Disorder
- Axis III, No Diagnosis

Comment

This patient's treatment failed because of his lack of motivation and cooperation. The first indication of problems was his refusal to try a new antidepressant medication. He had an unusual ability to mislead the dual diagnosis treatment staff into thinking that he was making progress and recovering. It was also clear from his parents' reaction that they were not invested in his recovery and that they helped him avoid treatment by making up excuses for his nonattendance.

One of the most important lessons to be learned from this case is that this individual had an extensive history of failed treatment coupled with a chronic relapsing course and a powerful resistance to treatment. The prognosis in these cases is extremely poor. Nothing, including treatment with antidepressants, altered the course of his illness because he was not committed to his own recovery. Such individuals are essentially untreatable, except perhaps in long-term residential programs.

Case 4

Patient T was a 16-year-old female in the eleventh grade. At admittance, she stated, "I've been messing around with drugs a little too much....My grandfather, older brother, and father have been touching me....I cut my wrists and overdosed." The cutting had occurred in Houston 3 weeks prior to admission. The patient also stated after she returned from Houston that she had been taking "white crosses" (amphetamine). Her parents stated that the other reasons for her current admission were that she was having severe mood swings, she was out of control, and she was extremely oppositional.

The patient related a 4-year history of substance use, which began when she took her father's pain pills from the medicine cabinet. She then switched to Valium, white crosses, and marijuana, which she stole from her older brother. She stated that she had drunk between half and three-quarters of a fifth of vodka or tequila or three to four six-packs of beer in a 5–6 hour period. She had been drinking heavily 6 days prior to admission although she had claimed to have stopped drug abuse since her suicide attempt.

The patient also related several depressive symptoms, including a 1½–2-year history of difficulty falling asleep; decreased appetite; an 8-pound weight loss; feeling helpless, hopeless, worthless, sad and blue, and down in the dumps; and wanting to cry. These symptoms had culminated in her suicide attempt. She acknowledged hearing the voice of a friend who had died 1 year previously. She repeated her claim that she had been sexually molested by her grandfather, her father, and her brother; she claimed they would rub her breasts and genitals but that no intercourse had occurred, although it was attempted.

Mental status examination was negative except for the previously mentioned auditory hallucinations. The patient showed no evidence of drug or alcohol withdrawal and all of her laboratory testing was within normal limits. She quickly stabilized and did well. However, her parents requested discharge after the alleged sexual abuse was reported. In view of the past suicide attempts and the allegations of sexual abuse, it was believed that the she should continue her evaluation in a hospital setting. The child abuse authorities insisted that she remain and receive treatment. Over the next few days she insisted that she was not depressed and had no suicidal ideation. She refused to participate in the dual diagnosis program and did not engage in any therapeutic activities. She was released from treatment against medical advice when she was no longer a threat to herself or others. Both the patient and her parents were told that the chances of relapse under these conditions were extremely high. They were also told that the patient could return for further treatment under the proper conditions.

At discharge the patient's final diagnosis was

- Axis Ia, Substance (cannabis, benzodiazepine, alcohol) Induced Mood Disorder
- Axis Ib, Posttraumatic Stress Disorder (secondary to sexual abuse)
- Axis Ic, Possible Bipolar Disorder
- Axis Id, Polysubstance (alcohol, cocaine, cannabis) Abuse
- Axis Ie, Conduct Disorder
- Axis If, Cannabis Abuse
- Axis Ig, Benzodiazepine Abuse
- Axis Ih, Amphetamine Abuse
- Axis Ii, Alcohol Abuse
- Axis II, No Diagnosis
- Axis III, No Diagnosis

Comment

This patient's treatment was sabotaged by her parents' failure to encourage her to complete treatment. In fact, her discharge was precipitated by her allegations of sexual abuse. Because of the patient's serious suicide attempts, severe substance abuse, and her chaotic and contradictory stories, it was decided to wait until the situation could be further clarified. When she was no longer dangerous to herself or others and it was clear that she would gain no benefit from further treatment, she was released to her parents. Sadly, she was essentially untreatable because neither she nor her parents acknowledged her illness or her need for further treatment. Her prognosis was extremely guarded.

Conclusion

Untreatable substance-abusing adolescents do exist. They can be very difficult to care for. They can wreak havoc in a treatment program and can enrage treatment staff. For these reasons, it is important to identify these individuals and remove them from the program as quickly as possible. In addition, the mere consideration of untreatability should prompt a complete reevaluation of the patient, focusing on what treatable disorders were overlooked or misdiagnosed. If the reevaluation determines that the adolescent is not treatable, discharge should rapidly ensue.

However, these adolescents should never be discharged in haste or anger and must be discharged into a safe environment. This requires informing the parents, legal authorities, and sometimes the child abuse authorities. No adolescent should ever just be shown the door.

Reference

American Psychiatric Association: Diagnostic and Statistical Manual of Mental Disorders, 4th Edition. Washington, DC, American Psychiatric Association, 1994

Index

Page numbers printed in **boldface** refer to tables or figures.

Abstinence
  aftercare and, 159–160
  recovery versus, 254
  treatment programs and, 149
  12-step treatment and, 206
Abuse, physical and sexual, as risk factor, 16, 22
Abuse, substance. *See* Substance abuse
Accreditors, treatment planning and, 142
Achenburg Child Behavior Checklist (CBCL), 131
Acknowledgement, 12-step treatment and, 210–214
Activity therapy, 180–181
Addiction. *See also* Substance dependence
  adult, 38
  avoiding addicting medications, 96
  drug use and abuse versus, 267–268
  as level of use, 135, 137–138
  questionable. *See* Questionable addictions
ADHD. *See* Attention-deficit/hyperactivity disorder (ADHD)
Admissions, treatment, 9–10
Adolescents
  development of. *See* Development, adolescent
  diagnostic criteria for substance-abusing, 60–61, 63–64. *See also* Diagnosis
  families of. *See* Family; Parents
  identifying substance-abusing, 55–58
    legal system and, 57
    parents and, 56
    peer groups and siblings and, 58
    primary physicians and, 57, 92–93
    psychiatrists, psychologists, social workers, psychiatric nurses, and counselors and, 58
    school system and, 56
  interviews with, as part of evaluation, 105–107
  medical evaluation of substance-abusing. *See* Medical evaluation
  profiles of, and family treatment, 241–242
  spiritual evaluation of family and, 107
  spirituality and, 231. *See also* Spirituality
  substance use among younger, 7–8. *See also* Epidemiology
  12-step techniques to engage, 207. *See also* 12-step treatment
  substance abuse by. *See* Substance abuse
  untreatable. *See* Untreatable adolescents

Adults. *See also* Parents
  addiction in, 38
  comorbidity in, 69–70
  diagnostic criteria for
    DSM-III-R definitions, 61–62
    DSM-IV definitions, 62–63
  lack of guidance from, 267
  separation of adolescents from, 169
Affective disorders. *See also* Psychiatric disorders
  comorbid, 75–76
  depression. *See* Depression
  emotional problems, 9
  family history of, 115
  medication usage and case examples of, 195–199
Aftercare
  behavior modification and, 176
  managed care and, 148
  outpatient treatment and, 159–160
Age
  as diagnostic issue, 51, 52, 65
  of initiation of use as risk factor, 14–15
Aggression
  alcohol use and, 41
  comorbid disruptive behavior disorders and, 72, 74
  comorbid suicidal behavior and, 76–77
  inpatient programs and, 182–183
  as risk factor, 15–16
Agonist prevention therapy, 192
AIDS/HIV
  intranasal abuse and, 36, 45
  intravenous abuse and, 38
  testing for, 95, 108
Alateens, 259. *See also* 12-step treatment
Alcohol
  abuse of, 40–41
  annual use of, 6
  anxiety disorders and, 77–78
  comorbidity and, 79–80
  current/daily use of, 6
  definition of alcoholism, 135
  detoxification and risk management with, 189
  gender, race/ethnicity, and regional comparisons of use of, 9
  genetic/family factors and use of, 20–21
  lifetime use of, 3
  quantity of use of, 7
Alcoholics Anonymous, 47, 110, 116, 117, 148, 205. *See also* 12-step treatment
Alienation, 16
American Association of Partial Hospitalization Child and Adolescent Special Interest Group, 150
American Society of Addiction Medicine (ASAM)
  criteria, 103, 131–132, 165
  Patient Placement Criteria, 103
Amotivational syndrome, 100
Amphetamines
  abuse of, 42–43
  ecstasy, 43, 124–125
  lifetime use of, 4–5
  as medications, 187
  methamphetamine. *See* Methamphetamine
  perceived availability of, 8
Amyl nitrate (poppers), routes of abuse of, 39
Anabolic steroids
  intramuscular injection of, 38
  as questionable addiction, 46
Angel dust. *See* Phencyclidine hydrochloride (PCP)
Anger, missed diagnoses and staff, 274
Annual use trends, 2, 5–6
Anorexia nervosa, 48, 79

Antagonist prevention therapy, 191–192
Antidepressants, 193
Antisocial behavior, 15–16. *See also* Conduct disorders
Anxiety disorders, comorbid, 77–78
Assessment. *See* Diagnosis
Athletes, anabolic steroids and, 38, 46
Attention-deficit/hyperactivity disorder (ADHD)
  comorbid, 72–74
  medication and, 187, 194
  as risk factor, 16–17
  suicidal behavior and, 77
  symptoms of, and substance abuse, 100
Atypical depression, 12-step treatment case example of, 219
Availability of substances, perceived, 8
Axis V subscales, 144

Barbiturates
  abuse of, 41–42
  perceived availability of, 8
Beck Depression Index, 81
Behavior
  comorbid disruptive behavior disorders, 9, 72–74
  correlates of substance abuse. *See* Behavioral correlates
  diagnosis and, 23, 104–105
  management of, in inpatient programs, 174–177
    behavior modification, 175–177
    environmental control and, 114
    unit freeze and, 177
  predicting. *See* Predicting phase of family treatment
  suicidal. *See* Suicidal behavior
Behavioral correlates, 9, 15–20. *See also* Comorbidity
  ADHD, 16–17. *See also* Attention-deficit/hyperactivity disorder (ADHD)
  Conduct disorders, 15–16. *See also* Conduct disorders
  expectations, 18
  peer influences, 17–18. *See also* Peer groups
  psychiatric disturbances, 19. *See also* Psychiatric disorders
  school performance, 17
  self-esteem, 18–19
  suicidal behavior, 19–20. *See also* Suicidal behavior
Behavior modification, 114, 168–169, 175–177
Beliefs
  as risk factors, 18
  spiritual evaluation and, 107. *See also* Spirituality
Benzodiazepines
  abuse of, 41–42
  as medications, 189
Berkson's bias, 70
Binge drinking, 7, 9
Biopsychosocial diagnostic summaries, 143
Bipolar disorder, 12-step treatment case example of, 211–213
Blood tests, 95, 108–109, 110
Boot camps, 161–162
Brain chemistry and drug of choice, 65
Brain delivery systems, 36. *See also* Routes of abuse
Brothers, diagnosis and, 58
Bulimia
  and depression, 12-step treatment case example of, 220–221
  as food/eating disorder, 48, 79
  as risk factor, 19

Cannabis products, 40
  hashish, 40

Cannabis products *(continued)*
- marijuana, 40. *See also* Marijuana

Case examples
- discharging untreatable adolescents, 277–284
- medication usage, 195–202
- psychiatric and substance abuse evaluation, 116–125
- 12-step treatment, 211–214, 216–218, 219, 220–221

Case management. *See* Treatment planning and case management

Child Behavior Checklist, 81–82, 151

Child-parent relationships as risk factors, 21. *See also* Parents

Cigarettes. *See* Tobacco

Cleveland Criteria, 103

Clinical implications
- of adolescent development, 271
- of comorbidity, 82–83

Clinician diagnostic techniques and skills, 53–55. *See also* Mental health professionals
- clinician qualities, 54–55
- gathering of data, 53–54
- intuition and, 65–66

Clonidine, 190

Cocaine
- abuse of, 43–45
- cocaine hydrochloride, 44
- crack cocaine, 44–45
- lifetime use of, 5
- perceived availability of, 8

Cocaine Anonymous, 110, 148–149, 178, 205. *See also* 12-step treatment

Cocaine hydrochloride, routes of abuse of, 44

Coexisting problems. *See* Behavioral correlates; Comorbidity

Cognitive omnipotent decisions, 260

Combinations of drugs, detoxification and risk management for, 191

Committee on Managed Care, 145

Communication, medical treatment and, 96

Community-based programs, 148–149

Comorbidity, 69–83
- adolescent development and, 270–271
- assessment and, 80–82
- clinical implications of, 82–83
- common psychiatric disorders and, 72–79
  - anxiety disorders, 77–78
  - disruptive behavior disorders, 72–74
  - eating disorders, 78–79
  - mood disorders, 75–76
  - suicide, 76–77
- development of substance abuse and, 79–80
- emotional problems and, 9
- family treatment diagnostic issues and, 243
- inpatient programs and, 182
- medication usage and, 193–195
- relapse and, 260
- relationships between coexisting substance abuse and psychopathology, 71
- research on, 69–70
- risk factors and, 15. *See also* Risk factors

Compensatory use, 135

Compulsion stage, 137–138

Concurrent review, 146

Conduct disorders
- ADHD and, 16–17
- comorbid, 72–72
- psychiatric evaluation and, 100–101
- as risk factors, 15–16
- 12-step treatment case examples of, 213–214, 216–217, 217–218

Confidentiality
  adolescent privacy versus parents' right to know, 55
  diagnostic interviews and, 106
  surveys and, 2
Continuum, substance abuse as, 133–134
Contracting
  discharge planning and, 181–182
  for outpatient treatment, 110
  for treatment, 138–139
  12-step treatment and, 207–208
Control, loss of, as diagnostic criteria, 62–63
Counselors
  diagnosis and, 58
  inpatient program staff, 172–173
  program directors, 171–172
Courts. *See* Legal system
Crack cocaine, 44–45
Crystal meth, 43
Current use trends, 2, 6

Daily use trends, 2, 6
Data
  clinician techniques and skills in gathering, for diagnosis, 53–54
  sources of epidemiological, 1–2
Day hospital, outpatient treatment and, 159
Day treatment
  considerations, 111–113
    possible withdrawal, 112
    psychotic symptoms, 112–113
    suicide, 112
  managed care and, 148
Decision tree method, 131
Defense mechanisms, 176
Definitions, diagnosis and confusing, 58–59
Denial, 55, 65, 242–243
Dependence. *See* Substance dependence
Depression. *See also* Affective disorders
  comorbid, 75–76, 116–118
  depressive mood as risk factor, 19
  family history of, 115
  marijuana-induced amotivational syndrome and, 100
  medication and, 187–188
  suicide and, 183
  12-step treatment case studies, 219, 220–221
Detoxification. *See also* Withdrawal
  diagnosis and, 66
  medication risk management and, 188–191
    alcohol and sedative hypnotics, 189
    drug combinations or unknown withdrawals, 191
    opiates, 189–191
  psychiatric diagnosis after, 114–115
Development, adolescent, 265–271
  adolescent profiles and, 242
  basic questions of substance abuse and, 265–266
  clinical implications of, 271
  developmental arrest as symptom, 101
  developmental stages of substance abuse and, 269–270
  drug use and abuse as not meaning certain addiction, 267–268
  dual and triple diagnosis and, 270–271
  effects of substance abuse on, 268
  evaluation and issues of, 101–102
  habilitation and, 170
  normal, 266–267
Development, inpatient program staff, 179–180
Development, substance abuse
  comorbidity and, 79–80
  as continuum, 133–134
  stages of, 269–270

Dextroamphetamine, 42, 187
Diagnosis, 51–67
abuse versus dependence, 51
abuse versus use, 14
adolescent criteria
life areas and adolescent criteria, 63–64
traditional stages-of-use definitions, 60–61
adolescent privacy versus parents' right to know, 55
adult criteria
DSM-III-R definitions, 61–62
DSM-IV definitions, 62–63
age, vulnerability to substance abuse, and, 65
assessment as first step of treatment planning, 130–131
assumptions, 52
clinician techniques and skills, 53–55
clinician qualities, 54–55
data gathering, 53–54
comorbidity and, 80–82
confusion of definitions of abuse, dependence, use, experimentation, and, 58–59
danger of missed, due to staff anger, 274
drug of choice and, 65
dual, 71, 99
dual and triple, and adolescent development, 270–271
family treatment issues, 243–245
as first step of treatment planning and,
genetics and, 64
identifying potential patients, 55–58
legal system and, 57
parents and, 56
peer groups and siblings and, 58
primary physicians and, 57
psychiatrists, psychologists, social workers, psychiatric nurses, counselors and, 58
school system and, 56
inpatient evaluation, 113–114
environmental control and, 114
inpatient urine testing and, 113
school and, 113
interviews and, 81–82
limitations of, 52–53
limitations of, and gender prevalence rates, 23
meaning of, 52
medical. *See* Medical evaluation
outpatient evaluation
limits of, 53, 111
outpatient treatment from, 155–156
psychiatric and substance abuse, 102–103
psychiatric and substance abuse. *See* Psychiatric and substance abuse evaluation
recommendations for, 65–67
relapse evaluation, 257
risk factors and, 13–15. *See also* Risk factors
Diagnostic Interview Schedule for Children (DISC), 81
Diagnostic Interview Schedule for Children and Adolescents (DICA), 81
Diagnostic summary of treatment plan, 143
Disapproval of substances, perceived, 8, 10
Discharge
planning, 181–182
of untreatable adolescents
risk management of, 275–277
as therapeutic, 274
Discipline, behavioral management and, 174

Discontinuance rates, 6
Disruptive behavior disorders, comorbid, 72–74
Disulfiram, 192
Documentation, treatment plan, 141–145
  aftercare and, 160
  common problems with, 142–143
  components of, 143–145
    diagnostic summary, 143
    problem list, 143–144
    treatment goals, 145
    treatment goals versus treatment modalities, 145
    treatment objectives, 144–145
Double thinking, 54
Dropouts, school, 17
Drug abuse education, 158–159
Drug chart, 12-step treatment, 208–210
Drugs, 38–45. *See also* Medication usage
  abuse of. *See* Substance abuse
  alcohol, 40–41. *See also* Alcohol
  amphetamines and other stimulants, 42–43; *See also* Amphetamines
    ecstasy, 43
    methamphetamines, 42–43
  cannabis products, 40
    hashish, 40
    marijuana, 40. *See also* Marijuana
  choice of, as developmental issue, 269–270
  choice of, as diagnostic issue, 61–62, 65
  cocaine, 43–44. *See also* Cocaine
    cocaine hydrochloride, 44
    crack cocaine, 44–45
  detoxification and risk management for combinations of, 191
  gateway, 133, 269
  hallucinogens, 45
  heroin and other opiates, 45. *See also* Opiates
  illicit. *See* Illicit drugs
  inhalants, 39–40. *See also* Inhalants
    amyl nitrate (poppers), 39
    nitrous oxide, 40
    volatile hydrocarbons, 39
  "look-alike drugs," 42
  perceived availability of, 8
  perceived harmfulness and disapproval of, 8
  phencyclidine hydrochloride (PCP), 5, 41
  routes of abuse of. *See* Routes of abuse
  sedative hypnotics, benzodiazepines, barbiturates, and methaqualone, 41–42
  testing for. *See* Testing, drug
  use of. *See* Epidemiology; Substance use
Drug Use Screening Inventory (DUSI), 131
DSM-III-R diagnostic criteria for adults, 52, 60, 61–62, 144
DSM-IV diagnostic criteria for adults
  adolescents and, 100
  definitions of, 59, 62–63
  diagnosis and, 51, 52
  levels of use and, 134
  recommendations, 65–66
  for substance abuse, **137**
  for substance dependence, **136**
Dual diagnosis
  comorbidity and, 71, 99
  inpatient programs and, 166
  medications and, 193
  relapse and, 260
Dysphoria, 37

Eating disorders. *See* Food/eating disorders

Ecstasy
abuse of, 43
in case example, 124–125
Education
drug abuse, for outpatient treatment, 158–159
inpatient staff specialists in, 173
parental, 246
Eighth graders, substance use among, 2, 7–8
Emergency departments, 156
Emotional development. *See* Development, adolescent
Emotional problems, 9. *See also* Affective disorders
Environmental factors
family as, 20
inpatient evaluation and, 114
inpatient treatment and, 169–170
peer groups. *See* Peer groups
Epidemiologic Catchment Area Study, 69–70
Epidemiology, 1–11
annual use, 5–6
changes in prevalence of adolescent substance use, 10–11
current use/daily use, 6
gender, race/ethnicity, and regional comparisons, 9
lifetime use, 2–5
alcohol, 3
amphetamines, 4–5
cocaine, 5
hallucinogens, 5
heroin and other opiates, 5
illicit drugs, 4
inhalants, 5
marijuana, 4
tobacco, 4
international prevalence, 10
perceived availability of substances and, 8
perceived harmfulness and disapproval of substances and, 8
quantity of use, 6–7
sources of data, 1–2
substance abuse treatment admissions, 9–10
substance use among younger students, 7–8
Essential therapies, outpatient treatment, 162
Ethnicity, use comparisons and, 9
Euphoria, 37
Evaluation. *See* Diagnosis; Medical evaluation; Psychiatric and substance abuse evaluation
Expectations as risk factors, 18
Experimentation
confusing definitions of abuse, dependence, use, and, 58–59
and continuum of substance abuse, 133–134
drug abuse education and, 158–159
experimental stage of substance use, 135
lack of drug knowledge and, 35
prevalence of use and, 11
rationalizations for, 13–14
sexual and physical abuse and, 22

Failure to respond to outpatient treatment, 160–161. *See also* Relapse; Untreatable adolescents
Family. *See also* Family treatment; Parents
assessment, comorbidity, and family history, 81
conduct disorders and, 16
contracting and, 138–139
diagnosis and information about, 106
genetics/family history and risk factors, 20–21

history of affective disorders, 115
inpatient programs and, 169
intervention and, 148
pathology of, 235–236
peer influences and, 18
siblings and diagnosis, 58
spiritual evaluation of adolescent and, 107

Family treatment, 235–252. *See also* Family; Parents
adolescent denial, 242–243
adolescent profiles, 241–242
diagnostic issues, 243–245
family pathology and, 235–236
family role in, 248
fathers and, 239–241
forming parenting partnerships, 250–251
habilitation versus rehabilitation, 248–249
inpatient programs and, 178–179
mothers and, 238–239
orientation to philosophy of, 246–247
parental education, 246
parental reassurance, 245–246
parental treatment, 250
parent gender issues, 237–238
parent profiles, 238–241
predicting behaviors phase of, 247–248
last outburst, 248
pretending cooperation, 247–248
use of guilt, 247
protocol for, 245
rationale for gender-specific, 236–237
settling-in phase of, 247
12-step treatment and, 218
value of, 252

Fathers, family treatment and, 237–238, 239–241. *See also* Family treatment; Parents
Females. *See* Gender
Follow-up studies, relapse and, 253–254
Food/eating disorders
comorbid, 78–79
as questionable addictions, 47–48
as risk factor, 19
Forgiveness, 12-step treatment and, 223
Freebase cocaine, 44–45
Freeze, unit, 177
Fundamentals of Psychiatric Treatment Planning (Kennedy), 141

Gambling, as questionable addiction, 47
Gamma-hydroxybutyrate (GHB, Georgia Home Boy), as questionable addiction, 46–47
Gas chromatography/mass spectrometry (GC/MS), 109
Gateway drugs, 133, 269
Gathering data for diagnosis, 53–54
Gender
comparisons of use and, 9
differences in, in substance use disorders, 22–23
parent issues of, 237–238
rationale for gender-specific family treatment, 236–237
Genetics. *See also* Family
as diagnostic issue, 64
and risk factors, 20–21
Goals, treatment, 145
objectives versus, 144–145
treatment modalities versus, 145
God, 12-step treatment and, 214–216, 218–219. *See also* Spirituality; 12-step treatment

Group therapy, 58, 140, 176, 178, 250
Guilt, family treatment and use of, 247

Habilitation
- inpatient treatment and, 170
- rehabilitation versus, 248–249

Habitual stage, 135, 137
Hallucinogens
- abuse of, 45
- lifetime use of, 5
- perceived availability of, 8
- physical symptoms of using, 105

Harmfulness of substances, perceived, 8, 10
Hashish, 40
Health care professionals. *See* Mental health professionals; Physicians
Hedonistic use, 135
Heritability studies, 20–21
Heroin
- abuse of, 45
- lifetime use of, 5
- perceived availability of, 8

Higher levels of care, outpatient treatment from, 157
HIV. *See* AIDS/HIV
Home contracts, 181–182
Homicide, 1
Homosexuality, 39
Honesty, 12-step treatment and, 221–222
Hospitalization, 149–151. *See also* Inpatient evaluation; Inpatient programs; Residential and partial residential care
Household surveys, 1–2
Huffing, 37, 39
Hydrocarbons, volatile, 37, 39
Hypnotics, sedative. *See* Sedative hypnotics

Ice (smokable methamphetamine), 43
Identification of substance-abusing adolescents, 55–58. *See also* Diagnosis
- legal system and, 57
- parents and, 56
- peer groups and siblings and, 58
- primary physicians and, 57, 92–93
  - importance of suspicion, 92–93
  - suspicion in different medical settings, 93
- psychiatrists, psychologists, social workers, psychiatric nurses, and counselors and, 58
- risk factors and, 13–15
- school system and, 56

Illicit drugs
- annual use of, 5–6
- gender, race/ethnicity, and regional comparisons of use of, 9
- lifetime use of, 4

Immunoassay techniques, 109
Impulsivity, suicidal behavior and, 76–77
Individual risk factors, 20–22
- genetics/family history, 20–21
- parent–child relationships, 21
- sexual and physical abuse, 22

Individual therapy, 178
Inhalants
- abuse of, 39–40
- amyl nitrate (poppers), 39
- annual use of, 6
- lifetime use of, 5
- nitrous oxide, 40
- testing for, 110
- volatile hydrocarbons, 39

Inhalation as abuse route, 37
Initiation of use, age of, 14–15
Injury, 1
Inpatient programs, 165–185
- activity and recreational therapies, 180–181

aggression and violence concerns, 182–183
behavioral management, 174–177
behavior modification, 175–177
unit freeze, 177
comorbid psychiatric disorders and, 182
discharge planning, 181–182
environmental change and, 114, 169–170
evaluation, 113–114
environmental control and, 114
inpatient urine testing and, 113
school and, 113
habilitation, 170
managed care and, 53, 165, 183–185
psychotherapies, 178–179
recidivism and, 185
school and, 180
setting up, 166–169
staffing, 170–173
leadership positions, 171–172
other staff, 172–173
outside physicians and therapists, 173
staff training and development, 179–180
suicide concerns, 183
transfer to outpatient treatment from, 157
12-step recovery and, 181
unitary rounds, 173–174
Instrumental use, 135
Insurance. *See* Managed care
Intensity, treatment, 140
Intensive treatment after school, 159
International use prevalence, 10
Intervention
assessment and effective, 130
as prevention effort, 23
as primary treatment, 148
12-step treatment and, 207
Interviews
with adolescents, 105–107
diagnostic, 81–82
lying and, 53
outpatient, 102–103
with parents, 103–105
Intramuscular injection as abuse route, 38
Intranasal abuse route, 36
Intravenous injection as abuse route, 38, 43
Intuition, diagnostic, 65–66
Iowa Conners Scale, 82

Juvenile justice system. *See* Legal system

Laboratory testing. *See also* Testing, drug; Urine tests
medical evaluation and, 92, 95
psychiatric evaluation and, 108–110
actual urine test, 109–110
imaginary urine test, 109
Lapses, 255
Last outburst, family treatment and, 248
Laughing gas, 40
Leadership positions in inpatient programs, 171–172
medical director position, 171
nurse manager position, 172
program director position, 171–172
Learning disabilities, 167, 173
Least-risk rules. *See* Risk management
Legal system
diagnosis and, 57
discharges and, 276
failure to respond to outpatient treatment and, 160–161
long-term treatment options in juvenile justice system, 161–162
boot camps, 161–162

Legal system *(continued)*
long-term treatment options in juvenile justice system *(continued)*
outdoor therapeutic programs, 161
motivational leverage and, 107–108
outpatient treatment from courts and juvenile justice system, 157–158
Length of inpatient stay, 132, 155, 183–184
Levels of treatment intensity, 140
Levels of use, 134–138
Leverage, motivation toward treatment and, 107–108, 160–161
Life areas as diagnostic criteria, 64
Life story, 12-step treatment, 208–210
Lifestyle changes, 149
Lifetime use trends, 2–5
alcohol, 3
amphetamines, 4–5
cocaine, 5
hallucinogens, 5
heroin and other opiates, 5
illicit drugs, 4
inhalants, 5
marijuana, 4
tobacco, 4
Locked units, 168
"Look-alike drugs," 42
Loss of control as diagnostic criteria, 62–63
Lying, 53, 54, 55, 56
Lysergic acid diethylamide (LSD)
abuse of, 45
lifetime use of, 5
perceived availability of, 8

Major relapses, 254–257
Males. *See* Gender
Managed care
diagnostic limitations of, 53
documentation and, 142
inpatient programs and, 165, 183–185
medical evaluation and, 93
treatment options and, 148
treatment programs and, 129–130, 151–152
utilization review and, 145
Management, utilization, 145–147
Marijuana
abuse of, 40
amotivational syndrome of, 100
in case examples, 119–125
current/daily use of, 6
lifetime use of, 4
perceived availability of, 8
substance abuse treatment admissions and, 10
Matching treatments. *See* Patient treatment matching
Mate tea, 36, 44
Medical director, inpatient program, 171
Medical evaluation, 91–97. *See also* Diagnosis
assessment of suspected substance abuse, 93–95
laboratory testing and, 95
physical examination and, 94
triage and referral and, 95
identification of substance abuse by primary care physicians, 92–93
importance of suspicion, 92–93
suspicion in different medical settings, 92
inpatient programs and, 166
lack of training in all specialties and, 92
medical treatment and, 96
avoiding addicting medications, 96
communication and, 96

recommendations, 97
referrals and, 91–92
Medical necessity, 146–147
Medical settings, suspected substance abuse in different, 93
Medical treatment, 96
avoiding addicting medications, 96
communication and, 96
Medication usage, 187–202
aggression, violence, and, 183
avoiding addicting medications, 96
in case examples, 195–202
after detoxification, 115
history and drugs of, 187–188
relapse prevention, 191–192
agonist prevention therapy, 192
antagonist prevention therapy, 191–192
noxious agent therapy, 192
risk management of, 188–195
detoxification and, 188–191
overdose and, 188
substance use as self-medication, 79–80
treatment of comorbid psychiatric disorders, 193–195
12-step treatment, 211
Meditation, 12-step treatment and, 223–224
Mental health problems. *See* Psychiatric disorders
Mental health professionals
clinician diagnostic techniques and skills, 53–55
clinician qualities, 54–55
gathering of data, 53–54
intuition and, 65–66
communication between physicians and, 96. *See also* Physicians
danger of missed diagnosis due to anger by, 274
inpatient program staff. *See* Staff, inpatient program
lack of training of, 92
outpatient treatment from, 156–157
parenting partnerships and, 250–251
Mentors, family treatment and, 236
Methamphetamine
abuse of, 42–43
lifetime use of, 5
Methadone, 190, 192
Methaqualone, 41–42
Methods for the Epidemiology of Child and Adolescent Mental Disorders (MECA), 70, 72, 75, 77
Methylenedioxymethamphetamine (MDMA, ecstasy), 43
Minnesota Multiphasic Personality Inventory (MMPI), 151
Minor relapses, 254–257
Modalities, treatment, treatment goals versus, 145
Monitoring the Future study, 2. *See also* Epidemiology
Mood disorders. *See* Affective disorders
Mood swing stages, 60
Moral development. *See* Development, adolescent
Moral inventory, 12-step treatment and, 219–221
Mortality, 1
Mothers, family treatment and, 237, 238–239. *See also* Family treatment; Parents
Motivation toward treatment, 107–108, 160–161
Mucous membranes and abuse routes, 36–37
Multidiagnosis, 71. *See also* Dual diagnosis
Multidisciplinary teams, 142–143

Narcotics Anonymous, 205. *See also* 12-step treatment

National Association of Addiction Treatment Providers (NAATP), 103
National Comorbidity Survey, 70
National Council on Alcoholism, 135
National Household Survey on Drug Abuse, 1–2
Necessity, medical, 146–147
Nitrous oxide, 40
Nonrecovering staff, 170–171, 180
Normative use, 134
No use contracts, 138–139
Novelty seeking, 16
Noxious agent therapy, 192
Nurse manager, inpatient program, 172
Nurses, diagnosis and, 58

Obesity, 47–48. *See also* Food/eating disorders
Objectives, treatment, 144–145
Odors, 168
Omnipotent thinking, 260
Opiates
  detoxification and risk management of, 189–191, 191–192
  intermuscular, 38
  lifetime use of, 5
  as medications, 188
  perceived availability of, 8
  routes of abuse of, 45
Oppositional defiant disorder, 72
Oral abuse route, 36
Oregon Adolescent Depression Project (OADP), 70
Orientation, parental, 246–247
Outburst, family treatment and last, 248
Outcome as factor in treatment planning, 132–133
Outdoor therapeutic programs, 161
Outpatient treatment, 155–163
  contracting for, 110
  from courts and juvenile justice system, 157–158
  essential therapies, 162
  evaluation and
    limits of, 53, 111
    outpatient treatment from, 155–156
    psychiatric and substance abuse, 102–103
  failure to respond to, 160–161
  from higher levels of care, 157
  levels of, 158–160
    aftercare, 159–160
    day hospital, 159
    drug abuse education, 158–159
    intensive treatment after school, 159
    residential and partial residential care, 159
  long-term options in juvenile justice system, 161–162
    boot camps, 161–162
    outdoor therapeutic programs, 161
  managed care and, 53
  from outpatient evaluations, 155–156
  from primary care physicians and mental health professionals, 156–157
  recommendations, 163
  after relapse, 158
  role of drug testing in, 162
  treatment matching and, 140–141, 158
  treatment planning and features of, 151
Overdose, medication risk management and, 188

Parents. *See also* Family; Family treatment

adolescent privacy versus right to know of, 55
diagnosis and, 56
discharges and, 276
drug use among, and ambivalence about adolescent use, 11
forming parenting partnerships, 250–251
gender issues of, 237–238
interview with, as part of evaluation, 103–105
marijuana use and, 40
parental risk factors, 16
parent–child relationships as risk factors, 21
profiles of, 238–241
treatment of, 250
Partial hospitalization guidelines, 150–151
Partial residential care, outpatient treatment and, 159
Partnerships, forming parenting, 250–251
Patient placement criteria, 131–132
Patient treatment matching
comorbidity and, 82
outpatient treatment and, 158
treatment planning and, 139–141
PCP. *See* Phencyclidine hydrochloride (PCP)
Peer groups
diagnosis and, 58, 106
family treatment and, 249
gender differences in substance abuse and, 22–23
influences of, as risk factor, 17–18
inpatient programs and, 169
relapse and, 260–261
Perceived availability of substances, 8
Perceived harmfulness and disapproval of substances, 8, 10
Permissiveness, parental, 21
Phencyclidine hydrochloride (PCP)
abuse of, 41
lifetime use of, 5
Phenylpropanolamine, 42
Physical abuse as risk factor, 16, 22
Physical examinations
medical evaluation and, 94
psychiatric evaluation and, 108
Physicians
clinician diagnostic techniques and skills, 53–55
clinician qualities, 54–55
data gathering, 53–54,
emergency department, and outpatient treatment, 156
inpatient programs and outside, 173
medical evaluation by. *See* Medical evaluation
primary care. *See* Primary care physicians
Physiological diagnostic criteria, 62–63
Planning, discharge, 181–182
Planning, treatment. *See* Treatment planning and case management
Point system, behavior modification, 175
Polysubstance abuse
case examples, 118–119, 124–125
DSM-IV criteria and, 63
Poppers (amyl nitrate), 39
Posttraumatic stress disorder (PTSD), 19, 22, 77–78, 216
Powerlessness, 12-step treatment and, 210–214
Prayer, 12-step treatment and, 223–224
Predicting phase of family treatment, 247–248
last outburst, 248
pretending cooperation, 247–248
use of guilt, 247
Predisposing factors. *See* Risk factors
Pregnancy, teenage, 1
Pretending cooperation, family treatment and, 247–248

Prevalence of use. *See* Epidemiology
Prevention efforts, 10–11, 13
Primary care physicians. *See also* Physicians
  communication between mental health professionals and, 96. *See also* Mental health professionals
  diagnosis and, 57. *See also* Medical evaluation
  identification of suspected substance abuse by, 92–93
    importance of suspicion, 92–93
    suspicion in different medical settings, 93
  lack of training of, and referrals, 91–92
  outpatient treatment from, 156–157
Primary-secondary paradigm of comorbidity, 71
Prior review, 145–146
Privacy. *See* Confidentiality
Problem list of treatment plan, 143–144
Profiles
  adolescent, 241–242
  parent, 238–241
    fathers, 239–241
    mothers, 238–239
Program director, inpatient program, 171–172
Psychiatric and substance abuse evaluation, 99–125. *See also* Diagnosis
  case examples, 116–125
  contracting for outpatient treatment, 110
  developmental issues, 101–102
  diagnostic problems and, 99–101
  guidelines for selecting day hospital or inpatient treatment, 111–115
    day treatment, 111–113
    elapsed time after detoxification before psychiatric diagnosis, 114–115
    inpatient evaluation, 113–114
  interviews with adolescents, 105–107
  interviews with parents, 103–105
  laboratory testing, 108–110
    actual urine tests, 109–110
    imaginary urinary tests, 109
  limits of outpatient evaluation, 111
  looking for motivational leverage, 107–108
  outpatient evaluation, 102–103
  physical examination, 108
  recommendations, 115–116
  spiritual evaluation of adolescents and families, 107
Psychiatric disorders
  alcohol abuse and, 41
  common comorbid, 72–79
    anxiety disorders, 77–78
    disruptive behavior disorders, 72–74
    eating disorders, 78–79
    mood disorders, 75–76
    suicide, 76–77
  diagnosing. *See* Psychiatric and substance abuse evaluation
  emotional problems, 9
  inpatient programs and, 166–167, 182
  medication usage and treatment of, 193–195
  medication usage case example of, 199–202
  relapse and, 260
  relationships between coexisting substance abuse and, 71
  as risk factors, 1, 19
  12-step treatment case examples of, 211, 218–219, 222
  volatile hydrocarbons and, 39

Psychiatric nurses, diagnosis and, 58
Psychiatrists
  diagnosis and, 58
  lack of training of, 92
  medical directors, 171
Psychoeducational groups, 250
Psychologists, 58, 156–157
Psychopathology. *See* Psychiatric disorders
Psychotherapies, inpatient program, 178–179. *See also* Therapies
Psychotic symptoms, day treatment and, 112–113
Public figures, drug use by, 11

Qualities, clinician, and diagnosis, 54–55
Quantity of use, 6–7
Questionable addictions, 45–48
  anabolic steroids, 46
  food/eating disorders, 47–48
  gambling, 47
  gamma-hydroxybutyrate (GHB, Georgia Home Boy), 46–47
  sexual activity, 47

Race, use comparisons and, 9
Rationalizations, 13–14
Reassurance, parental, 245–246
Recidivism, inpatient program, 185
Recovering staff, 170–171, 179–180
Recovery Book, The, 206
Recovery versus abstinence, 254
Recreational therapists, 172–173
Recreational therapy, 180–181
Rectum as route of abuse, 37
Referrals
  medical evaluation and, 91–92, 95
  patient progress and, 148
  by primary care physicians, 57
Regional use comparisons, 9
Regrouping phase of family treatment, 247–248
Rehabilitation versus habilitation, 248–249
Relapse, 253–262
  abstinence versus recovery, 254
  day treatment and, 111
  early remission and, 63
  evaluation of, 257
  follow-up studies and, 253–254
  frequency and commonness of, 257–258
  immediate treatment decisions after, 258–259
  inpatient program recidivism, 185
  legal system and, 160–161, 162
  minor and major, 254–257
  outpatient treatment after, 158
  pathways to, 259–261
  preventing, 191–192
    agonist prevention therapy, 192
    antagonist prevention therapy, 191–192
    noxious agent therapy, 192
    12-step treatment and, 215
  recommendations, 261–262
  status, 174, 177
  12-step treatment and, 206, 259
Relationships
  communication between physicians and mental health professionals, 96
  diagnostic interviews and, 105–106
  parent–child, as risk factors, 21
  parenting partnerships, 250–251
Religion versus spirituality, 230
Remission, 63
Residential and partial residential care
  guidelines for, 150–151
  managed care and, 148
  outpatient treatment and, 157, 159
Risk factors, 13–23
  assessment of suspected substance abuse and, 93–94

Risk factors *(continued)*
- behavioral correlates, 15–20
  - ADHD, 16–17
  - conduct disorders, 15–16
  - expectations, 18
  - peer influences, 17–18
  - psychiatric disturbances, 19
  - school performance, 17
  - self-esteem, 18–19
  - suicidal behavior, 19–20
- clinician data gathering and, 53–54
- comorbidity and, 82. *See also* Comorbidity
- gender differences in substance abuse disorders, 22–23
- identifying, 13–15
- individual, 20–22
  - genetics/family history, 20–21
  - parent–child relationships, 21
  - sexual and physical abuse, 22

Risk management, 188–195
- detoxification and, 188–191
  - for alcohol and sedative hypnotics, 189
  - for drug combinations or unknown withdrawals, 191
  - for opiates, 189–191
- discharges and, 275, 277–284
- overdose and, 188

Rounds, unitary, 173–174

Routes of abuse, 35–38. *See also* Drugs
- inhalation, 37
- intranasal, 36
- intravenous, 38
- mucous membranes, 37
- oral, 36
- smoking, 37
- subcutaneous/intramuscular, 38

Sabotage, 168, 274

Schedule for Affective Disorders and Schizophrenia for School-Age Children (K-SADS), 81, 131

School
- diagnosis and, 56
- discharges and, 276
- information from, and inpatient evaluation, 113
- inpatient programs and, 180
- intensive treatment after, 159
- performance at, as risk factor, 17
- surveys, 1–2, 15. *See also* Epidemiology

Screening, 80–81. *See also* Diagnosis

Second opinions, 95, 111

Sedative hypnotics
- abuse of, 41–42
- detoxification and risk management of, 189

Seemingly irrelevant decisions, relapse and, 261

Self-esteem as risk factor, 18–19

Self-help groups. *See* 12-step treatment

Self-medication, substance use as, 79–80

Serenity Prayer, 224

Serial contracting, 138–141

Serotonin re-uptake inhibitors (SSRIs), 193

Settings, suspected substance abuse in different medical, 93

Settling-in phase of family treatment, 247

Sexual abuse as risk factor, 22

Sexual activity
- adolescent development, substance abuse, and, 266–267
- amyl nitrate and, 39
- physical examinations and, 94, 108
- as questionable addiction, 47
- as risk factor, 14, 16
- sexually transmitted diseases, 1

Siblings, diagnosis and, 58

Skin popping, 38

Slips, 255

Smokeless tobacco, lifetime use of, 4

Smoking as abuse route, 37. *See also* Tobacco
Sniffing, 39
Social groups. *See* Peer groups
Social phobia, 77–78
Social workers
  diagnosis and, 58, 156–157
  inpatient program staff, 172
Spirituality, 229–233
  addressing, in treatment, 231–233
  controversial nature of, 229–230
  definitions of, in context of treatment, 230–231
  inpatient programs and, 167
  as issue for adolescents, 231
  recommendations, 233
  spiritual evaluation of patient and family, 107
  12-step treatment and, 214–218. *See also* 12-step treatment
Stabilization, 184
Staff, inpatient program, 170–173
  leadership positions, 171–172
    medical director position, 171
    nurse manager position, 172
    program director position, 171–172
  other staff, 172–173
  outside physicians and therapists, 173
  setting up inpatient programs and, 167–168
  staff training and development, 179–180
Stages of use, developmental, 269–270
Stages-of-use diagnostic criteria, 60–61, 66
Stepping stone hypothesis, 269
Step Workbook for Adolescent Chemical Dependence Recovery, 181, 208, 220
Steroids, anabolic, 38, 46
Stimulants, abuse of, 42–43. *See also* Amphetamines
Stress management, 170
Students, substance use among. *See* Epidemiology
Subcutaneous injection as abuse route, 38
Substance abuse
  addiction versus use and, 267–268. *See also* Addiction
  adolescent development and, 265–271
  comorbidity and. *See* Comorbidity
  confusing definitions of dependence, use, experimentation and, 14, 52–53, 58–59
  as continuum, 133–134
  dependence versus, 1, 51. *See also* Substance dependence
  diagnosis of. *See* Diagnosis
  drug education for, 158–159
  drugs of. *See* Drugs
  DSM-IV-TR criteria for, **137**
  family treatment of. *See* Family treatment
  inpatient programs for. *See* Inpatient programs
  as level of use, 135, 137
  medical evaluation and, 91–97
  medication usage. *See* Medication usage
  outpatient treatment for, 155–163
  parental, 104
  prevalence of, 1–11. *See also* Epidemiology
  predisposing factors for. *See* Risk factors
  psychiatric and substance abuse evaluation and. *See* Psychiatric and substance abuse evaluation
  questionable addictions, 45–48
    anabolic steroids, 46

Substance abuse *(continued)*
questionable addictions *(continued)*
food/eating disorders, 47–48
gambling, 47
gamma-hydroxybutyrate (GHB, Georgia Home Boy), 46–47
sexual activity, 47
relapse, 253–262
routes of, 35–38
spirituality and, 229–233
treatment planning and case management for. *See* Treatment planning and case management
12-step treatment for. *See* 12-step treatment
untreatable adolescents, 273–284
use versus, 14–15, 267–268. *See also* Substance use
Substance abuse units, 166–169. *See also* Inpatient programs
Substance dependence. *See also* Addiction
abuse versus, 1, 51. *See also* Substance abuse
confusing definitions of abuse, use, experimentation, and, 52–53, 58–59
DSM-IV-TR criteria for, **136**
as level of use, 138
physiological, 63
treatment options and definition of, 147
Substance misuse, 135
Substance use
abuse versus, 14–15, 267–268. *See also* Substance abuse
addiction versus abuse and, 267–268. *See also* Addiction
confusing definitions of abuse, dependence, experimentation, and, 52–53, 58–59
as level of use, 135
levels of, 134–138
prevalence. *See* Epidemiology
Suicidal behavior
alcohol use and, 41
comorbid, 76–77
as day treatment consideration, 112
inpatient programs and, 183
as risk factor, 19–20
substance abuse and, 1
Surveys, 1–2, 15
Suspicion
diagnosis and, 54–55, 56
in different medical settings, 93
environmental control and, 114
importance of, for primary care physicians, 92–93, 96

Tasks, developmental. *See* Development, adolescent
Teenage pregnancy, 1
Tenth graders, substance use among, 2, 7–8
Terminology, confusing diagnostic, 58–59
Testing, drug
laboratory. *See* Laboratory testing
by primary care physicians, 92–93
role of, in outpatient treatment, 162
urine tests. *See* Urine tests
Therapeutic discharge, 274
Therapies
inpatient program, 178–179
outpatient treatment, 162
Therapists. *See* Mental health professionals
Time after detoxification before psychiatric diagnosis, 114–115, 194–195
Time frames for substance abuse trends, 2–6
annual use, 2, 5–6
current use/daily use, 2, 6
lifetime use, 2–5
alcohol, 3

amphetamines, 4–5
cocaine, 5
hallucinogens, 5
heroin and other opiates, 5
illicit drugs, 4
inhalants, 5
marijuana, 4
tobacco, 4
Time-out status, 174
Tobacco
current/daily use of, 6
gender, race/ethnicity, and regional comparisons of use, 9
lifetime use of, 4
perceived harmfulness of, 8
quantity of use of, 7
Training
inpatient program staff, 179–80
lack of medical, 92, 156–157
Tranquilizers, 8
Treatment
admissions, epidemiology and, 9–10
inpatient. *See* Inpatient programs
matching
comorbidity and, 82
outpatient treatment and, 158
treatment planning and, 139–141
medical, 96
avoiding addicting medications, 96
communication and, 96
medication usage. *See* Medication usage
outpatient. *See* Outpatient treatment
planning. *See* Treatment planning and case management
spirituality and, 230–231, 231–233. *See also* Spirituality
Treatment planning and case management, 129–152
assessment as first step in treatment planning, 130–131
diagnosis and, 66–67
DSM-IV-TR criteria for substance abuse, **137**
DSM-IV-TR criteria for substance dependence, **136**
levels of use and, 134–138
managed care and, 129–130, 151–152
outcome as factor in, 132–133
outpatient evaluation and, 102–103
patient placement criteria, 131–132
patient treatment matching, 139–141
after relapse, 258–259
substance abuse as continuum, 133–134
treatment options and approaches, 147–151
intervention as primary treatment, 148
spectrum of, 148–151
treatment plan documentation, 141–145
common problems with documentation, 142–143
components of treatment plans, 143–145
use of contracting, 138–139
utilization review, 145–147
Trends. *See* Epidemiology
Triage and medical evaluation, 95
Twelfth graders, substance use among, 2. *See also* Epidemiology
12-step treatment, 205–225
contracting for outpatient treatment and, 110
drug chart and life story as preparation for step 1, 208–210
gambling and, 47
inpatient treatment and, 181
intervention, 207
patient treatment matching and, 140
questionable addictions and, 45, 47

12-step treatment *(continued)*
  relapses and, 255–256, 259
  sexual activity and, 47
  spirituality and, 230–231. *See also* Spirituality
  step 1, 210–214
    case examples, 211–215
    initial use of medications in, 211
    psychiatric issues in, 211
  step 2, 214–218
    case examples, 216–218
    psychiatric issues in, 216
  step 3, 218–219
    case example, 219
    psychiatric issues in, 218–219
  step 4, 219–221
    case example, 220–221
    psychiatric issues in, 222
  step 5, 221–222
    psychiatric issues in, 222
  step 6, 222
  step 7, 222
  step 8, 222–223
  step 9, 223
  step 10, 223
  step 11, 223–224
  step 12, 224–225
  success of, 205–206
  techniques to engage adolescents, 207
  as treatment option, 148–149
  written contracts, 207–208

Unitary rounds, inpatient programs and, 173–174
Unit freeze, inpatient programs and, 177
Unknown drug withdrawals, risk management and, 191
Untreatable adolescents, 273–284
  case examples, 277–284
  danger of missed diagnosis due to staff anger, 274
  reasons for classifying, 273–274
  recommendations, 284
  risk management of discharging, 275–277
  therapeutic discharge of, 274
Urine tests
  actual, 109–110
  contracting for, 110
  imaginary, 109
  inpatient, 113
  medical evaluation and, 95
  by primary care physicians, 57, 92
Use. *See* Substance use
Utilization review, 145–147

Vagina as route of abuse, 37
Violence. *See also* Aggression
  alcohol use and, 41
  inpatient programs and, 182–183
Volatile hydrocarbons, 37, 39
Vulnerability to abuse as diagnostic issue, 65

Waiting periods before readmission, 281
Warning signs, 15
Wilderness programs, 161
Withdrawal. *See also* Detoxification
  dangers of, 42
  day treatment and possible, 112
  risk management for unknown drug, 191
Written contracts. *See* Contracting

Younger students, substance use among, 7–8
Young People's Alcoholics Anonymous, 209. *See also* 12-step treatment

Zero tolerance, 14